RISK ASSESSMENT FOR HUMAN METAL EXPOSURES

RISK ASSESSMENT FOR HUMAN METAL EXPOSURES

Mode of Action and Kinetic Approaches

GUNNAR F. NORDBERG

Emeritus Professor, Umeå University
Department of Public Health and Clinical Medicine, Sweden

BRUCE A. FOWLER

Private Consulting Toxicologist, Adjunct Professor
Emory University, Rollins School of Public Health
and President's Professor of Biomedical Research
University of Alaska, Fairbanks

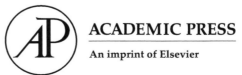

ACADEMIC PRESS

An imprint of Elsevier

Academic Press is an imprint of Elsevier
125 London Wall, London EC2Y 5AS, United Kingdom
525 B Street, Suite 1650, San Diego, CA 92101, United States
50 Hampshire Street, 5th Floor, Cambridge, MA 02139, United States
The Boulevard, Langford Lane, Kidlington, Oxford OX5 1GB, United Kingdom

Notices
Knowledge and best practice in this field are constantly changing. As new research and
experience broaden our understanding, changes in research methods, professional practices,
or medical treatment may become necessary.

Practitioners and researchers must always rely on their own experience and knowledge in
evaluating and using any information, methods, compounds, or experiments described
herein. In using such information or methods they should be mindful of their own safety and
the safety of others, including parties for whom they have a professional responsibility.

To the fullest extent of the law, neither the Publisher nor the authors, contributors, or editors,
assume any liability for any injury and/or damage to persons or property as a matter of
products liability, negligence or otherwise, or from any use or operation of any methods,
products, instructions, or ideas contained in the material herein.

Library of Congress Cataloging-in-Publication Data
A catalog record for this book is available from the Library of Congress

British Library Cataloguing-in-Publication Data
A catalogue record for this book is available from the British Library

ISBN: 978-0-12-804227-4

For information on all Academic Press publications visit our website at
https://www.elsevier.com/books-and-journals

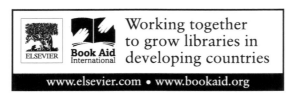

Working together
to grow libraries in
developing countries

www.elsevier.com • www.bookaid.org

Publisher: Andre Wolff
Acquisition Editor: Kattie Washington
Editorial Project Manager: Tracy Tufaga
Production Project Manager: Punithavathy Govindaradjane
Cover Designer: Victoria Pearson

Typeset by TNQ Technologies

I would like to dedicate my contributions to this book to my wife, Mary Jo Sexton, for her unwavering support over the years.
Bruce A. Fowler

CONTENTS

AUTHOR BIOGRAPHIES

Gunnar F. Nordberg, MD, PhD

Dr. Gunnar F. Nordberg is an emeritus professor at Umea University, Umea, Sweden, where he served as chairman of the Department of Environmental and Occupational Medicine for many years. He has also worked as a professor and chair at the Department of Environmental Medicine, Odense University, Denmark, and for the periods of a year at the International Agency for Research on Cancer, Lyon, France, the University of North Carolina, and the National Institute of Environmental Health Sciences, NC, USA. In his capacity as a university professor, he tutored many PhD and master students in environmental medicine, a number of them from countries around the world. He has published more than 280 papers in scientific journals and international handbooks. In addition, he authored, edited, or co-edited 24 scientific books and participated in international task groups evaluating risks of environmental agents, which resulted in 30 international books or reports. Some of these publications resulted from his activities as a chairman of the Scientific Committee on the Toxicology of Metals, International Commission on Occupational Health. He is presently the task group chairman of Cadmium Risk Assessment in the Toxicology and Risk Assessment Group of the International Union of Pure and Applied Chemistry. His scientific publications are mainly on toxicology and epidemiology of environmental agents, particularly metals and the application of such data for human risk assessment. He has coordinated EU projects on environmental epidemiology and toxicology of metals and participated as an active scientist in several such projects. He has been the principal investigator of many research projects funded by Swedish funding agencies and is presently actively involved in such research. He is one of the editors of a textbook in Swedish "Arbets-och Miljömedicin," latest (third) edition 2010 and chief editor, Handbook on the Toxicology of Metals, fourth edition, published in 2015 by Academic Press/Elsevier. He has extensive experience as an expert serving Swedish and international authorities, such as the Swedish National Board of Health (Socialstyrelsen); Japan Food Safety Agency; US Environmental Protection Agency; National Institute of Environmental Health Sciences; Agency for Toxic Substances and Disease Registry, USA; World Health Organization HQ; Geneva/International Program on Chemical Safety/WHO

Commission on Health and the Environment, Energy Panel; International Agency for Research on Cancer, Lyon, France; Europe/European Environment Agency, Copenhagen; European Medicines Agency, London; European Food Safety Authority, Parma, Italy.

Bruce A. Fowler, PhD, ATS

He is a private consulting toxicologist; co-owner of Toxicology and Risk Assessment Consulting Services (TRACS), LLC; adjunct professor, Emory University's Rollins School of Public Health, President's Professor, University of Alaska Fairbanks' Center for Alaska Native Health Research.

Dr. Fowler began his scientific career at the National Institute of Environmental Health Sciences prior to becoming director of the University of Maryland's system-wide program in toxicology and professor at the University of Maryland School of Medicine. He then served as Associate Director for Science in the Division of Toxicology and Environmental Medicine at Agency for Toxic Substances and Disease Registry. He is currently a private consultant and co-owner of Toxicology Risk Assessment Consulting Services (TRACS), LLC. In addition, Dr. Fowler serves as an adjunct professor, Emory University's Rollins School of Public Health and President's Professor of Biomedical Sciences, Center for Alaska Native Health Research at the University of Alaska Fairbanks. Dr. Fowler is an internationally recognized expert on the toxicology of metals and has served on a number of state, national, and international committees in his areas of expertise. These include the Maryland Governor's Council on Toxic Substances (chair), various National Academy of Sciences/National Research Council Committees, including the 1993 landmark NAS/NRC Report on "Measuring Lead Exposure in Infants, Children, and Other Sensitive Populations" for which he served as the committee chair. He has also served on a number of review committees of the National Institutes of Health, the USEPA Science Advisory Board, and the Fulbright Scholarship review committee for Scandinavia (Chair, 2000–01). In 2016, he became an Inaugural Member of the Fulbright 1946 Society and in 2018 became a member of the Fulbright Association Board of Directors. He has also served as a temporary advisor to the World Health Organization (WHO) and on working groups of the International Agency for Research Against Cancer for a number of toxicology and risk assessment issues. He is presently appointed as a member of the Joint FAO/WHO Expert Committee on Food Additives for the period 2016–20. Dr. Fowler has been honored as a fellow of the Japanese Society for the Promotion of Science, a Fulbright scholar, and Swedish Medical Research Council visiting professor at the Karolinska Institute, Stockholm, Sweden, and elected as a fellow of the Academy of Toxicological Sciences. His more recent awards include a CDC/ATSDR, Honor Award for Excellence in Leadership Award (2010), The US Pharmacopeia (USP) Toxicology Committee 2010—15 and the USP Elemental Impurities Panel, which received the 2014 USP Award for an innovative response to public health challenges (group award). He is currently appointed to the USP Nanotechnology Subcommittee 2015-. Dr. Fowler was previously elected to the Council of the Society of Toxicology (2005—07), the Board of Directors of the Academy of Toxicological Sciences (2006—09), and more recently, to the Council of the Society for Risk Analysis (2014—17). He is the Federal Legislative and National Active and Retired Federal Employees Association and (NARFE)-PAC chair for the Rockville Maryland Chapter of NARFE and is currently chair of the Federal Legislative Committee for the Maryland NARFE Federation. Dr. Fowler is the past president of the Rotary Club of North Bethesda, Maryland (2016—17) and was selected as Rotarian of the Year in 2015 for his work in developing a taxi-based program to help persons with disabilities gain independence via reliable transportation to work. Dr. Fowler is the author of over 260 research papers and book chapters dealing with molecular mechanisms of metal toxicity, molecular biomarkers for early detection of metal-induced cell injury, and application of computational toxicology for risk assessment. He has been the editor, co-editor, or author of 10 books or monographs on metal toxicology and mechanisms of chemical-induced cell injury, molecular biomarkers and risk assessment and computational toxicology. Dr. Fowler is currently focused on the global problem of electronic waste (e-waste) in developing countries. He serves on the editorial boards of a number of scientific journals in toxicology and is an associate editor of the journal Toxicology and Applied Pharmacology and a past associate editor of Environmental Health Perspectives (2007—16).

PREFACE

Risk Assessment for Human Metal Exposures: Mode of Action and Kinetic Approaches is a concise text describing current principles of risk assessment with a focus on mode of action, toxicokinetics, and toxicodynamics. In connection with the publication of the fourth edition of the Handbook on the Toxicology of Metals (Elsevier, Academic Press, 2015), the editors were approached by the publisher concerning the possibility to prepare a shorter text. The reason for this request was that the Handbook had expanded considerably compared with the size it originally had in its first edition (1 volume of totally 709 pages and the pages were considerably smaller than in the present fourth edition which is in 2 volumes, totally 1542 pages). Many students in the field of toxicology and environmental health, scientists in adjacent fields, as well as administrators dealing with risk assessment and risk science and others, for example, employees in metal industries, desiring an introduction to Risk Assessment of Human Metal exposures without the need for the detailed information in the Handbook, might be interested in a smaller book. This book summarizes the most important principles and presents summaries of data relevant for risk assessment of a selection of metals/metalloids, and we hope it will prove to be useful. Fourteen metals/metalloids and their compounds are briefly reviewed, including four well-investigated metals/metalloids (arsenic, cadmium, lead, and mercury), nickel, cobalt, and platinum as representatives of sensitizing metals/metal compounds and a few where the database is limited such as gallium, indium, palladium, and the lanthanides (lanthanum, cerium, and gadolinium). This book describes well-established concepts and principles in risk assessment, including mode of action, toxicokinetics, and toxicodynamics. In addition, it brings into discussion some recent new concepts such as "adverse outcome pathways," not much discussed in the Handbook, but increasingly used recently in risk assessment of toxic chemicals. The discussion considers how this and other concepts are used and gives examples for specific metals.

As indicated above, the Handbook on the Toxicology of Metals is a dominating basis of the present book, and the authors like to recognize the importance that it has served. One of the editors of the Handbook, who is not an author of the present book, is Monica Nordberg.

She participated in the initial discussions with the publisher but opted not to be an author of the present book. The authors are grateful for her continuous support and advice that she has given when we have written the texts of the chapters in this book.

Gunnar F. Nordberg
Bruce A. Fowler

Metal Exposures and Human Health—Historical Development, Current Importance, and Toxicological Concepts for Prevention

Abstract

Metallic elements constitute a large proportion of all existing elements. They are intrinsic components of the earth's crust and the environment, thus causing variable exposures of humans. Metallic macroelements occurring in high concentrations in human tissues play a key role in the practice of clinical medicine and are not included in the present book, which focuses in trace metals/metalloids, i.e., those metallic elements that occur in trace concentrations in human tissues. These metals are also those that have widespread use in various industrial processes and consumer products and such anthropogenic processes have increased human exposures. Many metallic chemical species such as inorganic and organic compounds of lead and mercury as well as inorganic compounds of arsenic and cadmium are recognized as toxic agents causing acute and chronic poisoning at high exposures. Epidemiological studies in recent decades have demonstrated that relatively low exposures in the general environment increase the occurrence of several diseases. The total worldwide exposure to metallic species makes an important contribution to the global burden of disease. This book deals with the risk and hazard assessment of human exposures to these metallic species. Such assessments are crucial in order to estimate the likelihood that existing exposures cause human disease or other adverse effects and for judging the need for societal action to reduce exposures. Some trace metals are essential for human life and well-being, and a minimum daily intake from food is required. For population groups with lower intakes, deficiency will result in disease states, also contributing to the global burden of disease. There is an obvious need to define exposures leading to toxicity or deficiency and to recommend preventive action. This chapter discusses, in an introductory way, historical developments in the field as well as current methods and exposure situations of importance for estimation of hazards and risks related to human metal exposures. It further draws attention to issues of current concern for hazard assessment, risk assessment, and prevention. The subsequent chapters of this book further develop these considerations.

Risk Assessment for Human Metal Exposures
ISBN: 978-0-12-804227-4
https://doi.org/10.1016/B978-0-12-804227-4.00001-7

1.1 INTRODUCTION

Metals are important constituents of the earth's crust. Approximately 70 elements in the periodic table are metals or metalloids occurring in the earth's crust. Human populations have been exposed to metals since antiquity, partly as a consequence of human activities and partly because metals are elements and have always been present in the environment. The present book focuses on trace metals/metalloids, i.e., those elements that occur in humans in trace quantities. The metallic macroelements sodium, magnesium, potassium, and calcium are not included here because there is a large clinical literature and there are many books on the clinical use of these elements in diagnosis and treatment of various diseases. An extensive compilation of existing data on toxicology and human health effects of trace metals/metalloids is available (Nordberg et al., 2015a), and the present book will not attempt to include this extensive amount of information. Instead, it will explain concepts important for risk assessment and give examples. There is increasing recognition of the fact that natural geological factors play an important role as determinants of human metal exposures and related health effects. Both deficiencies in the supply of essential metals such as iron and zinc and adverse effects related to exposures to toxic metals/metalloids like lead, mercury, cadmium, and arsenic can be a result of geological factors as discussed in the field of medical geology (Selinus et al., 2013). High exposures to metals in occupational settings giving rise to acute, subacute, and chronic poisoning has occurred in many countries in the past and still occurs because of accidents and/or inefficient control of industrial environments. Adequate documentation of health effects in humans and the use of all available evidence from experimental research at the molecular, cellular, and whole-organism levels are crucial for an assessment of risks related to human exposures to metallic compounds through diet, drinking water, and inhalation. Concepts of fundamental importance for risk assessment and prevention, defined a long time ago by the Task Group on Metal Toxicity (TGMT, 1976; see Section 1.5) are still important but may need to be refined and complemented based on recent advances in the toxicological sciences. In order to define exposures to toxic and essential metals that are optimal for human health, there is a need for models based on molecular initiating event (MIE), mode of action (MOA), and toxicokinetic-toxicodynamic (TKTD) data. Chapters 2 and 3 provide further explanation of these concepts, review current methods of their application and give examples of the use of related data for risk assessment. The MOA-TKTD models can serve as important instruments in risk assessment and in evaluating the causality of epidemiological findings. The evidence available for some metals (e.g., cadmium) provides good examples of how MOA-TKTD models can be efficiently used in risk assessment. There is a possibility to develop this experience when suggesting predictive modeling for exposures to metallic compounds where only more limited data are available and to employ these general principles for chemicals other than metallic compounds. We, the authors of this book, have a long-term commitment in this field and hope to contribute to widening the access to information and understanding of methods useful for risk assessment of human exposures to metals. We hope that the use of these methods will contribute to further definition and prediction of effects of environmental pollution by metals in order to curb the present worldwide impact of pollution on disease and premature death (Landrigan et al., 2018).

1.2 WIDESPREAD EXPOSURE TO METALS CONTRIBUTES TO GLOBAL BURDEN OF DISEASE

In the last century, the use of metals has expanded substantially and given rise to widespread exposure of humans. It has long been recognized that certain metals are important toxic agents that may cause acute and chronic poisoning in metalworkers and population groups with high exposures. Evidence presented in recent years indicates that low-level exposures to toxic metallic compounds may also contribute to the occurrence of several common diseases. The World Health Organization (WHO, 2009) has estimated that, on a global basis, 143,000 deaths and nearly 9 million disability-adjusted life years (DALYs; i.e., years of healthy life lost) were caused by lead exposure in 2004. Although lead exposure in the general population of many countries has decreased since 2004 because of the continued phaseout of lead in gasoline, several recent epidemiological studies (see Chapter 8) support the notion that low-exposure effects of lead occur in addition to those considered by the WHO (2009). It is therefore quite possible that an estimate of the present global burden of disease caused by lead exposure would arrive at the same or a greater number than the one estimated for exposures occurring in 2004 due to new sources of lead exposure and increases in the world population.

In addition to the estimates of lead-related disease and mortality, there are other well-documented effects that were not included in the WHO estimates of the global burden of disease noted above. This organization further summarized data (Pruss-Ustun et al., 2011), indicating 9100 deaths and 125,000 DALYs per year in Bangladesh from arsenic in drinking water and that mercury exposure (mainly methylmercury [MeHg]) through fish consumption causes cognitive deficits and mild retardation in a considerable number of children. An increased incidence of myocardial infarction has been reported in populations with a high intake of MeHg from fish and a low intake of polyunsaturated fatty acids. The public health impact of this observation of interaction between a nutritional factor and a toxic metal compound may be considerable. There is evidence for a role of relatively low occupational exposure to manganese, as well as exposure in the general environment, as a contributory factor to the increasing prevalence of Parkinson disease. There are potentially great consequences for metal exposures in early life as risk factors for neurodegenerative disorders later in life. Recent epidemiological evidence indicates a role for cadmium in the general environment in increasing the occurrence of renal effects and osteoporosis, as well as cardiovascular diseases (see Chapter 8). There is no doubt thus that exposure to toxic metals and their compounds represent important causal factors contributing to the global burden of disease. WHO (2009) estimated that deficient dietary intakes of essential metals in food, in a global perspective, cause 433,000 deaths and 15,580,000 DALYs from zinc deficiency and 273,000 deaths and 19,734,000 DALYs per year from iron deficiency.

The considerable global burden of disease caused by metals makes it obvious that there is a need for improved risk assessments leading to preventive action against existing exposures. It is also evident that there is a need for better predictive approaches in order to avoid the occurrence of adverse human health effects from new uses of metals in the future.

1.3 METAL POISONING—CLINICAL SYMPTOMS AND SIGNS IN OCCUPATIONAL AND ENVIRONMENTAL SETTINGS

Lead poisoning in workers has been known since antiquity. Greek physicians had identified lead colic and paralysis related to occupational exposures (Waldron, 1973). It has later been confirmed that gastrointestinal (lead colic), neurologic, and hematopoietic symptoms and signs are prominent in occupational lead poisoning (Chapter 8). In childhood lead poisoning, neurodevelopmental and hematopoietic symptoms and signs are prominent. Such poisoning occurred in the 1970s as a result of environmental exposures from lead paint, gasoline additives, and other sources.

Bronchitis and skin rashes may occur in workers inhaling arsenic trioxide. Tremor and neuropsychiatric symptoms may be caused by excessive exposure by inhalation of metallic mercury vapor. If, instead, inorganic mercury salts are inhaled, there may be renal damage, in severe cases leading to anuria. Neurologic symptoms with tunnel vision, ataxia, and speech and hearing difficulties occurred in the population of Minamata, Japan, after consumption of high doses of MeHg via contaminated fish (Minamata disease). Women exposed to MeHg during pregnancy gave birth to children suffering neurological diseases, including cerebral palsy in severe cases (Chapter 8, Section 8.9). Skeletal decalcification with multiple fractures, anemia, and kidney damage (itai-itai disease) was seen in Japan after long-term ingestion of high doses of cadmium through consumption of contaminated rice (Chapter 8, Section 8.3). These syndromes characterizing specific forms of metal poisoning were identified in the past, but cases may still occur accidentally or if there is failure of preventive measures.

The information on metal toxicity in humans is derived from industrial health, large-scale, severe episodes of poisoning via contaminated drinking water and food (MeHg, Cd, Pb) and recently from recognition of widespread occurrence of less obvious but adverse effects on large population groups. There are at least 20 metals or metal-like elements that can give rise to rather well-defined toxic effects in humans. For a few of these metals descriptions of their toxicological properties are given in Chapter 8. Information on other metals can be found in the Handbook on the Toxicology of Metals (Nordberg et al., 2015a). Arsenic, cadmium, lead, manganese, and mercury have been studied most thoroughly, but other metals are also of concern. Molybdenum brings about gout-like signs, and aluminum has been shown to have serious effects on the central nervous system (CNS) under certain circumstances. Antimony and cobalt may have effects on the cardiovascular system. Some organometallic tin compounds give rise to effects in the CNS and on the immune system. The latter type of effects are also known to be a result of exposure to platinum, palladium, and beryllium, in the latter case constituting the mechanism for development of chronic beryllium disease, a form of pneumoconiosis (Jakubowski and Palczinsky, 2015). Effects on the lungs in the form of pneumoconiosis can also arise after exposure to aluminum, antimony, barium, cobalt, indium, iron, tin, and tungsten or their compounds.

While most of the industrial and environmental exposures giving rise to the human health effects noted above have been controlled in the developed countries, there is an urgent need for preventive action in many developing and newly industrialized countries (Landrigan et al., 2015; Fowler et al., 2015a). Large population groups are still exposed to elevated levels of inorganic arsenic in drinking water in Bangladesh, until recently giving rise to classical symptoms of arsenic poisoning with typical skin manifestations (see above) and in the long term also several forms of cancer. In addition to these classical manifestations, there are adverse effects on the cardiovascular and nervous system and the fetuses of pregnant women (Fowler et al., 2015c; Rahman et al., 2009).

1.4 DETAILED INVESTIGATION IS REQUIRED FOR IDENTIFICATION OF ADVERSE EFFECTS AT LOW-LEVEL METAL EXPOSURES

What is it that makes exposure to metals a specific problem? Metals are elements and have been an intrinsic component of the environment to which humans and animals have adapted. A "natural exposure" to any metal may thus be harmless to human beings and other species. However, geological factors and widespread contamination from industrialization form an elevated general background exposure in some countries that give rise to adverse health effects among sensitive sections of the general human population.

In ancient times, clinical symptoms and signs of lead poisoning were known from high-level occupational exposures but adverse health effects of lower level exposures were unknown. In the Roman Empire such effects probably occurred in wide sectors of the general population including the upper classes. Later research has suggested that such effects were caused by the widespread use of lead. Lead pipes were used for distribution of drinking water, and lead was used in cups and vessels for food and drink. The Romans used "sapa" to improve the taste of wine that had gone sour. Sapa was sour wine, boiled in a lead pot, thus producing lead acetate or lead sugar. Adding it to sour wine improved the taste. Unidentified lead poisoning is a suggested contributing factor for the fall of the Roman Empire because of adverse effects on the brain and on reproduction. Widespread adverse effects of lead on humans caused by the use of lead additives to gasoline (Section 1.2 and Chapter 8, Section 8.8) is a more recent example of lead-related human health effects. Such adverse effects were unrecognized for decades, but are now decreasing subsequent to the discontinuation of this use of lead in most countries. The insidious lead toxicity caused by the use of lead in gasoline impacted mainly on young children. It was recognized gradually as a result of careful clinical and epidemiological investigations and increasing understanding of environmental exposure pathways and lead biokinetics.

The Minamata disease in Japan has already been mentioned. It occurred in the 1950s and 1960s because of factory discharges of mercury compounds into the sea in Minamata Bay in southern Japan. MeHg was taken up by fish used for human consumption, causing a severe neurological disease in adults and lower doses caused similar severe diseases including cerebral palsy in children of exposed pregnant women (see further Chapter 8, Section 8.9). In the 1960s, when it was discovered in Sweden that MeHg occurred in fish from Swedish lakes, an evaluation of risks was undertaken based on the available information from minamata disease in Japan in combination with information gathered in experimental animals (Berglund et al., 1971; Chapter 8, Section 8.9). In a few fishermen in Sweden, concentrations of mercury in blood were found in the same range as observed in the Japanese poisoning cases, but no clinical cases of poisoning were recorded in Sweden. Regulation of concentrations of mercury in fish for human consumption in combination with recommendations limiting consumption of lake fish among pregnant women was implemented in Sweden already in the 1970s and in other countries shortly thereafter partly as a result of additional evidence on the toxicity of MeHg (Chapter 8, Section 8.9). There was general regulation of mercury in food in the European Union (EU) in 2001 and a ban on export of mercury from EU in 2008. The United Nations Environment Program (UNEP) launched the "Minamata Convention" in 2013, which is signed by an increasing number of nations, presently more than 100. It focuses on protection from anthropogenic emissions of mercury. All these preventive measures on a global scale were initiated by careful, detailed investigation and adequate risk assessment.

Some metals are required for human health (essential metals) because they have a biological function, for example, in many enzymes. In areas where food consumption is based on local produce, and where the levels of some minerals are low for geological reasons, deficiencies may occur. On the other hand, excessive intakes of essential metals may occur, for example, by the misuse of elevated doses of preparations intended as dietary supplements. The need for detailed investigations and to define an acceptable range of oral intakes (AROIs) has been recognized by WHO/International Programme on Chemical Safety (WHO/IPCS, 2002; see also Chapter 6).

Recent large epidemiological studies have reported statistical associations between low-level human metal exposures, for example, the higher quartile of background exposures and adverse health effects like neurodevelopmental deficiencies in children, increased risks of cancer, renal dysfunction, osteoporosis, and cardiovascular diseases in adults.

It is an important and challenging task to collect and display relevant information that is crucial for prevention of adverse effects from metal exposures on human health and the focus of this book is on methods and examples of risk assessments that form a basis for such prevention.

1.5 PERSPECTIVES ON HISTORICAL DEVELOPMENT OF CONCEPTS USED IN RISK ASSESSMENT OF METAL EXPOSURES—ROLE OF THE SCIENTIFIC COMMITTEE ON THE TOXICOLOGY OF METALS

After World War II, lists of allowable concentrations of substances in workroom air were published. There were, however, substantial differences between values promulgated in the United States and in Russia creating a need for reconciliation. As a consequence of decisions taken by the International Commission on Occupational Health (www. icohweb.org), an evaluation of values for mercury and its compounds in the working environment was made at a symposium held at the Karolinska Institutet (KI) in Stockholm in 1968 (Friberg et al., 1969). One recommendation from this symposium was to form a group of scientists experienced in the toxicology of metals. During the 16th congress of International Commission on Occupational Health (ICOH) in Tokyo in 1969, the Scientific Committee on the Toxicology of Metals (SCTM) was formed as one of the subgroups under ICOH. Lars Friberg was the first chairman of this committee and later both of the present authors have had the privilege to serve as chairs. Since the 1970s, the SCTM of the ICOH has been actively engaged in developing and applying toxicological concepts for use in risk assessment of human metal exposures. The Task Group on Metal Accumulation (TGMA, 1973) emphasized the importance of knowledge regarding metal uptake, disposition and metabolism for an understanding of metal toxicology. The TGMT (1976) defined relationships between critical concentrations in cells and organs and defined the *critical organ* as the particular organ that first attains its critical concentration and exhibits the *critical effect* under specified circumstances of exposure and for a given population. Under continuous exposure, the organ that first attains its critical concentration is also the organ that attains this concentration at the lowest external exposure. This terminology has later been confirmed by the International Union of Pure and Applied Chemistry (Nordberg et al., 2004a; Duffus et al., 2007, 2017).

The *critical concentration* (in a cell or organ) is the concentration of a substance at and above which adverse functional changes, reversible or irreversible, occur in a cell or organ.

The *critical organ concentration* is the mean concentration of a substance in the critical organ when the substance reaches its critical concentration in the most sensitive type of cell in the organ. The critical organ concentration varies among individuals in a population and a critical concentration value thus should be specified whether it is the average value for the population or a lower value, representing, for example, the 5% most sensitive individuals in a population. This concept has been named *population critical concentration (PCC)*, for example, PCC-5 is the concentration, giving rise to an effect in 5% of individuals in a population. The understanding is that the lowest external exposure giving rise to adverse effects in any organ should be avoided by applying these concepts. By using PCC-5, for example, 95% of individuals in a population will be protected from the adverse effects identified as the critical effect (Friberg and Kjellstrom, 1981).

The critical effect thus is the effect that occurs at the lowest dose and is related to the critical concentration in the critical organ. Occurrence of the critical effect in the most sensitive part of the population is an important starting point for preventive measures. The critical effect concept is presently used not only by Swedish Agencies but also by, for example, the US Environmental Protection Agency.

The mentioned concepts have been widely used in metal toxicology and in risk assessments, for example, in the Environmental Health Criteria Documents published by WHO/UNEP International Program on Chemical Safety (WHO/IPCS, 1992—cadmium and other criteria documents). Nordberg (1992) have also noted application of these approaches in relation to carcinogenesis. Further discussion of the use of these concepts in risk assessment will be given in Chapter 3, where a number of recent refinements and additional concepts like MIE, mode/mechanism of action, and TKTD data as well as adverse outcome pathways (AOPs) in risk assessment will also be described.

Considerable efforts were devoted to cadmium toxicology in Friberg's research group in the 1960s. When it was recognized, in 1968, that itai itai disease in Japan was related to cadmium exposure, there was exchange of information between Japanese and Swedish scientists, and joint epidemiological studies in the contaminated area in Toyama prefecture in Japan were carried out. Cadmium was also of interest to the US Environmental Protection Agency, and the group at KI was contracted to write a resource document "Cadmium in the Environment "(Friberg et al., 1971). The risk assessment concepts developed within the SCTM were applied and a consensus meeting on important issues for the risk assessment of cadmium was organized by the SCTM in Bethesda, MD, in 1978 (Fowler, 1979). The important role for cadmium toxicology of the small sulfur-rich protein metallothionein was one of the reasons why the SCTM sponsored a conference on that protein in Zurich, Switzerland (Kagi and Nordberg, 1979). A follow-up conference on metallothionein and cadmium nephrotoxicity was held in Research Triangle Park, NC, in 1983 (Goyer et al., 1984). A book reviewing available evidence relevant for risk assessment of cadmium at that time was published in 1985 (Friberg et al., 1985).

An international conference on environmental arsenic was co-sponsored by the SCTM and held in 1976 in Bethesda, MD (Mahaffey and Fowler, 1977). The risks for skin cancer from exposures to inorganic arsenic were identified and the need for preventive measures was pointed out.

An international workshop on permissible levels for occupational exposure to lead was held in Amsterdam (Zielhuis, 1977).

Another consensus document of importance in metal toxicology was the one issued by the Task Group on Metal Interactions (TGMI, 1978), which focused on factors influencing dose—response relationship of metals. Considerations of various types of combined action of metal exposures like independent action, synergism, and antagonism were an important part of this document. In Chapter 6, these types of joint action of metals will be described and discussed.

As a result of the agreements reached in these consensus documents, it was considered of value to compile the Handbook on the Toxicology of Metals, first edition published in 1979, second edition in 1986, third edition in 2007, and the latest fourth edition in 2015 (Nordberg et al., 2015a).

Further important consensus documents were those on carcinogenesis (Belman and Nordberg, 1981), reproductive and developmental toxicity of metals (Clarkson et al., 1983, 1985), biological monitoring (Clarkson et al., 1988; Nordberg and Skerfving, 1993), and "Immunotoxicity of metals and immunotoxicology" (Dayan et al., 1990). Considerable uncertainty in chemical determination of concentrations in biological media made it necessary to apply strict quality assurance and quality control (QAQC) programs for meaningful application of biological monitoring. The TRACY program (Vesterberg et al., 1988) employed strict criteria in their evaluations of published data (Vesterberg et al., 1993). Such strict QAQC programs are still crucial for successful biological monitoring (Smith and Nordberg, 2015). In collaboration with WHO and the SCTM and supported by the EU-INCO DC program, epidemiological studies of metal contaminated areas in China were conducted and the results reported in a symposium jointly organized by the SCTM and other organizations (Nordberg et al., 2004b). Health risks related to cadmium and inorganic arsenic exposures were in the focus of discussions. Additional studies have later contributed further to our knowledge about health effects of cadmium (Chapter 8, Section 8.3).

The following sections consider further issues of current concern in toxicology and epidemiology of metals and their compounds and will summarize a number of cross-cutting research areas for metals that are discussed in much greater detail in subsequent individual chapters.

1.6 CURRENT LONG-TERM LOW-LEVEL EXPOSURES AND RELATED HEALTH EFFECTS

Metals are an intrinsic component of the environment and humans are exposed to varying degrees from natural sources. In addition, there are anthropogenic exposures as a result of widespread contamination of the environment due to the industrial use of metals. Variation in natural exposure in combination with additional exposures caused by metal-related manufacturing and the use of metal-containing commodities give rise to adverse health effects in sensitive subsections of the human population. Essential metals are required for human life, and in some areas where food production is based on local produce and where concentrations of essential metals are low for geological reasons, deficiencies may occur. The impact of geological factors on human health, considered by the science of "medical geology," is recently attracting increasing attention (Selinus et al., 2013). Recent large epidemiological studies have reported statistical associations between low-level human metal exposures, for example, the higher quartile of background exposures, and adverse health effects in susceptible subsections of the general population. Such effects are sometimes unexplained but may be due to special sensitivity determined by deficiencies or low intakes of essential nutrients. Special sensitivity determined by genetic factors has been shown for beryllium. Persons with a specific variant of the human lymphocyte antigen (HLA) system were more prone to developing a chronic lung disease (chronic beryllium disease or berylliosis) after exposure to low concentrations of beryllium in air (Jakubowski and Palcziynski, 2015).

1.6.1 Neurotoxicology of Metals

Neurotoxic effects of exposure to lead (Pb), and mercury (Hg) and its compounds are well established, and evidence has become available in the last decades that low-level exposures in children may cause adverse effects on cognition and behavior (Chapter 8). Neurotoxic effects of manganese (Mn) are also well established. Other metals known to cause neurotoxicity in humans are aluminum, arsenic, copper, and thallium (Lucchini et al., 2015). Increasing recognition of adverse health effects from Pb and Hg has initiated preventive action by banning or limiting certain uses of these metals. It is necessary to emphasize that it is important to avoid using Mn and other neurotoxic metals in a way that causes widespread dispersion in ambient air. As stated in the Declaration of Brescia, the avoidance of such new applications of the metals is of fundamental importance in protecting humans from potential adverse health effects (Landrigan et al., 2007). It is also obvious that there is a need to find out more about the toxicology of other metals now suggested as replacements for the known toxic metals being phased out. Because of the possibility of adverse effects in children from low-level exposure to lead and MeHg occurring in sections of the general population in several countries, further limitations of existing exposures are needed as pointed out in the Declaration of Brescia 2007 (Landrigan et al., 2007). In addition to the concern for adverse effects in fetuses and children, the possible role of neurotoxic metals as contributing factors for the increasing occurrence of neurodegenerative diseases is an important issue.

1.6.2 Cardiovascular Disease Related to Metals

Exposure to inorganic arsenic and lead are established causative agents for cardiovascular disease. There is also evidence indicating an effect of cadmium and mercury (Sjogren et al., 2015). Increased oxidative stress, inflammatory responses, and changes in coagulation activity are pathophysiological changes relevant to atherogenic disorders, and such changes are suspected to be induced by all these metal exposures. Epidemiological evidence is available for an increased occurrence of myocardial infarction in population groups with slightly elevated intakes of MeHg and a low dietary intake of polyunsaturated fatty acids (Chapters 6 and 8). Cardiomyopathy has been associated with excess intake of arsenic, cobalt, and iron as reviewed by Sjogren et al. (2015), who also gave a detailed review on other aspects of metal exposures and cardiovascular diseases.

1.6.3 Kidney Effects of Exposure to Metals

Metals may affect the renal glomerulus or the tubules. The latter type of effect is the most frequently encountered lesion induced by metal exposures. This lesion gives rise to increased urinary excretion of minerals, sugars, amino acids, and low-molecular-mass proteins. The most important nephrotoxic metals are lead, cadmium, and inorganic mercury. Acute nephrotoxic effects are sometimes seen as side effects when metal compounds (e.g., gold, platinum, and antimony compounds) are used in the treatment of certain diseases. Far more common is long-term exposure, via diet, drinking water, or occupational exposure. Such, long-term exposure to cadmium sometimes causes chronic kidney disease and in some cases development of end-stage renal disease with uremia. Further details concerning renal effects of cadmium, lead, and mercury and their compounds are given in Chapter 8. A detailed review also including other metals is given by Barregard and Elinder (2015).

1.6.4 Cancer Induced by Metal Exposures

Recognition of the role of metals as causative agents for cancer is of ever-increasing public health importance. Evidence based on epidemiological, experimental, and mechanistic data has existed since the 1980s, providing conclusive evidence that some metals and their compounds cause cancer according to evaluations by the International Agency for Research on Cancer (IARC). Chromium and nickel were the first metals to be classified as carcinogens by the IARC. During the 1980s, animal studies with inorganic arsenic confirmed existing epidemiological evidence, and inorganic arsenic was classified as a human carcinogen by IARC (2006). On the basis of the convincing evidence for arsenic carcinogenicity in humans and the fact that arsenic is released from gallium arsenide in animals in vivo, this compound has been classified as a human carcinogen (IARC, 2006). For beryllium, results of epidemiological studies confirmed earlier experimental evidence of carcinogenicity. Cadmium can contribute to the development of lung cancer and probably also to cancer of the prostate and other parts of the urinary tract. During the 1980s, long-term studies in rats inhaling cadmium chloride showed a remarkable dose-related incidence of lung cancer at low exposure levels. Cadmium and its compounds are classified as carcinogenic to humans by the IARC (2012). Lead and its inorganic compounds have been evaluated by the IARC and are classified as probable human carcinogens based on a combination of human and animal data (IARC, 2012; Ward et al., 2010).

The experience with these metals emphasizes the importance of carefully evaluating the consequences in humans of exposures to metals proven to be carcinogenic in animals. Cobalt compounds and antimony trioxide are examples of metal compounds considered to be possible human carcinogens mainly on the basis of animal data. A few metal and metalloid derivatives have shown chromosomal effects in vitro and in vivo, as well as point mutations in cellular assays including human fibroblasts. However, for most of the carcinogenic metals and their compounds, epigenetic mechanisms are considered of importance in their carcinogenicity. The carcinogenicity of some metal compounds and inorganic arsenic is further discussed in Chapters 4, 5, and 8. A more complete review of carcinogenicity of metals, metalloids, and their compounds is given by Laulicht et al. (2015). Davidson et al. (2015) have also reviewed molecular mechanisms of metal carcinogenicity.

1.6.5 Reproductive and Developmental Effects of Metal Exposures

Prenatal effects are known to occur in humans as a result of exposures to lead, MeHg, and inorganic arsenic. The effects of a toxic metal may sometimes mimic deficiency of an essential metal. Because of an efficient placental barrier function, cadmium does not penetrate into the fetus but instead causes an effect on the fetus probably as a result of a secondary zinc deficiency. Cadmium levels have been found to be high in the placenta; high cadmium levels most likely block the transfer of zinc through the placenta. Reproductive and developmental effects are not well documented in humans after exposures to other metals, but such effects have been observed in animals after exposure to large doses of cadmium, indium, lithium, nickel, selenium, and tellurium (Clarkson et al., 1985). The review on Epidemiological Approaches to Metal Toxicology by Grandjean and Budz Jorgensen (2015) pointed out difficulties experienced when performing epidemiological studies regarding these effects in humans.

1.7 ISSUES OF CURRENT CONCERN FOR HAZARD ASSESSMENT, RISK ASSESSMENT, AND PREVENTION

To collect and display relevant information that is crucial for the prevention of adverse effects of metal exposures on human health is important and challenging. This book summarizes some principles and gives a few examples of such information. A more complete treatise may be found in the Handbook on the Toxicology of Metals (Nordberg et al., 2015a). The following sections consider issues of current concern in toxicology and epidemiology of metals and their compounds and will summarize a number of cross-cutting research areas for metals. The basic questions are: To what extent are we able to define relevant human exposures and can we estimate the risks posed by these exposures? Can we suggest precautionary measures to avoid adverse human health effects?

1.7.1 Expanding Global Industrial Use of Metals

Natural processes such as the erosion of surface deposits of metal minerals, volcanic activity, as well as human activities such as mining, smelting, fossil fuel combustion, and the industrial application of metals may give rise to human exposure to metallic elements. The modern chemical industry is based largely on catalysts, many of which are metals or metal compounds. The production of plastics, such as polyvinyl chloride, involves the use of metal compounds, particularly as heat stabilizers. Plating and the manufacture of lubricants are still more examples of the industrial use of metals. The industrial and commercial uses of most of the metals are continuously increasing, although, because of the recognition of the toxicity, there is a leveling off for cadmium and there has been a decrease in the global use of mercury (USGS, 2017; Chapter 8). In the development of advanced technology materials, new applications have been found for the most familiar and the somewhat less familiar metallic elements. Most notable are their uses in the development and production of semiconductors, superconductors, metallic glasses, magnetic alloys, and high-strength, low-alloy steel and most recently in nanotechnology (IARC, 2006, 2010; Karlsson et al., 2015). Many other uses and also discharges from non-metal-producing activities such as electricity production from coal combustion may increase both the amount of metals and the distance over which they are being discharged into the human environment. The distance from the source of metal emissions to their environmental sinks can sometimes be more than 1000 km for airborne transport. When metals are transported along aquatic and terrestrial routes, they often enter into the food chain. Furthermore, the use and disposition of new technological equipment increase electronic waste (E-waste); if not recycled in appropriate waste-handling systems, metals/metalloids used in electronic devices can expose humans directly or through ecological pathways (Fowler, 2017).

1.7.2 Toxicity of Metallic Nanoparticles

Nanotechnology is a rapidly growing field. A large number of new materials containing metals or metal oxides have been developed with widely varying properties. Some of these materials have medical uses implying human exposures, and several others can cause exposure in manufacturing and some in end uses. Nanotoxicology is the new discipline investigating the interactions of nanomaterials with biological systems. It is based on traditional particle and fiber toxicology adapted and modified to consider the special properties of nanomaterials. Nanoparticles have a tendency to agglomerate in air, changing deposition and uptake patterns in the respiratory tract (further description given in Chapter 2). After uptake, nanoparticles in biological fluids will be covered by a biocorona that influences their biological properties. Metallic nanoparticles can exert their biological action either in a direct way or through release of metal ions. Direct interaction with biomolecules is possible; for example, 1.4-nm gold particles are toxic to DNA, probably because of interaction with the major groove in the DNA structure. Larger gold particles are less toxic. There is a large and expanding field of science characterizing the biological and toxicological properties of nanomaterials. Hazard ranking of such materials uses in vitro studies and mathematical modeling (Karlsson et al., 2015). The present book gives only a few examples of lung deposition patterns (Chapter 2) and risk assessments of nanomaterials. Iavicoli et al. (2016) present a more complete review of the effects of nanoparticles on the renal system.

1.7.3 Environmental Mobilization Processes

Long-range transport of air pollutants from combustion of fossil fuels not only contributes to the metal load to ecosystems but also alters the mobility of metals. Increased exposure to aluminum, cadmium, lead, and mercury is well recognized to be the result of long-range transport of air pollutants and the occurrence of acid rain (see Bjerregaard et al., 2015 "Ecotoxicology of Metals: Sources, Transport, and Effects on the Ecosystem"). Such emissions now have decreased considerably both in North America and Europe compared to the situation a few decades ago. These releases, however, are still increasing in other parts of the world where there is increased industrialization. The acidification of soil and lakes, caused by precipitation of sulfur and nitrogen oxides, still remains a problem and will take a long time to resolve, even if emissions decreased. These environmental changes have increased the possibility of adverse effects of metals in the environment due to increased bioavailability by acidification. Increasing acidity of surface waters, including lakes, caused by acid precipitation and changed forestry and agricultural practices means increased mobility of metallic compounds, thus increasing human exposures (Nordberg et al., 1985; Moldan et al., 2013). Natural events, such as hurricanes and flooding, are highly likely to be amplified by global warming and will increase the mobility of metals. Such increased mobility is seen, for example, for mercury in forestry in Sweden and for lead in flooding in New Orleans. Increased exposure may occur by means of increased concentrations of metallic compounds in drinking water and/or food. Small children may further be exposed by direct ingestion of contaminated sand and soil. Although this book is primarily concerned with human health effects resulting from excessive exposure to metals and their compounds, it should be recognized that metals might also have deleterious effects on other animal species and plants. Such effects may lead to modification of an entire population or species assembly in an ecosystem. Such effects of metals may be of great significance to human life and should be considered in the total evaluation of environmental pollution by metals and their compounds (Bjerregaard et al., 2015). It is difficult to rid the environment of a metal with which it has been contaminated. Two striking examples are mercury in the bottom sludge of lakes and cadmium in soil. In addition, several metals and metalloids may undergo methylation during their environmental and biological cycles (e.g., arsenic, gold, palladium, platinum, selenium, tellurium, thallium, and tin), but mercury is the only metal currently known to undergo biomagnification in food chains. MeHg concentrations in marine fish have increased from the mid-1900s, probably because of anthropogenic emissions (see Chapter 8, Section 8.9.3.1). It is obviously of great importance to understand the ecological cycles of metals to evaluate potential threats to human health from the consumption of food and drinking water. There are still considerable gaps in our knowledge in this scientific field (Andersen et al., 2015). The worldwide environmental contamination by the metals cadmium, lead, and mercury has added to the natural cycles of these metals. Despite efforts to limit their use, there is increasing epidemiological evidence that the present background exposure affects human health and contributes to the global burden of disease (Section 1.2). The WHO in Southeast Asia (WHO, 2005) expressed concern for metal exposure in developing countries. An example is transference of the manufacture of lead products to developing countries, where child labor increases the exposure of children to lead. There is still a need for improvements of working and environmental conditions in many developing countries (Fowler et al., 2015a).

1.7.4 Toxic Metals in Food and Oral Intake; Other Intake Routes

The classical environmental disease outbreaks of Minamata disease caused by oral intake of MeHg in fish and itai-itai disease from cadmium in rice has already been mentioned (Sections 1.3 and 1.4). In rice-growing countries in Asia, it has been the custom for farmers to depend, to a great extent, on locally grown products and if there is local contamination with metallic pollutants, it may lead to considerably elevated oral intakes with adverse effects even if all the classical environmental disease symptoms are not displayed. Osteoporosis and renal tubular dysfunction (but not osteomalacia) thus have been shown to occur in cadmium-contaminated areas of China (Nordberg et al., 2002) and adverse effects on brain development in children (but not cerebral palsy) have been shown to be related to increased intake of MeHg in the Faroe islands (Grandjean et al., 1997). Drinking water is sometimes a significant source of oral exposure. The extensive exposure to arsenic through groundwater contaminated by geological occurrence of arsenic in Bangladesh and West Bengal has already been mentioned. Other metals causing exposure through drinking water are aluminum, iron, uranium, and sometimes cadmium, copper, lead, and manganese. Whether or not local contamination exists, ingestion of metals via food and drinking water is ordinarily the main pathway of exposure for the general population (Fowler et al., 2015b). Risks for humans from such exposures from arsenic, lead, cadmium, and mercury are reviewed in Chapter 8.

Dermal uptake of inorganic metallic compounds is usually low, but for organometallic compounds, it can be high and has caused substantial, sometimes lethal, doses (Nierenberg et al., 1998). Inhalation is usually the most important occupational exposure route. Ambient air, except in the vicinity of an emission source, does not usually contribute significantly to the total exposure. Contaminated air may pollute soil and water secondarily resulting in contaminated crops and vegetables, thus causing oral human exposure through food. A route of exposure that must not be forgotten is the inhalation of tobacco smoke, which contains a number of metals, including cadmium, nickel, arsenic, and lead. Cadmium in tobacco smoke will often contribute a considerable proportion of the body burden of Cd in smokers. In areas where tobacco is grown and soils are contaminated by cadmium, substantial exposure may occur through smoking. Such exposure was reported by Cai et al. (1995) in an agricultural area in China where soils have been contaminated by cadmium-containing tailings from an ore dressing plant at a tungsten mine. Data have been presented showing that external metal contamination of cigarettes in industries where exposure to metals already occurs through air may increase the workers' inhalation dose of metals by several folds (IPCS 1992). Smoking, therefore, should not be allowed in occupational environments where metals are handled.

1.7.5 Metal Exposure by Release From Implanted Medical Devices

Exposure to metals usually takes place by the routes mentioned in the fore-going paragraph. Exposure can also be a result of release from implanted medical devices such as dental amalgam restorations, metallic neurological implants, metallic cardiovascular implants, and metallic joint replacement prostheses. This is the subject of a review by Brown et al. (2015), pointing out the importance of assessing the biocompatibility of such devices and the need for monitoring of releases of metals to systemic circulation. The shape of the devices and their composition in combination with the mechanical forces acting on them after they have been implanted in the human body are factors determining the likelihood of releases of wear debris and metal ions. There are case reports of adverse effects from metals, for example, cobalt, released from medical devices, but the few available epidemiological studies are small and difficult to interpret. Risk assessment of such releases follow the same principles as those used for other human exposures but starts from measured levels of metals in biological monitoring media such as blood and urine (see Chapter 8, Section 8.4).

1.7.6 Toxicokinetics and Dosimetry

As mentioned above, dermal uptake of inorganic metallic species is usually low, but high uptake may occur for organometallic species (see Section 1.7.4). Uptake into the body after exposure by the oral and inhalational routes is governed by a set of partly known processes. The uptake of inhaled gases and particulate aerosols has been described by a fairly well-established general model. The uptake of ingested metallic ionic species is less well characterized but can be modeled for specific metallic compounds. A toxicokinetic model may be set up involving data on the absorption, distribution, biotransformation, and excretion of a given metallic species. Basic considerations on toxicokinetic models are given in Chapter 2. One example is MeHg (Chapter 8). Almost 100% of ingested MeHg is taken up systemically from the gastrointestinal tract. The accumulation may be described by a one-compartment model, indicating that exchange between the different organs is considerably faster than excretion of the metal. The biological half-time is 33—189 days (see Chapter 8, Section 8.9). The toxicokinetics of cadmium is more complicated and an appropriate model is more difficult to establish. Some facts are well recognized, however. The absorption of cadmium from food will average around 5% in men and 10% in women (see Chapters 2 and 8). Absorption of cadmium after inhalation may vary between 10% and 50%, depending on particle size distribution. In long-term, low-level exposures, several series of autopsy data have shown that approximately one-third of the total body burden may be in the kidneys and about half in the kidneys and liver together. With higher exposure, proportionally more cadmium would be found in the liver. For cadmium, the biological half-time in humans is estimated to be 10—30 years. This long half-time may be related to the fact that cadmium is the most potent inducer of the synthesis of metallothionein, a high-affinity metal-binding protein (Nordberg, 1984, 1998; Nordberg and Kojima, 1979; Nordberg and Nordberg, 2002; Chapter 2). With constant exposure, such long biological half-times imply that accumulation will take place over an entire lifetime. A physiologically based multicompartment model has been developed to describe the behavior of cadmium (Nordberg and Kjellstrom, 1979; Chapters 2 and 8). This model has been further developed and generated values compared to the National Health and Nutrition Examination Survey data in the United States (Choudhury et al., 2001; Chapter 2). It has been possible to estimate the daily intake required to reach the critical concentration of cadmium in the kidney cortex and population risks for renal dysfunction (Diamond et al., 2003; Friberg et al., 1985; Kjellstrom and Nordberg, 1978; Nordberg et al., 2018). The European Food Safety Agency (EFSA) used a one-compartment model for cadmium when estimating cadmium intakes corresponding to biomonitoring data (EFSA, 2009). Using the toxicokinetic model for MeHg, the concentration in the brain may be calculated based on information about concentrations in the brain leading to poisoning; risk may be calculated at various oral intakes. These models for cadmium and MeHg have also been used in National Health criteria documents and in the Health criteria documents by WHO/IPCS (Berglund et al., 1971; Nordberg and Strangert, 1985; Task Group on Metal Toxicity (TGMT), 1976; WHO/IPCS, 1990, 1991, 1992). These estimates are in good agreement with directly observed associations between exposure, concentrations in organs, and effects. Toxicokinetic models have also been published for inorganic lead and for chromium compounds (see Chapter 2). There is a great need to set up appropriate toxicokinetic models for other metals, but in most cases, adequate data are not available. Clarkson et al. (1988) (see also Chapter 2) advanced this issue and presented kinetic/metabolic models for those metals seen as the most important at that time. The concept is important and should be applicable for further improvement of existing models and for metals of interest in the future.

In risk assessment, the acceptable exposure for a specific metallic compound can be estimated either from observations of dose—response relationships derived from external exposures or from an understanding of the tissue levels in organs or in biological monitoring media that are related to development of adverse health effects. The ability to utilize biomonitoring data for risk assessment purposes has been enhanced by the development of computer modeling techniques capable of delineating forward and reverse dosimetry relationships. *Forward dosimetry* is an estimation of internal exposures from measurements of external exposure in studies characterizing chemical toxicity; *reverse dosimetry*, sometimes called *dose reconstruction*, is an estimation of environmental exposures consistent with measured biological monitoring data. In Chapter 2, Section 2.8, examples are given of how these risk assessment tools can be used (see also Ruiz et al., 2010).

1.7.7 Essential Metals: Deficiency and Toxicity

Metals integrated in biological structures or in ionic form are found in all living organisms and play a variety of roles. They may be structural elements, stabilizers of biological structures, components of control mechanisms (e.g., in nerves and muscles), and, in particular, activators or components of redox systems. Thus, some metals are essential elements, and their deficiency results in the impairment of biological functions. A considerable global burden of disease is related to deficiencies of zinc and iron (see Section 1.2). Essential metals, when present in excess, may be toxic (Chapter 6). Gastrointestinal irritation occurs if high levels of ionic iron, zinc, or cadmium are ingested. Essential metals may also give rise to systemic toxicity if exposure is excessive (e.g., molybdenum gives rise to a gout-like disease). Metal toxicity is explainable on the basis of interference with cellular biochemical systems. Metals often interact at important sites such as the sulfhydryl (SH) groups of enzyme systems. They may also compete with other essential metals as enzyme cofactors or at competitors for common transporters. Whether deficiency or toxicity occurs depends on the daily oral intake. An AROIs exists between intakes which are too low and give rise to deficiency and intakes which are too high and give rise to toxicity, and it is important to define this range (see further description in Chapter 6).

1.7.8 Biological Monitoring

Biomonitoring or biological monitoring, using concentrations of metals in urine, blood, or hair as dose indicators, has been increasingly used in recent years (see Chapters 2 and 3). When interpreting such data, an appropriate toxicokinetic model (see above) is of great value because it will depict the relationships between concentrations in indicator media and concentrations in critical organs and in the body as a whole. The usefulness of such an approach was pointed out in a consensus document by the SCTM a long time ago (Clarkson et al., 1988) and some advances have been made (see foregoing section and Chapter 2). For MeHg, blood levels, particularly red cell levels, are valuable for assessing the concentration of MeHg in the CNS, as well as in the body as a whole. As a rule, urinary levels cannot be used because the excretion of MeHg in urine is extremely small, the main excretion route being the bile (Chapter 8). For cadmium, the situation is more complicated. In long-term, low-level exposures, urinary levels on a group basis give an indication of the concentration in the kidneys and the total body burden. In individual cases, caution must be exercised because of wide individual variations and, in the range of background values, an influence of diuresis (even after standardization by creatinine) and normal variation in urinary proteins may exist (Chapter 8). When the critical level of cadmium has been reached in the kidney cortex, tubular proteinuria occurs and cadmium excretion through urine increases simultaneously. Under such conditions, the cadmium concentration in urine no longer reflects the total body burden. Blood levels may be useful for evaluating recent exposure and sometimes for estimating the body burden. The biological half-time of cadmium in blood is considerably shorter than that in the kidneys or in bone tissue (Chapter 8).

1.7.9 Interactions Among Metals and Gene—Environment Interactions

The joint action of two or more metals and further the impact of other factors such as nutrients and host factors can substantially change dose—response relationships. Interactions constitute a subject on which more and more attention is being focused. This matter has been discussed at several international symposia (Fowler, 2005; Nordberg, 1978; Nordberg and Andersen, 1981; Nordberg and Pershagen, 1984) and is reviewed by

Nordberg et al. (2015b) and in Chapter 6. The protective effect of polyunsaturated fatty acids on cardiac toxicity of MeHg has already been mentioned and is an example of an interaction of considerable practical interest. Another example is the ability of selenium to decrease the toxicity of MeHg. Age seems to be an interaction factor of particular importance at both early and late stages of life. There are many data which indicate that the absorption of both cadmium and lead is substantially higher in young age groups than in old age groups. On the other hand, geriatric populations may be at increased risk of metal toxicity due to reduced plasticity of major organ systems such as the brain and kidney (Fowler, 2013). There are also apparent marked gender differences with regard to uptake of cadmium that persist over a broad age range (Ruiz et al., 2010). Children are more susceptible than adults to the development of neurotoxic effects of lead (see Chapter 8). By means of recent methods for identification of genetic variation in populations, the role of genetic polymorphisms is currently being examined in relation to metal toxicology (Broberg et al., 2015). It is obvious that such interactions occur frequently and can both increase and decrease the toxicity of metals. For example, there are data to support the conclusion that the risk of chronic beryllium disease developing is considerably increased among persons belonging to a specific genetic HLA variant.

1.7.10 Application of MOA TKTD Models, AOPs, or Other Systems Toxicology Approaches to Risk and Hazard Assessment of Metal Exposures

Previous sections of the present chapter (e.g., Section 1.5) mentioned the concepts of MOA, TKTD modeling, MIE, and AOP. The present section will briefly introduce these concepts; Chapters 3 and 4 give further explanation.

Previous text in the present section of this chapter pointed out the importance of toxicokinetics and dosimetry for risk assessment. When combined with an understanding of toxicodynamics, a TKTD model may be developed. Toxicodynamics describe the mechanism of action or the MOA of a toxic agent, how the agent causes tissue damage, and under what conditions in terms of tissue concentration and time of tissue exposure/dose that adverse effects occur. The interference by lead (Pb) on the heme synthesis pathway in the bone marrow is a good example of knowledge on the mechanism of action giving rise to the adverse effect—anemia—frequently observed in the past among workers in the lead industry (see further Chapter 3). Knowledge of the MOA and the tissue levels of cadmium related to the induction of dysfunction of the tubular part of the kidney, when combined with toxicokinetic knowledge, allowed the description of a TKTD model for cadmium exposure and kidney dysfunction. Risk assessments related both to occupational cadmium exposures and environmental exposure have used this TKTD model (see Chapters 5, 7, and 8). The Organisation for Economic Co-operation and Development described an AOP for allergic contact dermatitis caused by sensitizing chemical agents (Chapter 3). This AOP describes penetration into the skin of the sensitizing agent, the MIE in the skin, and the further molecular events leading to hypersensitivity. Chapter 3 discusses the use of this AOP in risk assessments of skin exposures to nickel in the general population. Further refinements of the AOP seem necessary for precise quantitative predictions of skin exposures causing sensitization in humans (see also Chapter 8, Section 8.10).

1.7.11 Applied Hazard- and Risk Assessment—Preventive Action and Management

Applied risk assessment covers the translation of exposure and toxicological data into risk assessments and applies this information into preventive measures and/or regulatory action. The term hazard assessment usually implies a qualitative or semiquantitative estimate of dose—response relationships, while risk assessments include quantitative observations or estimates of dose—response. Risk assessments should focus on the most susceptible part of the population and consider the type of risks, critical versus noncritical effects, threshold versus nonthreshold effects, and the severity of the critical effect. Chapter 7 gives further aspects on applied risk assessment, including risk management.

Risks to the health of humans may result from exposure to metals in industrial and general environments. The crucial questions are: which safety margins are needed and which ones are available. These questions are not easy to answer, but epidemiological evidence has been increasing in the last decades (see Chapter 8) demonstrating that for some metallic species, safety margins are very small or nonexisting in population groups with certain habits or life styles. If we consider MeHg, we know that MeHg exposure causes early developmental effects. Risks of such effects may result from the regular consumption of fish such as pike, tuna, shark, and swordfish by pregnant women. Risk assessments have resulted in restrictions of MeHg levels in food both in the United States and in the EU. Some countries (e.g., Sweden) have high concentrations of MeHg in lake fish because of acid rain, and thus a program is in effect, informing women of childbearing age to avoid fish high in MeHg. The global production and use of mercury has decreased considerably from 1975 to 1995. Efforts are being made on an international scale to further limit the use of mercury and to decrease human exposure to mercury and its compounds in the framework of the Minamata Convention 2013. The global cycling of mercury is nevertheless continuing because of emissions from coal-fired power plants, artisanal gold mining, degassing from the earth crust, and the oceans. These emissions are difficult to control (see further discussion in Chapter 8). MeHg concentrations in the mentioned fish species therefore still remain high and advisories about the safe amount of such fish that can be consumed by pregnant women still are warranted.

The slow development and recognition of knowledge about the neurodevelopmental toxicity of lead and MeHg in humans was noted by Grandjean and Landrigan (Grandjean and Landrigan, 2006), delaying societal preventive action. These scientists pointed out the lack, at present, of adequate data for a risk assessment of neurodevelopmental effects of a number of other neurotoxic metals and metal compounds such as aluminum, bismuth, ethylmercury, inorganic mercury, manganese, tellurium, thallium, and tin compounds. Considerable efforts are thus required to fill the gaps in knowledge.

As already mentioned, in the last couple of decades, high-level arsenic exposures of large population groups have occurred in Bangladesh and parts of India (West Bengal) because of the use of drinking water with high levels of inorganic arsenic. These exposures occurred in spite of existing knowledge about the toxicity of inorganic arsenic, but the high levels of arsenic in water were not discovered when these sources of bacteriologically safe water were established. In the last decade, extensive epidemiological studies have documented widespread adverse health effects in the exposed populations including increased occurrence of skin lesions, skin cancer, spontaneous abortion, increased perinatal mortality, and decreased birth weight. Adverse health effects have been documented at exposure levels previously believed to be safe. Measures have been taken to control exposures but are not yet fully implemented (Rahman et al., 2009).

To establish health criteria for exposure standards is an important task that is being increasingly recognized and structured at national and international levels. One issue of great interest is the dose—response relationship for cancer. While in the past, linear dose—response extrapolation was applied, for example, for carcinogenic effects of inorganic arsenic exposures, recent epidemiological observations have documented such relationships down to low exposure levels. Discussions have long been devoted to the question of whether it would be advisable to apply the philosophy of collective dose to some chemical substances, including metals. According to this concept, which is used in radiation protection, any emission, for example, from a coal-fired power plant, is considered to involve a certain degree of risk even if the effects may be remote both geographically and with respect to time, and may occur only when a simultaneous exposure from a number of other sources takes place. These and other aspects on risk assessment are discussed further in the following chapters of this book. Risk assessment concerning human health has been refined and improved by introducing new methods such as assessing benchmark dose, identifying new biomarkers, and by differentiating assessments by speciation of metals (Chapter 8; WHO/IPCS, 2006).

In conclusion, we hope that this first chapter has served to provide the reader with a historical perspective on the evolution of risk assessment for metallics and why this field remains of great public health importance in both developed and developing countries. We also hope the following chapters on current and evolving risk assessment approaches for metals will aid persons new to this major area of public health in developing their own thinking. It is clear that toxic metals have created human health problems for thousands of years and will likely continue as major issues due to new exposure paradigms and increased scientific understanding of adverse low-dose effects.

REFERENCES

Andersen, M., et al., 2015. Nature 517 (7534), 356–359.

Barregard, L., Elinder, C.G., 2015. Renal effects of exposure to metals. In: Nordberg, G.F., Fowler, B.A., Nordberg, M. (Eds.), Handbook on the Toxicology of Metals. Academic Press/Elsevier (Chapter 17).

Belman, S., Nordberg, G., 1981. Environ. Health Perspect. 40, 3.

Berglund, F., et al., 1971. Nord. Hyg. Tidskr. (Suppl. 4)

Bjerregaard, P., Andersen, C.B.I., Andersen, O., 2015. Ecotoxicology of metals: sources, transport, and effects on the ecosystem. In: Nordberg, G.F. (Ed.), Handbook on the Toxicology of Metals, fourth ed. Academic Press/Elsevier (Chapter 21).

Broberg, K., Engstrom, K., Ameer, 2015. Gene-environment interactions for metals. In: Nordberg, G.F., Fowler, B.A., Nordberg, M. (Eds.), Handbook on the Toxicology of Metals. Academic Press/Elsevier (Chapter 12).

Brown, R.P., et al., 2015. Toxicity of metals released from implanted medical devices. In: Nordberg, G.F., Fowler, B.A., Nordberg, M. (Eds.), Handbook on the Toxicology of Metals, fourth ed. Academic Press/Elsevier (Chapter 5).

Cai, S., Yue, L., Shang, Q., et al., 1995. WHO Bull. 73, 359.

Choudhury, H.T., et al., 2001. Toxicol. Environ. Health Part A 63, 321.

Clarkson, T.W., Nordberg, G.F., Sager, P., 1983. Reproductive and Developmental Toxicity of Metals. Plenum Press, New York.

Clarkson, T.W., et al., 1985. Scand. J. Work Environ. Health 11, 145.

Clarkson, T.W., Friberg, L., Nordberg, G.F., et al., 1988. Biological Monitoring of Toxic Metals. Plenum Publishing Co., New York, p. 317.

Davidson, T., Ke, Q., Costa, M., 2015. Selected molecular mechanisms of metal toxicity and carcinogenicity. In: Nordberg, G.F., Fowler, B.A., Nordberg, M. (Eds.), Handbook on the Toxicology of Metals. Academic Press/Elsevier (Chapter 9).

Dayan, A.D., et al., 1990. Immunotoxicity of Metals and Immunotoxicology. Plenum Press, New York, London.

Diamond, G.L., et al., 2003. J. Toxicol. Environ. Health A 66, 2141.

Duffus, J., et al., 2007. Pure Appl. Chem. 79, 1153.

Duffus, J.H., Templeton, D.M., Schwenk, M., 2017. Comprehensive Glossary of Terms Used in Toxicology. RSC Publishing.

EFSA (European Food Safety Authority), 2009. EFSA J. 980, 2.

Fowler, B.A., 1979. Environ. Health Perspect. 28, 1.

Fowler, B.A., 2005. Toxicol. Appl. Pharmacol. 206, 97.

Fowler, B.A., 2013. Cadmium and aging. In: Weiss, B. (Ed.), Aging and Vulnerabilities to Environmental Chemicals. Royal Society of Chemistry, Cambridge, pp. 376–387.

Fowler, B.A., 2017. Electronic Waste: Toxicology and Public Health Issues. Elsevier Publishers, Amsterdam, p. 84.

Fowler, B.A., et al., 2015a. Metal toxicology in developing countries. In: Nordberg, G.F., Fowler, B.A., Nordberg, M. (Eds.), Handbook on the Toxicology of Metals. Academic Press/Elsevier (Chapter 25).

Fowler, B.A., et al., 2015b. Toxic metals in food. In: Nordberg, G.F., Fowler, B.A., Nordberg, M. (Eds.), Handbook on the Toxicology of Metals. Academic Press/Elsevier (Chapter 6).

Fowler, B.A., et al., 2015c. Arsenic. In: Nordberg, G.F., Fowler, B.A., Nordberg, M. (Eds.), Handbook on the Toxicology of Metals. Academic Press/Elsevier (Chapter 28).

Friberg, L., Kjellstrom, T., 1981. In: Bronner, F., Colburn, J.W. (Eds.), Disorders of Mineral Metabolism I: Trace Metals. Academic Press, New York, pp. 317–352.

Friberg, L., et al., 1969. Arch. Environ. Health 19, 891.

Friberg, L., Piscator, M., Nordberg, G., 1971. Cadmium in the Environment. CRC Press, Cleveland, Ohio, p. 166.

Friberg, L., Elinder, C.-G., Kjellstrom, T., et al., 1985. Cadmium and Health, a Toxicological and Epidemiological Appraisal, 2 vols. CRC Press, Boca Raton, Florida.

Goyer, R., et al., 1984. Environ. Health Perspect. 54.

Grandjean, P., Budz Jorgensen, 2015. Epidemiological approaches to metal toxicology. In: Nordberg, G.F., Fowler, B.A., Nordberg, M. (Eds.), Handbook on the Toxicology of Metals. Academic Press/Elsevier (Chapter 13).

Grandjean, P., Landrigan, P.J., 2006. Lancet 368 (9553), 2167–2178.

Grandjean, P., et al., 1997. Neurotoxicol. Teratol. 19, 417.

IARC, 2006. Monograph. In: Cobalt in Hard Metals and Cobalt Sulfate, Gallium Arsenide, Indium Phosphide and Vanadium Pentoxide, vol. 86. IARC, Lyon, France.

IARC, 2010. Monograph. In: Carbon Black, Titanium Dioxide Talc, vol. 93. IARC, Lyon, France.

IARC, 2012. Monograph. In: Arsenic, Metals, Fibres and Dusts, vol. 100C. IARC, Lyon, France.

Iavicoli, I., et al., 2016. Crit. Rev. Toxicol. 46, 490.

Jakubowski, M., Palcziynski, 2015. Beryllium. In: Nordberg, G.F., Fowler, B.A., Nordberg, M. (Eds.), Handbook on the Toxicology of Metals. Academic Press/Elsevier (Chapter 30).

Kagi, J.H.R., Nordberg, M., 1979. Metallothionein. Birkhauser Verlag, Basel.

Karlsson, H.L., et al., 2015. Toxicity of metal and metal oxide nanoparticles. In: Nordberg, G.F., Fowler, B.A., Nordberg, M. (Eds.), Handbook on the Toxicology of Metals. Academic Press/Elsevier (Chapter 4).

Kjellstrom, T., Nordberg, G.F., 1978. Environ. Res. 16, 248.

Landrigan, P., et al., 2007. Am. J. Ind. Med. 50, 79.

Landrigan, P.J., et al., 2015. Principles for prevention of the toxic effects of metals. In: Nordberg, G.F., Fowler, B.A., Nordberg, M. (Eds.), Handbook on the Toxicology of Metals. Academic Press/Elsevier (Chapter 24).

Landrigan, P.J., et al., 2018. Lancet 391 (10119), 462−512.

Laulicht, F., et al., 2015. Carcinogenicity of metal compounds. In: Nordberg, G.F., Fowler, B.A., Nordberg, M. (Eds.), Handbook on the Toxicology of Metals, fourth ed. Academic Press/Elsevier (Chapter 18).

Lucchini, R., et al., 2015. Neurotoxicology of metals. In: Nordberg, G.F., Fowler, B.A., Nordberg, M. (Eds.), Handbook on the Toxicology of Metals, fourth ed. Academic Press/Elsevier (Chapter 15).

Mahaffey, K.R., Fowler, B.A., 1977. Environ. Health Perspect. 19, 165.

Moldan, F., et al., 2013. Ambio 42, 577.

Nierenberg, D.W., et al., 1998. N. Engl. J. Med. 338, 1672.

Nordberg, G.F., 1978. Environ. Health Perspect. 40, 3.

Nordberg, M., 1984. Environ. Health Perspect. 54, 13.

Nordberg, G.F., 1992. Application of the 'critical effect' and 'critical concentration' concept to human risk assessment for cadmium. IARC Scientific Publications No 118. In: Nordberg, G.F., Alessio, L., Herber, R.F.M. (Eds.), Cadmium in the Human Environment: Toxicity and Carcinogenicity, pp. 3−14.

Nordberg, M., 1998. Talanta 46, 243.

Nordberg, G.F., Andersen, O., 1981. Environ. Health Perspect. 40, 65.

Nordberg, G.F., Kjellstrom, T., 1979. Environ. Health Perspect. 28, 211.

Nordberg, M., Kojima, Y., 1979. In: Kagi, J.H.R., Nordberg, M. (Eds.), Metallothionein. Birkhauser Verlag, Basel, pp. 41−135.

Nordberg, M., Nordberg, G.F., 2002. In: Sarkar, B. (Ed.), Handbook of Heavy Metals in the Environment. Marcel Dekker, Inc., New York, pp. 231−269.

Nordberg, G.F., Pershagen, G., 1984. Toxicol. Environ. Chem. 9, 63.

Nordberg, G.F., Skerfving, S., 1993. Scand. J. Work Environ. Health 19 (Suppl. 1), 140.

Nordberg, G.F., Strangert, P., 1985. Scope and J. In: Vouk, V., Butler, G.C., Hoel, D.G., et al. (Eds.), Methods for Estimating Risk of Chemical Injury: Human and Non-human Biota and Ecosystems. Wiley Publishers, Chichester, New York, pp. 477−491.

Nordberg, G.F., et al., 1985. Environ. Health Perspect. 63, 169.

Nordberg, G., et al., 2002. Ambio 31 (6), 478.

Nordberg, M., et al., 2004a. Pure Appl. Chem. 76, 1033.

Nordberg, M., et al., 2004b. Biometals 17, 483.

Nordberg, G.F., Fowler, B.A., Nordberg, M., 2015a. Handbook on the Toxicology of Metals, fourth ed. Academic Press/Elsevier.

Nordberg, G.F., et al., 2015b. Interactions and mixtures in metal toxicology. In: Nordberg, G.F., Fowler, B.A., Nordberg, M. (Eds.), Handbook on the Toxicology of Metals, fourth ed. Academic Press/Elsevier (Chapter 11).

Nordberg, G.F., et al., 2018. Pure Appl. Chem. 90, 755.

Pruss-Ustun, A., Vickers, C., Haefliger, P., et al., 2011. Environ. Health 10, 9.

Rahman, A., et al., 2009. Am. J. Epidemiol. 169, 304.

Ruiz, P., et al., 2010. Toxicol. Lett. 198, 44.

Selinus, O., Alloway, B., Centeno, J.A., et al., 2013. Essentials of Medical Geology. Springer, Dordrecht.

Sjogren, B., et al., 2015. Cardiovascular disease. In: Nordberg, G.F., Fowler, B.A., Nordberg, M. (Eds.), Handbook on the Toxicology of Metals, fourth ed. Academic Press/Elsevier (Chapter 16).

Smith, D.R., Nordberg, M., 2015. General chemistry, sampling, analytical methods and speciation. In: Nordberg, G.F., Fowler, B.A., Nordberg, M. (Eds.), Handbook on the Toxicology of Metals, fourth ed. Academic Press/Elsevier (Chapter 2).

TGMA (Task Group on Metal Accumulation), 1973. Environ. Physiol. Biochem. 3, 65.

TGMI (Task Group of Metal Interactions), 1978. In: Nordberg, G.F. (Ed.), Environ. Health Perspect. 25, 1.

TGMT (Task Group on Metal Toxicity), 1976. In: Nordberg, G.F. (Ed.), Effects and Dose-Response Relationships of Toxic Metals. Elsevier, Amsterdam, pp. 7–111.

USGS, 2017. Mineral Commodity Summaries, p. 135.

Vesterberg, O., et al., 1988. Fresenius Z. Anal. Chem. 332, 556.

Vesterberg, O., et al., 1993. Scand. J. Work Environ. Health 19 (Suppl. 1), 19–26.

Waldron, H.A., 1973. Med. Hist. 17, 391–399.

Ward, E.M., et al., 2010. Environ. Health Perspect. 118, 1355.

WHO, 2009. Global Health Risks: Mortality and Burden of Diseases Attributable to Selected Major Risks. www.who.int/healthinfo/global_burden_disease/.

WHO Regional Office for South-East Asia, New Delhi, 2005. Environmental Health Impacts from Exposure to Metals. Report of an Interregional Workshop. Simla, India.

WHO/IPCS, 1990. Methylmercury. Environmental Health Criteria Document 101. WHO, Geneva.

WHO/IPCS, 1991. Inorganic Mercury. Environmental Health Criteria Document 118. WHO, Geneva.

WHO/IPCS, 1992. Cadmium. Environmental Health Criteria Document 134. World Health Organization, Geneva, Switzerland.

WHO/IPCS, 2002. Principles and Methods for the Assessment of Risk from Essential Trace Elements. Environmental Health Criteria 228. World Health Organization, International Program on Chemical Safety, Geneva.

WHO/IPCS, 2006. Elemental Speciation in Human Health Risk Assessment. EHC 234. WHO, Geneva.

Zielhuis, 1977. Int. Arch. Occup. Environ. Health 39, 59.

CHAPTER TWO

Exposure, Internal Dose, and Toxicokinetics (TK)

Abstract

This chapter not only describes the main routes of human exposure to metals and metallic compounds in drinking water, food, and ambient and workroom air but also exposure of the skin and internal exposures from metals in medical devices. Interesting scientific developments in recent years have contributed to our understanding of uptake mechanism. The disposition of nanoparticles in the lung is now an area of considerable interest and the subject of current research efforts. This chapter gives special attention to the processes of deposition, clearance, and absorption of inhaled gases and airborne particles in the respiratory tract. Our understanding has increased in recent years of deposition and absorption mechanisms in the gastrointestinal tract, which are also included in this chapter. Specific carriers and ion channels intended for endogenous substances and essential elements play a role in the transfer also of nonessential metals and metallic compounds through cell membranes and are important for uptake in body organs. This chapter considers available knowledge on the uptake, transport, and excretion of metallic nanoparticles. Fecal excretion of several metals occurs after enterohepatic circulation, i.e., the initial uptake and excretion through the liver and bile and the partial secondary uptake in the intestine, with a proportion excreted in feces. The roles of intestinal microflora in methylating/demethylating metallic compounds are increasingly recognized. For methylmercury, such processes are important for excretion of generated inorganic mercury in feces. Accumulation of metals in the kidney and urinary excretion depends on protein binding of metals in blood plasma. The best example is the binding of cadmium to the small sulfur-rich protein metallothionein. A quantitative description of the total body turnover of metals is possible by toxicokinetic models. Such models are often helpful in developing calculations of predicted dose—response relationships. Other chapters deal with these uses of the models.

2.1 INTRODUCTION; TERMINOLOGY

Concentrations of metallic compounds in exposure media such as air, drinking water, or food determined by chemical analyses or estimated from information concerning emissions usually forms the basis for exposure

Risk Assessment for Human Metal Exposures
ISBN: 978-0-12-804227-4
https://doi.org/10.1016/B978-0-12-804227-4.00002-9

measurements or estimates. A description of exposure to the metal compound that is under consideration is a very important component of risk assessment. Such an exposure assessment in combination with the results of dose—response analysis forms the basis for risk characterization (Chapter 7).

There have been attempts to distinguish the terms "exposure" from "dose," but there is still no general recognition of such special usage. In occupational and environmental health, the term *exposure* means that a person or group of persons are in contact with one or more chemical agents such as a metal or its compounds; sometimes this term is reserved for the external contact between the human being and the environment (*external exposure*). This is the focus of the International Programme on Chemical Safety Document 214, jointly published by the World Health Organization, International Labour Organization, and United Nations Environment Programme (IPCS, 2000), concerning the role of human exposure assessment in identifying and defining actual or anticipated (external) exposures in human populations. This can be a complex endeavor, requiring analysis of the many different aspects of contact between people and hazardous substances (IPCS, 2000). However, in cell biology, the term *exposure* often describes the in vitro exposure of cells and subcellular organelles to solutions of metal compounds. In such instances, *exposure* means the concentration of a chemical agent that reaches the cells or cell organelles (Duffus et al., 2007). The term *dose* originates from pharmacology and means the amount of drug given to a patient. According to the International Union of Pure and Applied Chemistry (Duffus et al., 2007), the *dose* is the total amount of a substance administered to, taken up by, or absorbed by an organism, organ, or tissue. The proportion of the given dose that is absorbed systemically is the *absorbed dose*, also named *internal dose* (see Duffus et al., 2007, 2009). By transfer, usually through blood, a fraction of the internal dose reaches the critical organ (see Chapter 1, Section 1.5 and Chapter 3 and Appendix). The concentration of a metal compound in the critical organ is of considerable interest in risk assessment of metal exposures, as discussed further in Chapter 3. The assessment of metal exposure and dose thus primarily encompasses the contact between human beings and metals in the surrounding media such as air, drinking water, food, and media in contact with the skin but may also include estimation of internal dose and accumulation in critical organs. This chapter will deal with exposure and dose assessment in this broader setting. The European Chemicals Agency (ECHA, 2009) uses the term *dose descriptor* for specific dose information such as the no-observed-adverse-effect level used as a basis (or point of departure [POD]) for deriving ECHA-specific dose descriptors (see dose—response estimates, Chapter 5).

The *exposome* is a relatively new concept. According to Wild (2012), "The concept of the exposome was developed to draw attention to the critical need for more complete environmental exposure assessment in epidemiological studies; environment is defined in this context in the broad sense of 'non-genetic.' The exposome, therefore, complements the genome by providing a comprehensive description of lifelong exposure history. Remaining focused on the element of application (to epidemiology) is a key to ensuring that the exposome is translated from concept to utility for better delineating the causes and prevention of human disease." The term "exposome" is the measure of all of the exposures of an individual in a lifetime and of how those exposures relate to health (CDC/NIOSH, 2017). All considerations given in the present chapter, thus, are included in the "exposome" concept, but in addition, the concept implies a desire to develop new "omics" technologies for efficient and wide studies of many different (internal) exposures that may interact with or modify target molecules important for the expression of a toxic effect.

As a basis for metal toxicology, it is important to understand how metals and their compounds move from the source to the site of action (or target site) in the human body and what mechanisms are involved. Knowledge of the chemical species of metals is of fundamental importance for such understanding. In exposure media such as food, drinking water, or air, metallic elements and metalloids usually occur in the form of compounds. Inorganic compounds are most common such as salts and salt-like products, but complexes (coordination compounds) and organometallic compounds also occur. Dissolved in water, the metallic compounds dissociate into metal ions, mostly cations. In some cases, oxoanions, for example, permanganate ions (MnO_4^-), occur. Events taking place in the ecosystem are sometimes of considerable importance for the concentrations of metallic species to which humans are exposed, for example, the conversion of inorganic mercury into methylmercury (see Section 2.3.2 below). Bjerregaard et al., (2015) presented a review also of other such events, not covered in the present chapter, which focused on the mechanisms and factors of importance for the uptake and distribution of metals in various media and biota in the environment to which humans are exposed. Airborne metals occur most frequently as aerosols, and metal particles inhaled into the respiratory tract can initiate adverse health effects both in the lungs and, after transport, in other organ systems. This chapter also discusses other absorption routes and factors governing the distribution and excretion of metals. The Task Group on Metal Accumulation (TGMA, 1973) discussed fundamental routes and processes of importance, for the uptake, disposition, accumulation, and excretion of metals. Many of these considerations are still valid, but the subsequent decades have contributed a lot of additional knowledge making up a large part of this chapter (Elder et al., 2015).

2.2 EXPOSURE

2.2.1 General Considerations

An *exposure assessment* provides a description of the exposure, often taken as external exposure, by exposure route and its distribution in time and space. Concentration of the metal/metalloid or its compounds in inhaled air, drinking water, food, or media contacting the skin describes exposure in quantitative terms. Direct measurements or estimates by modeling form the basis for such quantitation. Mathematical models may describe concentrations in exposure media based on knowledge of emissions of pollutants into air or water. Such models are often available as computer software for application in risk assessment, for example, the European Union System for the Evaluation of Substances. Other models used in relation to the Registration, Evaluation, Authorisation and Restriction of Chemicals (REACH) legislation are the Advanced REACH Tool (ART) and "Stoffen-manager" (Landberg, 2018). Actual measurements of concentrations of metals and their compounds in air are also performed both in the general environment and, particularly, in workroom air. Environmental monitoring programs register and report concentrations of metals in drinking water and recreational waters. Monitoring programs often include industrial emissions and other point sources releasing metals into the environment. Variable concentrations of metallic elements occur in drinking water and food. The daily oral exposure dose (or orally applied dose) (see IPCS, 1999) or *daily oral intake* of a metal is the amount of metal taken into the gastrointestinal tract on a daily basis. Section 2.2.2 describes how it is estimated.

The major sources of exposure to metals for humans are air, food, and drinking water. Air is especially important for occupational exposures, although the skin may also be exposed and both food and drink may be indirectly contaminated. All the three exposure sources can be important for the general population. In heavily industrialized regions and areas of high traffic density, air may well be an important route of exposure to certain metals.

Water can be the dominant exposure source in geographical areas where metals such as arsenic or uranium are naturally present in soils and rock formations. Food can be the major exposure source under a variety of circumstances, including accidental contamination and dietary habits. High natural background exposure may also occur, for example, to methylmercury in populations that are dependent on fish or marine mammals for their major source of protein. Infants and children may experience different degrees of exposure from air, water, or food compared with adults. Differences in intake per kilogram body weight are twofold higher for air, threefold higher for water, and sixfold higher for food in children compared to adults. The twofold difference for air is because, despite the lung volume being lower in newborns, the alveolar surface area is larger per kilogram body weight. In addition, the higher frequency of breathing in newborns gives a greater penetration and higher uptake of inhaled substances than in adults. It is not clear how nose breathing, which is more frequent in early life, affects these factors. The differences for food and water relate to greater hand-to-mouth exploratory behavior, enhanced absorption, and retention of nutrients, and a larger intake of calories and water per unit body weight for infants and children than for adults.

Exposure to metals may also occur by the dermal route, but only limited systemic uptake occurs for some metals and inorganic metallic compounds. The uptake is substantial for some organometallic compounds (see Section 2.3.1). Contact with nickel and chromium causes uptake in the skin and related immunological responses.

Another route of human exposure is through implanted medical devices such as hip and knee replacements made of cobalt, chromium, molybdenum, or titanium alloys. Various factors influence the degree of metal release such as the composition of the device and its design (metal-on-metal or other design) as well as the extent to which the adaptation of a prosthetic device is successful. At sufficiently high doses of released metallic particles or compounds, adverse effects may occur at the site of implantation, in target tissues distant to the implant site, or both. As a result, it is necessary to assess the potential local and systemic toxicity of metal ions and metallic wear debris released from implanted medical devices. Brown et al. (2015) reviewed adverse health effects associated with metal release from implanted neurological, cardiovascular, and orthopedic devices. These authors emphasized the importance to characterize the form of metallic exposure (particulate vs. ionic) and valence of the compound released from the device. They also pointed out the need to estimate the dose of the compound released from the device using biomonitoring data and the need to account for local effects at the implant site as well as systemic effects on target organs distant to the implant. Chapter 8, Section 8.4, further describes this important route of exposure to metal compounds for those who have such implants containing cobalt. Other unusual routes of exposure not covered by this chapter are hemodialysis with water contaminated with aluminum and other medical therapeutic procedures (see Sjogren et al., 2015 "Aluminum"; Gerhardsson and Kazantzis, 2015 and Chapter 8, Section 8.1).

2.2.2 Exposure Through Food and Drinking Water

Human exposure to metal compounds in the general environment is usually greater through food and drink than through air. Even in occupational circumstances, exposure to metals by ingestion may be of importance, although absorption after inhalation is usually of primary importance in industry. Metals and their compounds occur naturally in food and drinking water because they are intrinsic components of the Earth's crust and of various biota.

Determinations of the amount of metallic species in portions of food of the same composition as those consumed, i.e., the so-called *double portion method* is the most accurate method to measure the gastrointestinal intake of metallic compounds. Another method is to use records of consumption and determinations of metal concentration in various foodstuffs. In epidemiological studies, this method is often used. A *food frequency questionnaire* provides information on the consumption of various food items and this information in combination with information on metal concentrations in various food items obtained by chemical analyses makes it possible to calculate daily intakes. For metals with limited uptake in the gastrointestinal tract, by determinations of the amount of metal in feces, this latter method has been successfully used, for example, for cadmium (see Chapter 8).

Depending on geological variation, and agricultural and ecological processes, there are great geographical differences in metal intake among populations living in various parts of the world. Globalization of food sources, coupled with the application of metal-contaminated fertilizers and irrigation water sources has increased the importance of foodborne exposures to metallic compounds in both developed and developing countries.

Increased metal content occurs in crops harvested from fields fertilized with metal-rich waste water (Mahmood and Malik, 2014) or sewage sludge.

Some countries have therefore regulated the agricultural use of such sludge. In addition, phosphate fertilizers, which are widely used in agriculture, could contain some undesirable metals (e.g., cadmium). Furthermore, the acidification of soils by various processes including the application of certain fertilizers as well as acid rain can increase the uptake of certain metals (e.g., cadmium) in crops (Nordberg et al., 1985). In Europe, sulfur emissions are now controlled, but such emissions and related acid rain may occur in other parts of the world. There is a decreased input of cadmium into the soil subsequent to regulation of cadmium in phosphate fertilizers. Processes that take place in the environment sometimes transform a metal compound discharged into the environment into other chemical species. A well-known example is biomethylation and biomagnification of mercury in aquatic environments (see later this section and Chapter 8). Exposure of children to metals often takes place in ways that differ from those of adults. Exposure of infants and children to lead is a well-documented example. Infants and toddlers who crawl or play close to floors can be exposed to lead dust and even to larger particles released from indoor lead paint or entrained into the house from exterior paint and contaminated soils (see also Chapter 8, Section 8.8).

A striking example of drinking water contamination is inorganic arsenic in drinking water wells in large areas of Bangladesh, involving the exposure of millions of people and causing increased morbidity and mortality (see Chapter 8, Section 8.2).

In some instances, industrial processes have added substantially to environmental exposures, particularly in areas close to the source of emission or in the case of accidental release. A now classic example of local pollution contaminating the food supply is the outbreak of methylmercury poisoning in fishermen and their families who ate fish caught in a large ocean bay in Minamata, Japan (see also Chapter 8, Section 8.9). A chemical plant discharged mercury in various chemical forms into the bay. This plant used a mercury compound as a catalyst. Methylmercury was bioaccumulated in the aquatic food chain to such an extent that consumption of fish from the bay resulted in cases of severe poisoning and even fatalities. Neurological deficits occurred in children born in this area whose mothers had consumed contaminated fish. This disease, named "Minamata disease," was the starting point for toxicological and epidemiological investigations of methylmercury in other parts of the world (see Chapter 8, Section 8.9).

There are examples that the identification of risks for adverse health effects from human exposures to metallic compound has resulted in measures to reduce metal contamination. Documented decreases in population exposure are the reductions after the removal of lead from fuel and from food cans, as well as decreased cadmium intakes after restrictions on cadmium in fertilizers.

2.2.3 Exposure by Inhalation

In air, metals may occur as aerosols and, in some instances, as vapor. Particles in ambient air from combustion sources are often composed of a mixture of carbon compounds and metals. Vapor or fumes of metals often form small particles through the mechanisms of condensation or nucleation. Very small particles rapidly accumulate into larger particles by agglomeration. Mechanical forces on solid materials break them down into large particles, representing the largest particles in aerosols. The size distribution of larger size or intermediate-size particles in aerosols is often log-normal. Airborne particles aerosolized from the Earth's crust or by attrition of materials are generally greater than 1 μm in diameter and may contain high percentages of aluminum, magnesium, and iron, as well as specific metals from wear of metal objects. Particles formed from burning fossil fuels are generally of submicrometer size and are more highly enriched in transition metals and others such as chromium, cobalt, nickel, copper, zinc, arsenic, selenium, vanadium, cadmium, manganese, and lead (EPA, 2004). The role of vapor pressure in environmental transport of some metals may be considerable. While most metals have low vapor pressure at ambient temperatures, elemental mercury has a high vapor pressure. Evaporation of mercury vapor is more efficient from the continents than from the oceans (see Chapter 8, Section 8.9).

The release of mercury vapor from dental amalgam restorations constitutes a special case. Chewing and brushing of teeth gives rise to the release of small amounts of mercury, partly in the form of mercury vapor and partly as ionic mercury. This release can contribute significantly to the exposure of the general population to mercury vapor (see Chapter 8, Section 8.9). Norouzi et al. (2012) found a positive correlation between mercury levels in breast milk and the number of amalgam fillings in the mother. Chapter 8 further discusses possible health risks related to such intakes.

Natural and man-made sources contribute metal-containing aerosols to the atmosphere. A number of metals occur in the particles emitted from coal-fired power plants. Emission control systems remove a major proportion of particle fly ash, but, depending on the source of the coal, the emitted fly ash may contain different concentrations of lead, cadmium, zinc, arsenic, and other metals. Co-combustion plants (i.e., combined municipal waste and fossil fuel combustion) can offer additional challenges. Surface reactions on particles during the combustion process can alter the emission of toxic elements such as arsenic and selenium (Seames et al., 2002). With oil-fired power stations, the predominant metals in the emitted aerosols are vanadium and nickel, which are contained in oil, but they also may emit mercury (Boylan et al., 2003). A few countries still use lead additions to petrol (tetraethyllead), which was widely used in many countries in the past. It gives rise to air pollution in the form of lead-containing aerosols, particularly in cities and along highways. Most countries have banned the use of lead additives to petrol, and in some of these countries, an organo-manganese compound (methylcyclopentadienyl manganese tricarbonyl) is used to improve the octane rating of petrol, and increased exposure to manganese aerosol is likely to occur.

There are many occupational environments with elevated concentrations of metals in aerosol form, for example, in welding, soldering, mechanical manufacturing, and mining and smelting. Mercury exposures often occur in vapor form, for example, occupational exposure to mercury vapor occurs among dentists and dental technicians using mercury amalgam.

Increasing amounts of nanomaterials are used and possible adverse effects from human exposures are of concern. Difficulties in describing exposures in a way that is relevant from a risk perspective relates to the dose metric for inhaled metallic nanoparticles. As described in detail elsewhere (Karlsson et al., 2015), the surface area of particles in an aerosol seems better related to the occurrence of adverse pulmonary manifestations of airborne nanoparticles than the dose in terms of micrograms per cubic meter in air.

When there is exposure through inhalation, measurements of the metal or its compound in air in combination with estimations of lung ventilation volume and time of exposure and workload forms the basis for calculating the inhaled dose. Depending on the purpose of the study, there are different types of sampling procedures for estimating air levels of chemical substances such as area sampling and personal sampling. If source identification is important, then stationary sampling may be preferred, whereas the choice is personal sampling if an estimate of inhaled doses of individuals is desired (IPCS, 2000).

2.3 DEPOSITION AND ABSORPTION

2.3.1 General Considerations Including an Introduction to Skin Deposition

This section will focus mainly on the two major routes of entry into the body: inhalation and oral ingestion, but the text below also gives an introductory brief consideration of dermal uptake.

Hostynek (2003) reviewed deposition of metals and their compounds on skin and absorption through the skin. The issue has received renewed attention in recent years due to the use of nanoscale metals/metal oxide particles in cosmetics and sunscreens. Factors such as variations in chemical form, appropriateness of the in vitro or in vivo models, and appropriateness of study design (e.g., failure to address the in vivo fate of metal species that penetrate the outermost layers of skin) make it difficult to make conclusions regarding the importance of the transdermal exposure route in the total absorption of metals. The cell turnover and the growth pattern of normal skin, i.e., the continuous migration of cells from the basal layer toward the epidermal surface limits the absorption of metals through the skin. Nevertheless, there are reports of significant uptake through the skin, for example, for organic and inorganic thallium compounds and for cobalt in the hard metal industry. Compounds of aluminum, copper, chromium, lead, and mercury, for example, may penetrate skin to varying degrees (Hostynek, 2003). Skin exposure is also important in skin sensitization. For example, skin penetration with sensitization of T lymphocytes to beryllium leads to subsequent disease resulting from inhalation exposure and the immunological response (Tinkle et al., 2003). Sensitization to nickel and chromate also takes place mainly by dermal exposure; it is also a persistent problem for individuals with occupational exposures. Reports exist of rare instances of fatal outcomes from skin absorption of organometallic compounds (Nierenberg et al., 1998).

When a metal or metal compound enters into the lung by inhalation or into the gastrointestinal tract through food and drinking water, deposition of the metal or its compound initially occurs on surface areas of the walls of the airways or in the mucosa of the gastrointestinal tract. The amount deposited depends on the physical characteristics of the aerosol or the chemical form of the metal in food and drinking water. After deposition has taken place, transfer takes place of a certain fraction of the deposited amount through the walls of the lung or gastrointestinal tract into the systemic circulation. The physicochemical properties of metals in exposure media, such as air, food, and water, play an important role in determining the extent of their absorption into the body.

2.3.2 Deposition and Absorption After Ingestion

When ingested, metallic compounds in food and drink enter the gastrointestinal tract. Fig. 2.1 describes the various routes for these substances.

Initially, deposition occurs in the respiratory tract of inhaled metallic compounds. Subsequently, mucociliary clearance (see Section 2.3.4.1) transfers part of the deposited amount to the gastrointestinal tract. Metallic compounds also enter the gastrointestinal tract via secretion in the bile

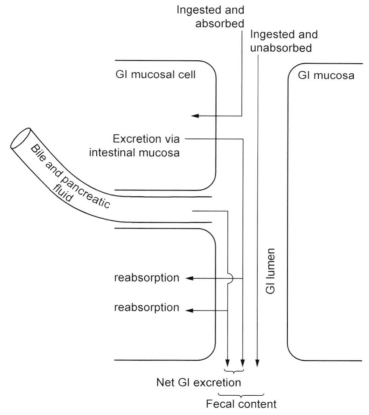

Figure 2.1 Routes for ingested metal absorption. Ingested metal is either absorbed or it passes unabsorbed through the gastrointestinal tract (GI). Metal may be excreted through intestinal mucosa and may subsequently be partly reabsorbed; the remaining part passes into feces. Excretion of metal may occur through bile and pancreatic fluid and is subsequently either reabsorbed or excreted into feces. When reabsorbed, it participates in enterohepatic circulation. Net GI excretion is the part of GI excretion that is not reabsorbed but is excreted in the feces. Fecal content is the sum of net GI excretion and unabsorbed metal.

and pancreatic fluids or through the intestinal mucosa. Subsequent reabsorption of metals secreted in bile amounts to an enterohepatic cycle, discussed later. Metallic compounds may be absorbed and sequestered inside intestinal mucosal cells but return to the intestinal tract when the cells exfoliate. The lifespan of an enterocyte is only a few days. Because of the high rate of intestinal cell turnover, this process can prove to be an important limiting factor for absorption into the bloodstream. Not illustrated in Fig. 2.1 is the role of intestinal microflora which are capable of inducing methylation and demethylation, as well as changing the oxidation state of metal. The metabolic interaction between metals and intestinal microflora may affect the degree of intestinal absorption and fecal excretion of the metal. Depending on the source, metals enter the fluids of the gastrointestinal tract in elemental form or as inorganic or organometallic compounds. The chemical form in which the metal occurs is of great importance because absorption can be entirely different for different compounds of the same metal. This is particularly so when inorganic and organometallic compounds of the same metal are compared. Methylmercury, for example, is almost completely absorbed (approximately 90%—100% absorption), whereas inorganic mercury (II) salts are absorbed to an extent of 10% or less. Another consideration with regard to exposure to metals through the gastrointestinal route is the physical form of the metal. In food, metal or metal compounds may sometimes occur as particles of various sizes mixed with other components of food. Whereas the particle size is not as important as it is in the case of the lung, it may sometimes greatly affect solubility and subsequent absorption. In addition, nonmetal compounds present in food may influence the uptake of metallic compounds from food and such interactions are important considerations when evaluating metal exposures through food. Knowledge about the chemical compounds of metals in foodstuffs is, therefore, of great importance. Established analytical methods can achieve some degree of speciation of metals, for example, by distinguishing between the methylated and inorganic forms.

Important toxicological differences exist for various forms of arsenic in food, organic forms like arsenobetaine being much less toxic than trivalent inorganic arsenic (Chapter 8, Section 8.2).

In the case of methylmercury, an instrumental method identified methylmercury bound to cysteine residues in fish meat protein (Harris et al., 2003). Immunochemical and chromatographic methods have detected cadmium in the form of cadmium—metallothionein in human and animal tissues (Nordberg et al., 2012; Nordberg and Kojima 1979).

A chemical may be absorbed from the gastrointestinal lumen by passive diffusion or by specialized (metabolism-dependent) transport systems. In addition, paracellular migration may contribute to transport into the lumen. With respect to absorption by passive diffusion, the lipid solubility of the molecule and its ionization are important (see reviews by WHO, 1978; Lehman-McKeeman, 2013). The pH of the unstirred surface mucus layer that adheres to the intestinal epithelium reflects the presence and activity of acid/base transporters in the apical membrane of the enterocytes. Surface pH determines the degree of ionization and thus the rate of absorption of weak acids and bases; it is slightly alkaline or neutral in the duodenum, slightly acidic in the jejunum, and neutral in the ileum and the large intestine (Allen and Flemström, 2005; Flemström and Kivilaakso, 1983; Seidler et al., 2011). Furthermore, diseases affecting intestinal electrolyte transport and mucosal paracellular permeability to ions, such as celiac disease and cystic fibrosis, may increase or decrease the surface pH. Inorganic salts of metals are usually not lipid soluble and are poorly absorbed by passive diffusion. For absorption of metallic compounds to occur, it is, in most instances, necessary that they are dissolved in the luminal fluids of the gastrointestinal tract; subsequently, they may be bound to molecules that facilitate their absorption. Absorption mechanisms for some essential metal ions may serve to transfer nonessential metals into the body. Examples are thallium salts (Leopold et al., 1969; Blain and Kazantzis, 2015) and cadmium ions; the latter metal ion is transported by divalent metal transporter 1 (DMT-1), which also transports iron and other divalent essential metals (Tallkvist et al., 2001) (see also Chapter 8, Section 8.3). Persons with low iron stores or iron deficiency have an enhanced intestinal cadmium uptake. A likely explanation is the upregulation of DMT1. Bridges and Zalups (2017) discussed a possible role of DMT1 and other transporters in mediating the uptake of divalent mercury. The presence or absence of suitable transport systems probably explains the large differences in gastrointestinal absorption of inorganic salts of metals from less than 10% for ionized cadmium, indium, tin, and uranium to almost complete absorption (90%—100%) for water-soluble inorganic salts of arsenic, germanium, and thallium. As mentioned, the solubility in the fluids of the gastrointestinal tract is important; for obvious reasons, this is most obvious for readily absorbable soluble metal salts. The dose level often influences the proportion of an oral dose of a metal salt that is absorbed. For many essential metals (e.g., copper, iron), small doses are more efficiently absorbed than larger doses. This is because homeostatic mechanisms—absorption and excretion—serve to keep concentrations of these metals at physiological levels. For nonessential metals (e.g., cadmium), there is contrasting evidence (i.e., small doses are absorbed to a lesser degree than moderate ones) (Engstrom and Nordberg, 1979a). For both essential and nonessential metals (e.g., iron, cadmium), excessive doses affect the integrity of the gastrointestinal mucosa, with a subsequent increase in uptake. For inorganic compounds of several metals (cadmium, cobalt, iron, lead, and mercury), gastrointestinal absorption is greater in newborn or young animals than in adults (Engstrom and Nordberg, 1979b). The high pinocytotic activity of the immature intestinal mucosa or greater (paracellular) leakiness of the epithelium in newborn animals is a possible explanation. One of the important contributory factors to childhood susceptibility to lead exposure in the home is the high rate of intestinal absorption. The composition of the diet is of concern because components such as ascorbic acid, phytate, and other metals may have a great influence on absorption (see Nordberg et al., 2015b "Interactions and Mixtures in Metal Toxicology"). The transfer of metals from the intestinal lumen into mucosal cells is not always associated with transport further into the organism (i.e., systemic uptake). Binding of metals by the low-molecular-weight protein, metallothionein, in the mucosa and subsequent loss by mucosal shedding is considered as an important mechanism in the homeostatic regulation of systemic uptake of an essential metal such as zinc (Nordberg and Kojima, 1979; Richards and Cousins, 1976). High oral doses of zinc induce metallothionein synthesis in mucosal cells and block copper uptake by the intestinal mucosa. The clinical use of this mechanism serves to avoid tissue accumulation of copper in patients with Wilson disease (see Ellingsen et al., 2015, "Copper"). A homeostatic mechanism for iron implies that iron is stored in intestinal cells bound to ferritin. Some metal particles are ingested in food or drinking water or swallowed following respiratory tract clearance, and a small proportion (0.1%–0.5%) of the ingested dose undergoes particle size-dependent systemic uptake as shown for gold nanoparticles by Schleh et al. (2012).

2.3.3 Deposition and Absorption After Inhalation

The chemical form, size, shape, density, and in vivo solubility of airborne metallic particles determine their fate and effects. These physicochemical characteristics, as well as the inhalation mode, determine the extent to which deposition and retention of the particles will occur, and these factors, in turn, play a role in their toxicological effects in the lung and their systemic absorption (Oberdorster and Driscoll, 1997; Elder et al., 2015). Also for gases and vapors, deposition and absorption in the respiratory tract depends on their physicochemical properties.

2.3.3.1 Deposition and Absorption of Gases and Vapors

Deposition of gases and vapors occur throughout the respiratory tract. The penetration of metal vapors and gases into the airways and/or alveoli depends on their physicochemical properties, the respiratory tract structure, and the properties of the respiratory tract-lining fluid. Solubility in water is an important physicochemical property of a gas that affects its absorption. The higher the solubility in water, the higher up in the respiratory tract the gas will be absorbed. Vapors and gases of metallic compounds that are poorly soluble in water can reach the alveoli, where they can penetrate the air—blood barrier. Poorly soluble mercury vapor is one example: it is absorbed to a high extent in the alveolar region of the lung because of rapid diffusion through the alveolar membrane and because of the capacity of red blood cells to bind and oxidize mercury to mercuric mercury (see Chapter 8). Other less important factors that determine the efficiency of up-take of vapors and gases include the rate of air flow (increased absorption with increased airflow) and the concentration of the gas (Elder et al., 2015).

2.3.3.2 Deposition of Particles

The equivalent aerodynamic diameter determines the behavior of airborne particles greater than 0.5 μm in diameter. The aerodynamic diameter is equal to the diameter of a spherical particle of unit density (1 g/mL) with the same terminal settling velocity in air as the particle in question. Under 0.5 μm aerodynamic diameter, particle deposition is governed more by diffusion, with particles striking molecules of gas and impacting airway walls as a result of Brownian motion. For such particles, the Stokes diameter is the appropriate size description. For irregular particles, Stokes diameter is the diameter of a sphere with the same aerodynamic resistance and density. Unlike aerodynamic diameter, the Stokes diameter is independent of mass (EPA, 2004). The main mechanisms for particle deposition in the lung are impaction, sedimentation, and diffusion (review Elder et al., 2015). The effect of impaction increases with particle size and air velocity, and it is most important in the nose, throat, and the larger bronchi (i.e., where the velocity of the air is the highest). The effect of sedimentation increases with particle size and decreases with air velocity; it is most important in the smaller airways and the alveoli. The effect of diffusion is of importance for submicrometer particles, and the effect increases with decreasing particle size. Electrostatic effects are also important for particle deposition under some conditions. Electrostatic attraction between the particle charge and the charge on the epithelium increases the total deposition. The model of particle deposition presented by the International Commission on Radiological Protection (ICRP, 1994) predicts considerable deposition of small nanoscale particles in the nose and upper respiratory tract: 80%−90% of inhaled 1-nm particles in the nasopharyngeal region, 10%−20% in the tracheobronchial region, and almost nothing in the alveolar region of the lung at nose breathing (Fig. 2.2).

For 10-nm particles, 40%−50% of the inhaled amount will be deposited in the alveolar region (Fig. 2.2; Hofmann, 2011; Landsiedel et al., 2012). As mentioned in Section 2.2.3, nanoscale particles easily agglomerate in aerosols and deposition patterns change to the one representing the size of the aggregates. The deposition pattern displayed in Fig. 2.2 with a predominant deposition in the alveolar region is valid for particles up to a size of 100 nm (0.1 μm). For particles lager than 0.5 μm, the mass median aerodynamic diameter (MMAD) of an aerosol is important in determining the pulmonary deposition. Particles with an MMAD smaller than 5 μm have more potential than larger particles to penetrate to the gas-exchange region (alveoli) in humans (Fig. 2.2) and are thus termed *respirable particles*. Human nasal passages efficiently capture particles with an MMAD greater than 10 μm (Hofmann, 2011).

Fig. 2.3 shows the total deposition in relation to particle size.

Measurements of the size of particulate matter in ambient air uses the following terms: particulate matter with an MMAD less than 10 μm (PM$_{10}$; which is likely to penetrate beyond the upper airway filtering mechanisms and reach the thoracic region); particulate matter less than 2.5 μm (PM$_{2.5}$); and particulate matter less than 0.1 μm (PM$_{0.1}$). Deposition of the two latter categories occurs in the terminal bronchioles and alveoli, i.e., acinar deposition (Fig. 2.2), and such particles may cause systemic effects.

Workplace aerosols are classified as respirable particles (MMAD less than approximately 5 μm that can penetrate into and be deposited in the alveolar or gas-exchange region), thoracic particles (MMAD less than 10 μm that can penetrate to the thoracic airways and beyond), and inhalable particles (can be deposited anywhere within the respiratory tract). Technical specifications of sampling define the exact particle sizes included in these categories (ISO, 2012). However, the fact that particles do not penetrate beyond the upper

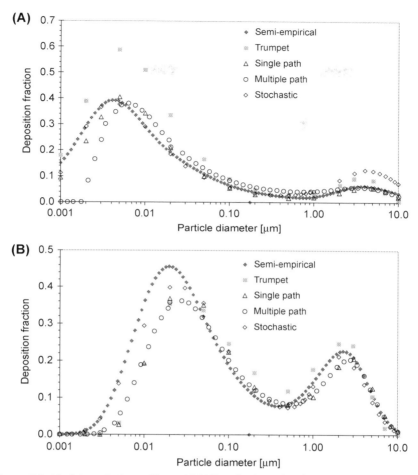

Figure 2.2 Model predictions of bronchial (A) and acinar/alveolar (B) deposition of unit-density particles ranging from 1 nm to 10 μm under nasal breathing conditions (ICRP, 1994), applying five different models: semiempirical (ICRP, 1994), trumpet, single path, multiple path, and stochastic as specified by Hofmann (2011). *From Hofmann, W., 2011. J. Aerosol Sci. 42 (10), 693–724.*

respiratory tract does not render them "safe"; soluble and insoluble compounds can cause diseases of the sinuses and irritation/inflammation of the upper respiratory tract. These general principles apply to all particles, whether metal or nonmetal.

The nose is an efficient filter not only of water-soluble gases but also of particles. It is a much more efficient filter than the mouth for particles of approximately 1 μm or larger. During heavy physical work, breathing

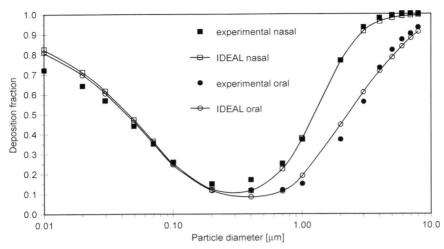

Figure 2.3 Comparison of total deposition predicted by the stochastic model IDEAL with the experimental data of Heyder et al. (1986) for a wide range of particle diameters (unit density) under nasal or oral breathing conditions: tidal volume, 1 L; respiration frequency, 15/min. *From Hofmann, W., 2011. J. Aerosol Sci. 42 (10), 693—724.*

through the mouth is necessary. Even during calm breathing, inhalation through the mouth occurs to some extent. The deposition fraction of particles increases further with exercise and is greater in subjects with mild asthma than in normal subjects. Total deposition varies in relation to particle size (Fig. 2.3). Deposition is less than one-third of the inhaled particle mass for unit density spherical particles 0.1—0.8 μm, and what is not deposited is exhaled.

The nose very effectively humidifies the inhaled air and the relative humidity is 98%—99% in the subglottic space. Hygroscopic particles can increase in size by increasing their water content and thus patterns of deposition changes. For example, after inhalation, particles of sodium chloride increase in diameter by seven times.

The theoretical models for particle deposition (e.g., ICRP, 1994) agree fairly well with experimental results (Figs. 2.2 and 2.3; Hofmann, 2011; Elder et al., 2015). The theoretical models give a good average estimate of deposition, but they do not take into account the large inter-individual differences that exist. The particle fraction deposited in the alveoli of the total deposition in the lung varies at least by a factor of two, even among young healthy male nonsmokers (see Hofmann, 2011; Elder et al., 2015).

2.3.3.3 *Clearance of Particles From the Respiratory System*

Particle clearance include absorptive (after in vivo dissolution) and nonabsorptive processes. Sneezing, nose wiping or blowing, mucociliary transport, dissolution and absorption into the blood or lymph, and endocytosis by phagocytes or epithelial cells all remove particles deposited in the nose or tracheobronchial regions. Dissolution and absorption into the blood or lymph, endocytosis by phagocytes or epithelial cells, or translocation into the systemic circulation are processes that remove particles deposited in the alveolar region. Particles deposited in that region can move to the interstitium, either as free particles or within phagocytic cells. Macrophages can also transport phagocytosed particles via lymphatic vessels to the lung-associated lymph nodes (see Elder et al., 2015). These clearance mechanisms apply broadly to all particle types, regardless of their chemical composition. Important considerations specifically related to metal-containing particles include their in vivo solubility and redox activity, the latter linked to the induction of inflammation (Zhang, 2012).

2.3.3.3.1 Tracheobronchial Clearance

Mucociliary transport is the mechanism of short-term particle clearance taking place in hours to 1—2 days. The upper airways, nasal passages, paranasal sinuses, auditory tube, and upper part of the pharynx have a ciliated epithelium, as do the lower airways from the lower parts of the larynx down to and including the terminal bronchioles. The cilia of the upper airways drive mucus backward and downward to the pharynx, and cilia of the lower airways drive mucus upward to the pharynx, after which it is swallowed. The lower layer of mucus, in which the cilia beat, consists of a low viscosity secretion (the sol layer) and the upper layer of a highly viscous secretion (mucus or gel layer). Complete elimination of the particles deposited in the most peripheral ciliated airways usually takes no more than 24 h (Camner and Philipson, 1978). If mucociliary transport is impaired, then the concentration of particles per unit surface area increases and the particles remain for a longer time in the lungs. Individuals with impaired mucociliary clearance often have chronic respiratory tract infections with bronchiectasis and obstructed airways. For example, subjects with congenital immotile cilia (primary ciliary dyskinesia) demonstrate delayed short-term (mucociliary) clearance (Moller et al., 2006; Elder et al., 2015). Short-term clearance can take up to 1 week in these subjects, but long-term clearance is not different from that in healthy subjects (Moller et al., 2006). Patients with impaired mucous production (e.g., cystic fibrosis) also exhibit delayed short-term particle clearance (Lindström et al., 2005). During acute infections with influenza A virus or mycoplasma pneumoniae, patients had markedly reduced mucociliary transport (Jarstrand et al., 1974). Some impairment persists even 5—15 months after the onset of mycoplasma infection. Patients with chronic obstructive pulmonary disease also have impaired mucociliary clearance (see Elder et al., 2015). Coughing is an effective elimination mechanism that seems to compensate for the reduced mucociliary transport. The average short-term effect of smoking cigarettes is increased mucociliary transport, but the average effect of long-term cigarette smoking is impaired mucociliary transport (Camner et al., 1972; Simet et al., 2010). However, some individuals who have smoked for 20—30 years do not have impaired clearance. Inhalation of environmentally and industrially relevant pollutants such as sulfur dioxide and sulfuric acid can also affect mucociliary transport (see Elder et al., 2015). Physical exercise increased bronchial clearance in healthy men, possibly via increased catecholamine levels during exercise.

2.3.3.3.2 Peripheral Lung Clearance and Translocation From the Respiratory Tract

Clearance from the airways of particles deposited distal to the ciliated epithelium, as well as some particles deposited on this epithelium, takes place more slowly. Mechanisms include dissolving particles in epithelial lining fluid, interstitial fluid, or phagocytic cells; transport by phagocytic cells (alveolar macrophages, polymorphonuclear leukocytes) to ciliated epithelium, lymphatics, or alveolar spaces; and translocation of solutes or solid particles out of the lung via the lymph or blood. Phagocytosis of particles by macrophages is most effective for those between 0.25 and 2 μm in diameter (see Elder et al., 2015). In addition, particles that have high length-to-width ratios can exhibit slower macrophage-mediated clearance, depending on their physicochemical properties such as in vivo solubility and durability. As mentioned previously, clearance by dissolution is one of the physical mechanisms involved in clearance from the respiratory tract. For the distal airways and alveoli, the balance of physical dissolution and phagocytosis defines solubility; readily soluble particles dissolve in lung-lining fluids faster than macrophage-mediated clearance occurs, while clearance of poorly soluble particles by phagocytic cells is faster than they dissolve in vivo.

In vivo solubility is of great importance for clearance following deposition in the lung. After instillation of cadmium compounds: cadmium chloride, cadmium sulfide, and cadmium oxide endotracheally into rat lungs, all three compounds had similar lung retention half-times, despite the difference in water solubility, with chloride being readily soluble and both sulfide and oxide being poorly soluble (see Chapter 8, Section 8.3). The compartmentalization in the lungs and systemic distribution (kidney, liver) of cadmium sulfide was different from that of cadmium oxide because of different in vivo solubility. Cadmium sulfide remained in lung tissue, in the timeframe of the study (30 days), while cadmium oxide distributed systemically.

While disease states (e.g., chronic inflammation) and inhaled toxicants may alter particle clearance from the peripheral lung due to perturbations in fluid flux or impaired phagocytic activity, chronic exposure to high concentrations of poorly soluble particles has been shown in rats and other rodent species to lead to their increased retention in the lungs. According to Morrow (1988), retention kinetics are altered when the lung particle burdens reach ∼1–3 mg/g lung tissue. Such "overloading" of macrophage-mediated clearance leads to fibroproliferative changes and tumor formation in rats (Heinrich et al., 1995; Warheit et al., 1997).

Uptake in and movement of phagocytic cells or the movement of free particles can translocate poorly soluble particles. Studies of particle translocation of inhaled poorly soluble nanosized (<100 nm) particles deposited in the alveoli showed that phagocytes do not efficiently take up particles of this size, and transport probably occurs without the involvement of the reticuloendothelial system (i.e., free particle transport). Data from humans exposed to technetium-99m-labeled ultrafine carbon particles via aerosol inhalation show that most (>95%) particles deposited in the alveolar region are retained there in the short term when leaching of the radiolabel is carefully accounted for (Moller et al., 2008; Wiebert et al., 2006; review Elder et al., 2015). Animal models reveal finer details about the specific translocation sites and amounts of translocated particles. Following endotracheal inhalation of radioactive aerosolized ultrafine iridium particles (very poorly soluble), translocation to secondary target organs such as the liver, spleen, kidney, heart, and brain was found to be ∼0.1%–0.2% of the total dose deposited in the respiratory tract (Kreyling et al., 2009; review Elder et al., 2015). Iridium appeared in these tissues within 24 h, and peak levels appeared 7 days after exposure. There was an inverse relationship between particle size and tissue accumulation (Kreyling et al., 2009). Gold appeared in the blood over a 7-day period following whole-body inhalation exposures to gold ultrafine particle aerosols (Takenaka et al., 2006). Deposition efficiencies are high for ultrafine/nanosized particles, as well as for large particles in the nasopharyngeal–laryngeal region, and particles deposited there may interact with and be transported via nerve axons that innervate the epithelium. The transport of particles takes place from the nasal epithelium to the ganglia of the trigeminus and to the olfactory nerve and olfactory bulb (review Elder et al., 2015). Particle physicochemical properties such as solubility, reactivity, agglomeration state, and in vivo solubility are of importance for translocation.

2.3.4 Total Absorption

Fig. 2.4 shows the pathways of metal absorption after inhalation or gastro-intestinal intake, including retention in the lung or intestinal compartment.

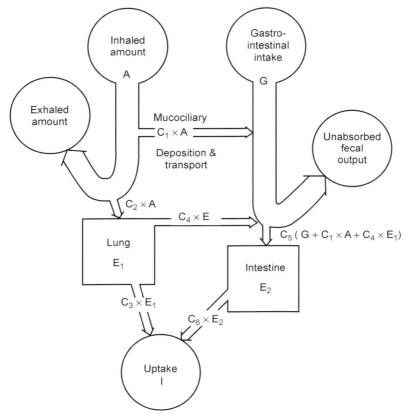

Figure 2.4 Pathways of metal absorption after inhalation or oral (gastrointestinal) intake and subsequent retention in the lung or intestinal compartment. Mathematical expressions for total absorption or uptake (I) and concentration or amount of metal retained in lung or gastrointestinal compartments are also given. *Modified from Nordberg and Kjellström (1979).*

Corresponding mathematical expressions for the total absorption (uptake, I) and concentration (amount) of metal retained in the lung (E1) or intestine (E2) are also given.

As mentioned in the previous sections, the mucociliary escalator transports particles deposited in the respiratory tract to the gastrointestinal tract. Uptake there, either shortly after inhalation or subsequently due to clearance from the small airways and alveoli, will be governed by the factors discussed in Section 2.3.2. It is important to remember that for the effects of metals that result from systemic uptake, several routes add to such uptake. These routes include metal that is absorbed directly through the lung via translocation or dissolution and the part that is absorbed after gastrointestinal translocation of inhaled particles, as well as those amounts of metal that are absorbed from the gastrointestinal tract from exposure through food and drink.

2.4 TRANSPORT, BIOTRANSFORMATION, AND DISTRIBUTION

Blood plasma is an important medium for transport of metallic compounds from the site of absorption into various body organs. Sodium ions are the dominating metal ions in plasma and provide an important part of its osmolality (Sterns, 2015). Potassium ions are dominating intracellularly. The sodium pump (Na^+/K^+ ATPase) excludes sodium from cells, exchanging it for potassium by active transport. While the macroelements Na, K, Ca, Mg, and P are very important for osmolality and acid–base balance, the trace elements, which are the subject of the present text, have a minor role.

The metal species that occur in blood plasma determine transport and distribution in the body. While the blood is the main transporting medium in the body, the lymph sometimes constitutes an important route, for example, from the lung into the blood circulation. There are very large differences in distribution among metallic compounds, i.e., transport to different organs of the absorbed dose as well as excretion varies a lot among metals and their compounds. A number of general factors are of importance for distribution. The protein-bound and *diffusible fraction* in the plasma, and interstitial and intracellular fluid; the rate of organ vascular perfusion; the rate of biotransformation; the permeability of cell membranes by the metal as it is present in plasma; and the availability and turnover rate of intracellular ligands for the metal are all of fundamental importance. Specialized transport processes are also operative. Protein binding to metal ions present in plasma and body organs varies greatly among metals. Germanium does not bind to plasma protein, but at least 99% of cadmium and mercury are protein bound. In plasma, transport of beryllium is in the form of a colloidal phosphate, adsorbed to plasma gamma globulin. Metals may also bind to proteins that normally handle essential metals, and, in some instances, protein binding may serve a transport function for the metal. For example, the plasma glyco-protein transferrin normally binds and transports iron(III), but it also binds indium(III), manganese(III), gallium(III), bismuth(III), and aluminum(III) (see Nordberg et al., 2015a).

The trace element most extensively investigated is probably iron. By far the largest proportion of body iron is present in hemoglobin in circulating erythrocytes. Oxidation of ferrous iron (II) easily takes place in blood plasma at its pH 7.4. The resulting ferric (III) ion has a very low solubility at such a pH and forms ferric hydroxide. However, only minute concentrations of ionic Fe (III) exist in plasma and specialized molecules and mechanisms present in human tissues take care of iron transport and storage. Transferrin binds iron (III) and transports it between the sites of absorption, storage, and utilization. The bone marrow uses iron for synthesis of hemoglobin. Ferritin is the storage protein for iron. In addition, to the mentioned three iron-binding proteins, there are more than 20 genes/proteins involved in iron metabolism (Ponka et al., 2015).

A slow release to blood plasma of cadmium bound to metallothionein (molecular weight 6500 Da) is of importance, for the selective uptake of filtered cadmium in the proximal tubules of the kidneys by tubular reabsorp-tion (Nordberg and Nordberg, 2000; Chapter 8, Section 8.3). The diffusible fraction in plasma is of special importance to renal accumulation and excre-tion. As discussed, glomerular filtration of the cadmium—metallothionein complex is an initial step leading to renal tubular uptake. Another example is the renal accumulation of uranium from plasma as a bicarbonate complex. The following section describes its renal accumulation and excretion. The term *diffusible fraction* does not necessarily imply that metals move from one body compartment to another by passive diffusion. Instead, the term stands for the small molecular weight or ultrafiltrable fraction that oftentimes includes small-molecular-mass compounds of the metal, transported by specific protein carriers. For example, Fig. 2.5 illustrates the structure of the arsenate and chromate oxyanions. Such structures mimic those of the endogenous anions phosphate and sulfate, respectively, and protein carriers for the endogenous anions transport oxyanions like arsenate and chromate across cell membranes.

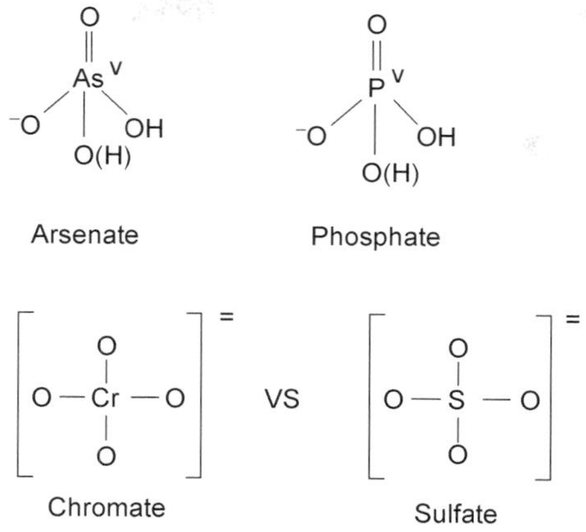

Figure 2.5 A diagrammatic comparison of the structures of arsenate and chromate with those of the endogenous phosphate and sulfate oxyanions, respectively.

This type of "ionic mimicry" also accounts for the transport of monovalent cations of thallium by potassium carriers and lithium by sodium carriers.

Transport of methylmercury—cysteine into the endothelial cells of the blood—brain barrier occurs by a process mimicking a natural substrate of the large neutral amino acid carrier (review Elder et al., 2015). Large neutral amino acids such as methionine inhibit the process. It is so selective that transport is only effective for the complex of methylmercury with the L optical isomer and not the D isomer. Thus, transport across the endothelial cells of the blood—brain barrier probably involves a stepwise process: (1) transport into the cell on the large neutral amino acid carrier, (2) the exchange of methylmercury from a cysteine thiol to a glutathione thiol because the latter is present inside the cell at much higher concentrations than cysteine, and (3) finally transport out of the cell on the glutathione carrier. A possible mimicry in which the methylmercury—cysteine complex is structurally similar to methionine may offer an explanation or a less-specific mimicry based on similarity with just the L (alpha) region of the amino acid part of the mercury-containing molecule, as suggested by Hoffmeyer et al. (2006). Methylmercury secretion into bile occurs by extrusion of methylmercury from cells as a complex with glutathione on the reduced glutathione carrier (Ballatori and Clarkson, 1983; review Elder et al., 2015).

Biotransformation, i.e., formation or breakdown of metal—carbon bonds or change of oxidation state of a metal in the biological system, is important for the toxicity of several metals. Examples are the impact on toxicity by change of oxidation state of chromium (see Langard and Costa, 2015) or mercury (see below, this section) and by the breakdown of methylmercury to inorganic forms of the metal (see below). After exposure to mercury vapor, transport of mercury to the brain occurs efficiently. The oxidation of mercury vapor to divalent mercuric mercury in the brain is important for expression of toxicity (see Chapter 8). Exposure to mercury vapor also exemplifies the importance of a rapid vascular perfusion for distribution. The rapid perfusion of the brain makes possible the transport of physically dissolved mercury vapor from the lungs to the brain before mercury is oxidized to mercury (II) in the blood (Nordberg and Serenius, 1969). The vapor penetrates the blood—brain barrier and is thereafter oxidized to mercury (II), which is "trapped" in the cells of the central nervous system, and there exerts its toxic effect. Hexavalent chromium is an example of transport into the cells followed by metabolic reduction to trivalent chromium that may induce mutations and ultimately carcinogenesis by its direct reaction with DNA (see Langard and Costa, 2015).

The toxicity of several metal compounds depends on methylation and/or demethylation processes. Methylation is involved in mediating the toxicity of arsenic in most animals and in humans (Chapter 8). Demethylation serves in the detoxification and elimination of mercury from animals and humans after exposure to methylmercury, as will be discussed in more detail in the next section. The breakage of one carbon—metal bond in tetraethyltin, on the other hand, yields a highly toxic metabolite (triethyltin) that is responsible for the toxic effects (Cremer, 1959), but mono- and diethyltin are less toxic than triethyltin (Ostrakhovitch, 2015). The metabolism of tetraethyl to triethyllead is a similar example (Cremer, 1958), because triethyllead is considered to be the toxic metabolite of tetraethyllead (Grandjean and Grandjean, 1984). Microsomal enzymes effect oxidative de-alkylation of these organometallic compounds.

2.5 EXCRETION

The most important excretory pathways are via the gastrointestinal tract and kidneys. In special cases, other processes of excretion such as salivary secretion, perspiration, exhalation, lactation, exfoliation of skin, loss of hair and nails, and bleeding, both as a significant means of elimination and as an index of exposure and body burden.

However, the present section deals only with the gastrointestinal and renal routes.

2.5.1 Gastrointestinal Excretion

Fig. 2.1 shows the routes for excretion of metals through the gastrointestinal tract. Active or passive processes may transport metallic compounds through the intestinal mucosa into the lumen of the gastrointestinal tract, effecting excretion into feces. Excretion of both inorganic mercury and cadmium occurs by this route, as indicated by autoradiographic studies (Berlin and Ullberg, 1963a,b). Another route of excretion that may be of considerable importance in certain cases is through cells of the intestinal mucosa that turns over rapidly and causes passive loss of metal by shedding into feces. Another main route of gastrointestinal excretion is from the liver through the bile and from the pancreas through pancreatic secretions.

Biliary excretion occurs for both inorganic and organometallic compounds of many elements (e.g., aluminum, arsenic, cadmium, cobalt, mercury, lead, and tellurium). Several chemicals and drugs influence the biliary excretion of metals (review by Elder et al., 2015). The liver plays an active role in the formation and secretion of methylmercury complexes, and factors affecting liver metabolism will influence biliary excretion. Metal compounds secreted in bile are reabsorbed to a variable extent further down the gastrointestinal tract and, consequently, become available for re-excretion in the bile. This process of biliary secretion followed by reabsorption in the biliary tree and intestinal tract is usually referred to as *enterohepatic circulation*. As discussed previously, many metals are secreted in the bile. Some degree of subsequent intestinal absorption is likely to occur. Thus, to varying degrees, enterohepatic recirculation does occur for many metals. Enterohepatic circulation occurs for methylmercury and ionic forms of arsenic, mercury, manganese, and lead. The process can be quite complex. Methylmercury is a well-documented example. Its secretion into the bile occurs as a complex with reduced glutathione. Animal data indicate that this first step is dramatically age dependent, being completely absent during the suckling period (Ballatori and Clarkson, 1992). The glutathione complex is hydrolyzed to its constituent amino acids by the enzyme gamma-glutamyltransferase/glutathione transpeptidase, as it passes down the biliary tree. Methylmercury is released as a complex with cysteine. As discussed in a previous section, the large neutral amino acid carrier transports this methylmercury complex across cell membranes. Some absorption back into the bloodstream takes place in the gallbladder and the remainder enters the intestinal tract where further reabsorption takes place across the mucosal cells. However, intestinal microflora present in the ileum and the large intestine also exposes methylmercury further down the intestinal tract. Microflora in the gut degrades methylmercury to inorganic mercury and such demethylation is a key step in the fecal excretion process. Changes in the diet or doses of antibiotic that affect the composition of gut flora also affect the fecal excretion rate of methylmercury in rodents and in humans (Rand et al., 2016). Inorganic mercury is poorly absorbed and passes directly into the feces. The process of biliary secretion followed by demethylation accounts for approximately 90% of the total elimination of methylmercury from the body. The process of enterohepatic recirculation preserves the body pool of bile acids. In clinical pharmacology, there are many studies describing such recirculation for drugs. The recirculation often gives rise to the appearance of at least two concentration peaks in the blood compartment: first, because of the initial dose of the drug, and second, because of enterohepatic circulation. The process is subject to genetic control, as well as to physiological changes associated with age and disease. The cycle can be broken and fecal excretion increased by oral doses of a nonabsorbable binding agent. There are successful tests in human poisoning cases of such resins, binding methylmercury in the gut and increasing excretion (Gerhardsson and Kazantzis, 2015).

2.5.2 Excretion Through the Kidneys

For many metals and their compounds, a considerable proportion of total excretion takes place through the kidneys into urine. This route is also important when the urinary concentration of metal is an index of body burden. An understanding of this excretory route may also make it possible to influence such excretion and thereby speed up the elimination of metals, thus providing a means for treatment of poisoning. The following overview summarizes some basic features and examples from the review by Elder et al., (2015), where specific references are given. Classical renal physiology states that the "ultrafiltrable fraction" in plasma is important for renal excretion. The complex physicochemical state of metals in blood, involving in some instances colloidal solutions and protein binding of various types, has to be considered to understand the renal excretory mechanisms. The glomerular ultrafiltrate contains various ions and compounds from plasma, ranging in size up to plasma albumin. Only a small proportion of plasma albumin appears in the glomerular filtrate, and proteins with larger molecules are retained in the blood. Macromolecules with relatively low molecular mass, such as inulin (5000 Da) and metallothionein (6500 Da), pass through the glomerular membrane. Metals bound to such small proteins are cleared from plasma into the tubular fluid. Some factors (e.g., changes in the concentration of some ions and other substances that occur normally in plasma) influence the filterable fraction of metal in plasma. Renal clearance and the ultrafiltrable fraction in plasma have been determined for a number of metals (Cr, Cu, Ni, Ra, Tl, U, and Zn). Often, renal clearance is lower than the calculated glomerular filtration, which may be explained by tubular reabsorption of a proportion of the metal present in tubular fluid. Cadmium is partly bound to metallothionein in blood plasma and glomerular filtration efficiently transfers this fraction to the tubular fluid. Subsequently metallothionein-bound cadmium is very efficiently reabsorbed in the renal tubule, and only a small fraction is excreted in urine. Beryllium is excreted in urine through tubular secretion. The role of tubular secretion or other forms of transtubular transport may be important for the renal accumulation and urinary excretion of mercury and lead. Changes in urinary pH give rise to changes in the urinary excretion of metals such as uranium and lead.

Uranium was the first and remains the most dramatic example of the influence of acid—base balance on renal accumulation and excretion of metal compounds. Uranium is present in plasma as the uranyl cation, UO_2^{2+}, partly protein bound and partly complexed with bicarbonate anions. The bicarbonate complex enters the proximal tubular fluid by filtration through the glomerulus. Dependent on the pH in the tubular fluid, the bicarbonate complex dissociates to release the uranyl cation that can then bind to proximal tubular cells. With higher concentrations of uranyl cations, there is damage to the resorptive mechanisms, as evidenced by the appearance of aminoaciduria. The undissociated bicarbonate complex is not absorbed and passes directly into urine. Pretreatment with sodium bicarbonate maintains a high pH in the tubular fluid such that little dissociation takes place and virtually all of the uranium passes into urine. Acidification by pretreatment with ammonium chloride results in a low tubular pH, almost complete dissociation of the complex, a large renal uptake, and a low level of uranium excretion. Urinary pH also affects the excretion of lead in urine.

The concentration of some amino acids such as cysteine and histidine may increase the filterable fraction of some metals (mercury, copper, or nickel). Several studies showed increased excretion of a number of metals because of exfoliation of tubular cells, cadmium being a well-known example. Thus, any agent that induces exfoliation of cells will increase the urinary excretion of metals accumulating in tubular cells. In contrast, acute renal failure will dramatically reduce the urinary excretion of metals.

2.5.3 Excretion Rate: Biological Half-Life (Half-Time)

A number of specific processes influence the rate of excretion or clearance of a metal compound from an organ or from the body as a whole. When the concentration gradient is the only governing process, it can be represented with reasonable accuracy by a single exponential function. According to the Task Group on Metal Accumulation (TGMA, 1973), the concentration in the organ under consideration may be expressed as:

$$c_t = c_0 \times \exp(-bt), \tag{2.1}$$

where c_t is the concentration in the organ at time t, c_0 is the concentration in the organ at time 0, b is the elimination constant, and t is time.

The biological half-life or half-time (i.e., the time it takes for the concentration to be reduced to half of its initial value) is then:

$$T1/2 = \ln 2/b, \tag{2.2}$$

where $T1/2$ is the biological half-time and $\ln 2$ is the natural logarithm of $2 = 0.693$.

The elimination of methylmercury from the human body fits reasonably well with Eq. (2.1).

Because the level of mercury in human hair is an excellent index of the level of methylmercury in the human blood and whole body, the elimination curve in human hair closely reflects the body burden. Fig. 2.6 shows the accumulation and elimination of mercury after intake of methylmercury in fish.

However, the use of the related one-compartment model for whole-body elimination of mercury after exposure to methylmercury may be an oversimplification because methylmercury is metabolized to inorganic mercury, which has a complicated metabolism. After exposure to metallic mercury vapor, inorganic mercury, probably bound to selenium, accumulates in the brain, from where it is eliminated very slowly, i.e., with a very long biological half-life. The concept of biological half-life is much used in evaluations of metal toxicity; this is further illustrated in the following section of this chapter, as well as in Chapter 8 on the various metals, where available data on the biological half-times are given. The biological half-life (half-time) varies greatly among metals. It is also different

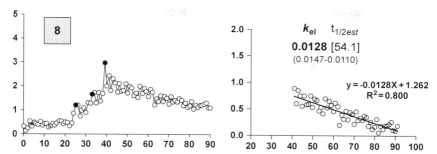

Figure 2.6 Experiment demonstrating the elimination of methylmercury from the body in a human volunteer (No. 8). Concentration of mercury in a single strand of hair was determined in relation to sulfur content in hair by laser ablation inductively coupled plasma mass spectrometry. Ordinate: natural logarithm of ratio Hg/S. Mercury (actually methylmercury) in hair increased after three fish meals on days 25, 35, and 40 (abscissa: days of experiment). Subsequent elimination according to a one-compartment model (see Section 2.6.1). Estimated $t_{1/2}$ 54.1 days. Derived elimination constant and equation describing the elimination phase indicated. The experiment was designed in order for the volunteers not to exceed the guideline for intake of methylmercury from fish according to the US Environmental Protection Agency. *Modified from Rand, M.D., et al., 2016. Toxicol. Sci. 149 (2), 385.*

in different tissues. For example, the half-life for cadmium is in the order of days to months in the blood but is 10–30 years in the kidney. When discussing half-life or half-time, it is customary to lump together various parts of the body that have the same elimination rate into one "compartment"; one may speak of, for example, the "soft-tissue compartment" or of a compartment with a half-life (half-time) of, for example, 5 days. Data on the half-time of a compartment may be obtained by actual measurements of elimination from that compartment after the termination of exposure, and in such a case, the anatomical structures comprising the compartment will be known. Such measurements may even be possible in humans through external scanning techniques after the ingestion or inhalation of substances labeled with radioisotopes and in some instances by in vivo neutron activation or in vivo X-ray fluorescence (see Chapter 3, Section 3.3.2).

When chemical analysis is used, it is usually necessary to limit the investigation to studies on the blood, urine, hair, and feces. As discussed later, knowledge of the population variance in excretion rates (biological half-lives) is essential for making a quantitative estimate of risk. This information is lacking for most metals, but for methylmercury, the best-studied example, we know that many factors influence the magnitude

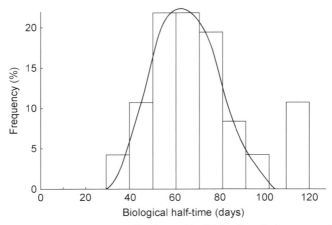

Figure 2.7 Population distribution of biological half-life of methylmercury obtained by segmental analysis of hair from persons exposed in Iraq. *From Shahristani and Shihab (1974).*

of biological half-life. Species differences cover a range of more than two orders of magnitude—from approximately 7 days in the mouse to more than 700 days in certain marine mammals. Half-lives were determined in humans exposed to high oral intakes in Iraq. The measurements gave an average value of approximately 70 days by means of segmental hair analyses. The bimodal distribution of values covered an approximately fivefold range—approximately 33—189 days (WHO, 1991; Fig. 2.7).

Lactating women—average half-life of 42 days—have significantly shorter half-lives than nonlactating adult women—average of 76 days (Greenwood et al., 1978). Recent measurements in nonlactating human volunteers (Fig. 2.6) consuming relatively low levels of methylmercury in fish in the United States found an average half-life of 44 days (Rand et al., 2016). The lower doses or other factors may explain the shorter half-life. Section 2.6 (below) describes and discusses the long half-life of 10—30 years for cadmium in the kidneys of humans.

2.6 TOXICOKINETIC MODELS

A quantitative description of the processes of absorption, distribution, biotransformation, and excretion of a chemical substance as a function of time constitutes a *toxicokinetic (or pharmacokinetic) model*. For pharmacologically active substances, the term "pharmacokinetic model" is used, and for toxic substances, the term "toxicokinetic model" is used. Such models, sometimes named *metabolic models*, may help us in a general manner to understand the occurrence of adverse effects of chemical compounds. These models may also be used together with toxicodynamic knowledge, particularly when critical concentrations in the critical organ can be estimated, to define exposures associated with a certain risk of adverse effects. In instances where this is possible, the toxicokinetic model constitutes a very important part of a total model for risk estimation. Such models may be of great value because they provide a means of calculating the expected dose—response relationships and may be helpful as a basis for risk assessment and setting exposure limits in the industrial and general environments (see Chapter 5). Toxicokinetic models may also serve a useful purpose by enabling the conversion of information about concentration in biomarker media (e.g., blood, urine) to intake and vice versa. However, the most important use of such models is to calculate the concentration in the critical organ (i.e., the most sensitive target organ—see Chapter 5 for further information) under various conditions of exposure. The following sections describe a basic one-compartment model as well as models that are more complex.

2.6.1 One-Compartment Model

The mathematical expression used in Section 2.5.3, where biological half-time/half-life was defined, also describes the *one-compartment model*. Eq. (2.1), in Section 2.5.3, describes the course of the elimination process from a compartment when there is no further influx (e.g., after a single dose). In this equation, c represents the concentration of metal in the compartment. The same mathematical expressions are also valid when the amount of metal in the compartment is studied. When additional doses are given at time intervals that are several half-lives long, the doses will not appreciably influence each other, and the concentration curve in the organ will take a course that is a repetition of the one after a single dose. When the interval between doses is shorter, there will be an accumulation of metal in the organ. This will also be the case if there is continuous exposure (Fig. 2.8).

Continuous exposure represents the greatest accumulation hazard and, therefore, deserves special attention. The accumulated amount (A) of metal in a compartment can be expressed mathematically as:

$$A = a/b[1 - \exp(-bt)] \tag{2.3}$$

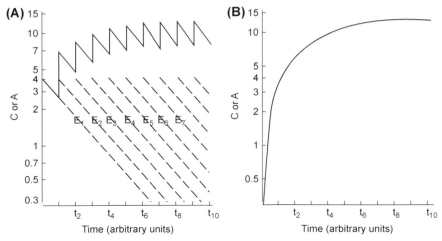

Figure 2.8 (A) Simulation of the cumulative plasma concentration. (C) of a chemical or amount (A) in the body after repeated administration or exposure. (B) Plasma or organ concentration in relation to time during continuous exposure. *(A) From WHO, 1978. Environmental Health Criteria, 6. WHO, Geneva.*

where A is the accumulated amount, a is the fraction of daily intake taken up by the organ, b is the elimination constant, and t is the time of exposure. At steady state:

$$A = a/b \qquad (2.4)$$

When t is sufficiently long (i.e., corresponding to five times the biological half-life or more), the steady state is considered to be reached from a practical point of view. These mathematical expressions are based on the assumption that intake and absorption are constant. If either intake or absorption changes systematically with age, type of exposure, period in time, etc., then the equation must be modified. Some examples of this will be given in the following text.

When describing the distribution and elimination of drugs and other chemical compounds including metallic compounds, the one-compartment model has been used extensively (WHO, 1978; Amzal et al., 2009). Chapter 3 discusses the use of the one-compartment model for calculations of expected concentrations in biomonitoring media and for estimating dietary intake from biomonitoring data. Chapter 5 includes description and discussion of dose–response calculations based on the one-compartment model as well as multicompartment models in toxicokinetic/toxicodynamic modeling.

2.6.2 Multicompartment Models and Physiologically Based Models

Many chemical compounds follow a more complex distribution and elimination patterns than the one described by the one-compartment model. It has long been recognized that an adequate and useful quantitative description of the toxicokinetics of many metals, including inorganic cadmium, lead, and mercury, requires multicompartment models (Task Group on Metal Accumulation, 1973; Task Group on Metal Toxicity, 1976; WHO, 1978).

Multicompartment models for these toxicologically important metals are also useful as a basis for interpreting data from environmental and biological monitoring programs and for calculating dose—response relationships (i.e., for toxicokinetic/toxicodynamic modeling).

For animal data, Cember (1969) developed a model for the retention and accumulation of inorganic mercury in the kidney. Elder et al. (2015) reviewed a number of models for accumulation of inorganic mercury, cadmium, or manganese in soft tissues of experimental animals, and they reviewed data on models for retention of strontium, barium, and radium in the bone.

For humans, both physiologically based (O'Flaherty, 1993) and compartment models have been developed and used in assessments of human uptake of lead from environmental sources (EPA, 2012). The O'Flaherty model of lead kinetics is based on an age-dependent approach to human growth and development and devotes special attention to bone turnover rates (MacMillan et al., 2015). Skerfving and Bergdahl (2015) describe a compartment model that includes an indication of the varying half-times of lead in human tissues. In blood plasma, the half-time is in terms of minutes; in soft tissues, in general, it is approximately 1 month; and in the cortical (compact) bone, it amounts to decades. Several aspects of human lead toxicokinetics have alternative mathematical descriptions. This is true for the relationship between exposure levels and blood lead levels and the relationship between bone lead, blood lead, and plasma lead.

The introduction of the concept of *physiologically based* models in metal toxicology occurred in the early 1990s. These models use information about physiological processes (e.g., bone formation and the incorporation of bone-seeking elements into the bone, as well as oxidation—reduction processes that change the oxidation state of metallic compounds in human body fluids).

All physiological processes that have an important impact on the toxico-kinetic model for the element under consideration are included in such models. Models developed for pharmacologically active substances are named physiologically based pharmacokinetic (PBPK) models. For toxicologically active substances, they are named physiologically based toxicokinetic (PBTK) models. Such modeling has been developed for the toxicokinetics of lead in humans (O'Flaherty, 1993, 1995) and for chromium toxicokinetics in humans after ingestion (O'Flaherty et al., 2001). These models, like the multicompartment models based on our knowledge of metal binding in plasma and tissues (see Section 2.6.2.1), both try (as much as possible) to use actual data and our current understanding of the metabolic and toxicokinetic behavior of metallic compounds in human tissues and body fluids. A multicompartment model for cadmium has been developed and applied to the interpretation of data on human cadmium exposure. This model for cadmium has been used for a long time with some modifications (see Section 2.6.2.1); it will, therefore, be used as an example of such a model (Choudhury et al., 2001; Fransson et al., 2014; Kjellstrom and Nordberg, 1978, 1985; Nordberg and Kjellström, 1979) and briefly described in the following section.

2.6.2.1 Description of a Multicompartment Model for Cadmium

Figs. 2.4 and 2.9 show the flow scheme describing the model. The first part of the model is identical to the general pathways for absorption described in Section 2.3.4 and Fig. 2.4.

The amount of cadmium transferred daily to the systemic circulation (daily uptake I) will be distributed among three blood compartments: B1, representing cadmium bound to albumin and other proteins (except metallothionein); B2, representing cadmium in erythrocytes; and B3, cadmium bound to metallothionein in plasma (Fig. 2.9). The amount of cadmium that can be bound to metallothionein directly in plasma (I2) is limited because the amount of circulating metallothionein is extremely small. Other binding sites in plasma are abundant, however, and it is assumed that cadmium not bound to metallothionein in plasma will instead be bound to these other binding sites (I1 = I − I2). The amount of cadmium reaching B1 will be further transferred to the various tissues in the body, and only a small proportion of the cadmium from these compartments will return to B1

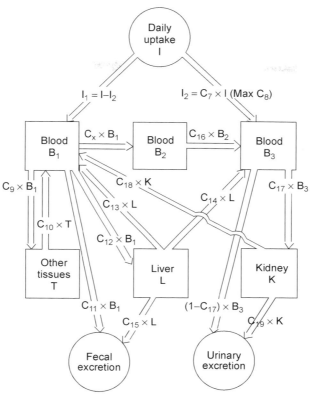

Figure 2.9 *Flow scheme describing the movement of cadmium among various compartments in humans.* After uptake (see Fig. 2.4), the amount of cadmium (Cd) taken up in the blood (I) is bound to metallothionein (I2). Because the amount of metallothionein available in the blood is limited, there is a maximum amount of binding. The remainder of the uptake is bound to high-molecular-weight proteins (mainly albumin) in plasma (I1 = I − I2). Cd bound to albumin in blood plasma is taken up by blood cells (B2), and the transfer coefficient is Cx. In blood cells, cadmium is bound to metallothionein; when blood cells turn over (C16), metallothionein-bound cadmium is released to the blood plasma (B3). Albumin-bound Cd in the blood plasma (B1) is in equilibrium with several other tissues (T) via transfer coefficients C9 and C10. A considerable proportion of B1 is transferred (C12) to the liver (L), and a small proportion C11 is excreted via the intestinal epithelium. In the liver, cadmium taken up from the blood plasma as bound to albumin will be bound to metallothionein, gradually released, and transferred (C14) to the blood plasma. Metallothionein-bound Cd (B3), because of its low molecular weight, will be efficiently transferred (C17) to the kidney (K). Urinary excretion results from a small proportion of B3 and from K. *From Nordberg and Kjellström (1979).*

because tissue binding is much stronger than binding to ligands in B1. Part of the cadmium in B1 will be excreted in the feces through the intestinal mucosa (C11 × B1). Part of the liver cadmium (C14 × L) will be released in the form of metallothionein to the blood (B3), and a very small proportion will be excreted in the bile (C15 × L). The kidney derives its cadmium content from the metallothionein fraction in plasma. A very minor part of B3 (approximately 5%) is transferred to urine. Because the renal tubular reabsorptive capacity diminishes with age, C17 is partly age dependent. The flow of cadmium among the compartments in the model described by Kjellstrom and Nordberg (1978) and Nordberg and Kjellström (1979) has been described by a series of equations. Choudhury et al. (2001) have described an improved mathematical approach that uses the same model for cadmium flow in the human body (Fig. 2.9). The equations describing intercompartmental transfers of cadmium were implemented as differential equations in Advanced Continuous Simulation Language (ACSL version 11), and improved growth algorithms and other adjustments were used. A Monte Carlo simulation propagates variability in daily intake through the model. On the basis of data concerning intake of cadmium in the US population, the levels of cadmium in urine in the US population were computed by this model. When comparing their results with those measured in a nationwide biomonitoring program in the US National Health and Nutrition Examination Survey II (NHANES II), they found good agreement in men, as shown in Fig. 2.10, whereas the urine cadmium values in women generated by the model were lower than those observed in NHANES II.

Data demonstrating a higher gastrointestinal absorption in women than men have been published since the Kjellström–Nordberg model was developed in the 1970s. Choudhury et al. used this information and adjusted the gastrointestinal uptake in women to 10% (instead of the 5% in both men and women, originally used by Kjellstrom and Nordberg, 1978). With this modification, Choudhury et al. (2001) found reasonably good agreement between the observed and model-generated values in females. Further calculations using a similar approach to the one used by Choudhury et al. have been presented by Ruiz et al. (2010). Fransson et al. (2014) employed slightly different computerized methods, using the Kjellstrom-Nordberg model as a basis and adapting the calculations to the most recent data on kidney accumulation in humans. Ruiz and Fowler (2015) discussed the predictions by the model in relation to the findings in NHANES II. Although there is a reasonably good agreement, there are differences in females of age

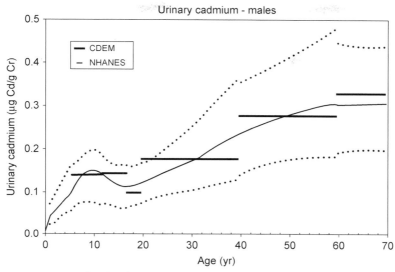

Figure 2.10 Urinary levels of Cd in relation to age in the US population and a comparison with values calculated by Choudhury et al. (2001). Horizontal bars represent uncertainty intervals of the measured values in the National Health and Nutrition Examination Survey (*NHANES*) biomonitoring of the US population. The *unbroken line* represents average values generated for different age groups when using the mathematical model (*CDEM*). The *dotted lines* represent upper and lower uncertainty levels of this calculation.

6–59 years, possibly due to overestimation of intakes used in the modeling. Software for toxicokinetic modeling is increasingly available. The MATLAB® programming environment is a useful tool for multicompartment and PBPK applications. Sasso et al. (2010) used this software in developing a Generalized Toxicokinetic Modeling System for Mixtures. This system was able to replicate the results of models that were optimized for specific metals such as the Kjellström-Nordberg model for cadmium. Chapter 5 describes the use of multicompartment models and PBTK models for estimating dose–response relationships when toxicodynamic information is available.

2.7 USE OF INDICATOR MEDIA FOR ESTIMATING CRITICAL ORGAN CONCENTRATION

To estimate the risk of poisoning for an individual or a group of individuals, it would be desirable to measure the dose at the site of effect (i.e., the concentration in the critical organ). In living individuals, this is seldom possible. It is more feasible to determine metal concentrations in other biological media such as blood, urine, or hair, these are often used as indicators of the concentration of the metal in the critical organ and, thus, provide an indication of the risk of adverse effects (reviewed by Santonen et al., 2015; see also Chapter 3).

When useful biological indicator media can be found, i.e., when metal concentrations in such media correlate accurately with the appearance of effects, biological monitoring may provide a more accurate means of evaluating the risk compared to measurement of exposure. Chapters 3, 4, and 5 further discuss biomonitoring as a means to estimate critical organ concentration/target dose and risk for adverse health effects.

REFERENCES

Allen, A., Flemström, G., 2005. Am. J. Physiol. 288, C1–C19.
Amzal, B., et al., 2009. Environ. Health Perspect. 117, 1293.
Ballatori, N., Clarkson, T.W., 1983. Am. J. Physiol. 244, G435–G444.
Ballatori, N., Clarkson, T.W., 1992. Am. J. Physiol. 262 (31), R761–R765.
Berlin, M., Ullberg, S., 1963a. Arch. Environ. Health 6, 586.
Berlin, M., Ullberg, S., 1963b. Arch. Environ. Health 7, 686.
Bjerregaard, P., Andersen, C.B.I., Andersen, O., 2015. Ecotoxicology of Metals — Sources, Transport, and Effects on the Ecosystem, pp. 425–459.
Blain, R., Kazantzis, G., 2015. Thallium. In: Nordberg, G.F., Fowler, B.A., Nordberg, M. (Eds.), Handbook on the Toxicology of Metals, fourth ed. Academic Press, Elsevier, Amsterdam, Boston.
Boylan, H.M., et al., 2003. J. Air Waste Manag. Assoc. (53), 1318.
Bridges, C.C., Zalups, R.K., 2017. Arch. Toxicol. 91, 63.
Brown, R.P., et al., 2015. Toxicity of metals released from implanted medical devices. In: Nordberg, G.F., Fowler, B.A., Nordberg, M. (Eds.), Handbook on the Toxcology of Metals, fourth ed., vol. 1. Academic Press, Elsevier, Amsterdam, Boston, pp. 113–122.
Camner, P., Philipson, 1978. Arch. Environ. Health 33, 181.
Camner, P., et al., 1972. Arch. Environ. Health 24, 82.
CDC/NIOSH, 2017. Workplace Safety and Health Topics. www.cdc.gov/niosh/topics/.
Cember, H., 1969. Am. Ind. Hyg. Assoc. J. 30, 367.
Choudhury, H., et al., 2001. J. Toxicol. Environ. Health A 63 (5), 321–325.
Cremer, J.E., 1958. Biochem. J. 68, 685.
Cremer, J.E., 1959. Br. J. Ind. Med. 16, 191.
Duffus, J.H., et al., 2007. Pure Appl. Chem. 79 (7).
Duffus, J.H., Templeton, D.M., Nordberg, M., 2009. In: IUPAC (Ed.), Concepts in Toxicology. RSC Publishing, Cambridge, p. 179.
ECHA, 2009. In: ECHA (Ed.), Guidance in a Nutshell Chemical Safety Assessment. ECHA, p. 22.
Elder, A., et al., 2015. Routes of exposure, dose and toxicokinetics of metals. In: Nordberg, G.F., Fowler, B.A., Nordberg, M. (Eds.), Handbook on the Toxicology of Metals, fourth ed. Academic Press, Elsevier, Amsterdam, Boston.
Ellingsen, D.G., et al., 2015. Copper. In: Nordberg, G.F., Fowler, B.A., Nordberg, M. (Eds.), Handbook on the Toxicology of Metals, fourth ed. Academic Press, Elsevier, Amsterdam, Boston.

Engstrom, B., Nordberg, G.F., 1979a. Toxicology 13, 215.

Engstrom, B., Nordberg, G.F., 1979b. Acta Pharmacol. Toxicol. 45, 315.

EPA, 2004. Air Quality Criteria for Particulate Matter (Final Report, 2004). www.epa.gov.

EPA, 2012. Air Quality: EPA's Integrated Science Assessments (ISAs). Integrated Science Assessment for Lead. U.S. Environmental Protection Agency, Washington, DC. EPA/ 600/R-10/075B.

Flemström, G., Kivilaakso, E., 1983. Gastroenterology 84, 787.

Fransson, M.N., et al., 2014. Toxicol. Sci. 141, 365.

Gerhardsson, L., Kazantzis, G., 2015. Diagnosis and treatment of metal poisoning: general aspects. In: Nordberg, G.F., Fowler, B.A., Nordberg, M. (Eds.), Handbook on the Toxicology of Metals, fourth ed., vol. 1. Academic Press, Elsevier, Amsterdam, Boston, pp. 488–505.

Grandjean, P.H., Grandjean, E.C., 1984. Biological Effects of Organolead Compounds. CRC Press, Boca Raton, FL.

Greenwood, M.R., et al., 1978. Environ. Res. 16, 48.

Harris, H.H., et al., 2003. Sci. Gov. Rep. 301 (5637), 1203.

Heinrich, U., et al., 1995. Inhal. Toxicol. 7, 533.

Heyder, J., et al., 1986. J. Aerosol Sci. 17, 811–825.

Hofmann, W., 2011. J. Aerosol Sci. 42 (10), 693–724.

Hoffmeyer, R.E., et al., 2006. Chem. Res. Toxicol. 19, 753.

Hostynek, 2003. Food Chem. Toxicol. 41, 327.

ICRP, 1994. Human respiratory tract models for radiological protection. Ann. ICRP 24.

ISO, 2012. In: International Standardization Organization (Ed.), Air Quality — Sampling Conventions for Airborne Particle Deposition in the Human Respiratory System. Geneva, Switzerland: ISO 13138, first ed. Geneva, Switzerland.

IPCS, 1999. Environmental Health Criteria, 210. In: IPCS (Ed.), Principles for the Assessment of Risks to Human Health from Exposure to Chemicals. WHO, Geneva.

IPCS, 2000. Human Exposure Assessment. Environmental Health Criteria, 214. World Health Organization, Geneva.

Jarstrand, C., et al., 1974. Am. Rev. Respir. Dis. 110, 415–419.

Karlsson, H.L., Toprak, M.S., Fadeel, B., 2015. Toxicity of metal and metal oxide nanoparticles. In: Nordberg, G.F., Fowler, B.A., Nordberg, M. (Eds.), Handbook on the Toxicology of Metals, fourth ed. Academic Press/Elsevier, Amsterdam, Boston, pp. 75–112.

Kjellstrom, T., Nordberg, G.F., 1978. Environ. Res. 16 (1–3), 248–269.

Kjellstrom, T., Nordberg, G.F., 1985. Kinetic Model of Cadmium Metabolism. In: Friberg, L., et al. (Eds.), Cadmium in the Environment, vol. 1. CRC Press, Boca Raton Fl, pp. 179–187.

Kreyling, W.G., et al., 2009. Inhal. Toxicol. 21, 55.

Landberg, H., 2018. The Use of Exposure Models in Assessing Occupational Exposure to Chemicals. Media Tryck, Lund University, Lund, Sweden.

Landsiedel, R., et al., 2012. Arch. Toxicol. 86, 1021.

Langard, S., Costa, M., 2015. Chromium. In: Nordberg, G.F., Fowler, B.A., Nordberg, M. (Eds.), Handbook on the Toxicology of Metals, fourth ed. Academic Press, Elsevier, Amsterdam, Boston.

Lehman-McKeeman, L.D., 2013. Absorption, distribution and excretion of toxicants. In: Klaasen, C.D. (Ed.), Casarett and Doull's Toxicology: The Science of Poisons, eighth ed. McGraw-Hill, New York (Chapter 5).

Leopold, G., et al., 1969. Arch. Pharmacol. Exp. Pathol. 263, 275.

Lindström, M., et al., 2005. Eur. Respir. J. 25, 317.

MacMillan, J.W., et al., 2015. Environ. Sci. Process. Impacts 17 (12), 2122.

Mahmood, A., Malik, R.N., 2014. Arabian J. Chem. 7, 91.

Moller, W., et al., 2006. Respir. Res. 7, 10.

Moller, W., et al., 2008. Am. J. Respir. Crit. Care Med. 177, 426.

Morrow, P.E., 1988. Fundam. Appl. Toxicol. 10, 369—384.

Nierenberg, D.W., et al., 1998. N. Engl. J. Med. 338, 1672.

Nordberg, G.F., Kjellström, T., 1979. Environ. Health Perspect. 28, 211.

Nordberg, M., Kojima, Y., 1979. In: Kagi, J.H.R., Nordberg, M. (Eds.), Metallothionein. Birkhauser Verlag, Basel, pp. 41—124.

Nordberg, M., Nordberg, G., 2000. Cell. Mol. Biol. (Noisy-Le-Grand, Fr.) 46, 451.

Nordberg, G.F., Serenius, F., 1969. Acta Pharmacol. Toxicol. 27, 269.

Nordberg, G.F., et al., 1985. Environ. Health Perspect. 63, 169.

Nordberg, G.F., et al., 2012. J. Trace Elem. Med. Biol. 26, 197.

Nordberg, G.F., Fowler, B.A., Nordberg, M., 2015a. Handbook on the Toxicology of Metals. Academic Press Elsevier, Amsterdam, Boston.

Nordberg, G.F., et al., 2015b. Interactions and mixtures in the toxicology of metals. In: Nordberg, G.F., Fowler, B.A., Nordberg, M. (Eds.), Handbook on the Toxicology of Metals, fourth ed. Academic Press, Elsevier, Amsterdam, Boston.

Norouzi, E., et al., 2012. Environ. Monit. Assess. 184 (1), 375.

Oberdorster, G., Driscoll, K., 1997. Environ. Health Perspect. 105 (Suppl. 5).

O'Flaherty, E.J., 1993. Toxicol. Appl. Pharmacol. 118 (1), 16—29.

O'Flaherty, E.J., 1995. Toxicol. Appl. Pharmacol. 131, 297.

O'Flaherty, E.J., et al., 2001. Toxicol. Sci. 60, 196.

Ostrakhovitch, E., 2015. Tin. In: Nordberg, G.F., Fowler, B.A., Nordberg, M. (Eds.), Handbook on the Toxicology of Metals. Academic Press, Elsevier, Amsterdam, Boston, New York (Chapter 56).

Ponka, P., Tenenbein, M., Eaton, J.W., 2015. Iron. In: Nordberg, G.F., Fowler, B.A., Nordberg, M. (Eds.), Handbook on the Toxicology of Metals. Academic Press, Elsevier, Amsterdam, Boston, New York.

Rand, M.D., et al., 2016. Toxicol. Sci. 149 (2), 385.

Richards, M.P., Cousins, R.J., 1976. J. Nutr. 106, 1591.

Ruiz, P., Fowler, B.A., 2015. Exposure assessment, forward and reverse dosimetry. In: Nordberg, G.F., Fowler, B.A., Nordberg, M. (Eds.), Handbook on the Toxicology of Metals, fourth ed. Elsevier Publishers, Amsterdam, pp. 141—153.

Ruiz, P., Mumtaz, M., Osterloh, J., Fisher, J., Fowler, B.A., 2010. Toxicol. Lett. 198, 44—48.

Santonen, T., et al., 2015. Biological monitoring and biomarkers. In: Nordberg, G.F., Fowler, B.A., Nordberg, M. (Eds.), Handbook on the Toxicology of Metals, fourth ed. Academic Press, Elsevier, Amsterdam, Boston, New York (Chapter 8).

Sasso, A.F., et al., 2010. Theor. Biol. Med. Model. 7, 17.

Schleh, C., et al., 2012. Nanotoxicology 6, 36.

Seames, W.S., et al., 2002. Environ. Sci. Technol. 36, 2772.

Seidler, U., et al., 2011. Acta Physiol. (Oxf.) 201, 3—20.

Shahristani, H., Shihab, K., 1974. Arch. Environ. Health 18, 342.

Simet, S.M., et al., 2010. Am. J. Respir. Cell Mol. Biol. 43, 635.

Sjogren, B., et al., 2015. Aluminum. In: Nordberg, G.F., Fowler, B.A., Nordberg, M. (Eds.), Handbook on the Toxicology of Metals, fourth ed., vol. 1. Academic Press, Elsevier, Amsterdam, Boston.

Skerfving, S., Bergdahl, I.A., 2015. Lead. In: Nordberg, G.F., Fowler, B.A., Nordberg, M. (Eds.), Handbook on the Toxicology of Metals, fourth ed., vol. 1. Academic Press, Elsevier, Amsterdam, Boston (Chapter 43).

Sterns, R.H., 2015. Disorders of plasma sodium—causes, consequences, and correction. N. Engl. J. Med. 372 (1), 55—65.

Takenaka, S., et al., 2006. Inhal. Toxicol. 18, 733—740.

Tallkvist, J., et al., 2001. Toxicol. Lett. 122, 171—177.

TGMA (Task Group on Metal Accumulation), 1973. Accumulation of toxic metals with special reference to their absorption, excretion and biological half-times. Environ. Physiol. Biochem. 3, 65—107.

Task Group on Metal Toxicity, 1976. In: Nordberg, G.F. (Ed.), Effects and Dose-Response Relationships of Toxic Metals. Elsevier, Amsterdam, pp. I—III.

Tinkle, S.S., et al., 2003. Environ. Health Perspect. 111, 1202—1208.

WHO, 1978. Environmental Health Criteria, 6. WHO, Geneva.

WHO, 1991. Mercury. Environmental Health Criteria, 118. World Health Organization, Geneva.

Warheit, D.B., Hansen, J.F., Yuen, I.S., et al., 1997. Toxicol. Appl. Pharmacol. 145, 10—22.

Wiebert, P., Sanchez-Crespo, A., Seitz, J., et al., 2006. Eur. Respir. J. 28, 286—290.

Wild, C.P., 2012. The exposome: from concept to utility. Int. J. Epidemiol. 41 (1), 24—32.

Zhang, H., 2012. ACS Nano 6, 4349—4368.

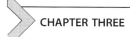

CHAPTER THREE

Biomonitoring, Mode of Action (MOA), Target Dose, and Adverse Outcome Pathways (AOPs)

Abstract

Risk and hazard assessments are crucial in order to estimate the likelihood of human disease or other adverse health effects resulting from existing human exposures to metals and their compounds on an individual or mixture basis. External exposures produce internal doses that produce the toxic dose at the site of action, named the target dose. The target organ that suffers toxicity at the lowest external exposure level is the *critical organ* and the adverse effect that occurs at the lowest external exposure is the *critical effect*. This effect is critical because it is crucial for preventive action (for definitions of concepts, see Appendix). It is thus important to try to estimate the target dose as accurately as possible. Unfortunately, it is seldom possible to measure this dose in living humans or animals. The concentration of the toxic metal species in the critical organ may be measured or estimated and is often a useful surrogate for the target dose. Biological monitoring (synonym: biomonitoring), for example, measurements of concentrations of metal compounds in tissues, blood, or urine, is often used as a basis for estimating target dose/concentration in critical organ. Toxicodynamics describes the mechanism or mode of action of toxicants, how they can cause tissue damage, and under what conditions in terms of tissue concentrations and time of tissue exposure/dose do adverse effects on tissue structure and function occur. When these conditions can be described in quantitative terms and when, in addition, a toxicokinetic model can be described, a quantitative toxicokinetic-toxicodynamic (TKTD) dose–response model can be set up and be used to predict relationships between exposure dose and the expected frequency of adverse health effects. A TKTD model may constitute a major part of an adverse outcome (AO) pathway describing the linking between a molecular initiating event and AO at the biological level of organization.

3.1 INTRODUCTION

For risk assessment, the exposure causing toxicity is important. Toxic effects occur in relation to the critical concentration in the critical organ or, more specifically, the target dose. Chapter 1 introduced and Appendix lists the definitions of the basic concepts of exposure, absorbed dose, critical organ, and critical effect as suggested by the Task Group of Metal Toxicity

Risk Assessment for Human Metal Exposures
ISBN: 978-0-12-804227-4
https://doi.org/10.1016/B978-0-12-804227-4.00003-0

(Nordberg, 1976; TGMT, 1976), later confirmed by other organizations (see Section 3.3.2). Modifying factors influence the relationship between exposure and toxicity. Chapter 1 already mentioned that The Task Group on Metal Interactions 1978 (TGMI, 1978) discussed early evidence on such modifying factors. Data that are more recent provide a considerable amount of additional evidence (see Chapter 6). Known modifying factors include age, nutritional status, gender, mixed exposures, and genetics. The influence on the risk of developing toxicity may occur at the molecular, cellular, organ, and whole organism levels of biological organization. Measurements of concentrations of metals and their compounds in biological media such as blood or urine (also named biomonitoring or biological monitoring) are often useful for estimating the absorbed dose in humans. Such biomonitoring performed by direct measurements of tissue levels in organs affected by a toxic metal compound has been performed in some instances, but usually biomonitoring data based on indicator media like blood and urine provide indirect estimates of uptake in the critical organ. The early considerations by the Task Group on Metal Accumulation, TGMA (1973), TGMT (1976), and Fowler (1979), emphasized the usefulness of measurements in biological media but pointed out some difficulties when interpreting obtained results. The book "Biological Monitoring of Toxic Metals" (Clarkson et al., 1988) summarized and discussed evidence concerning more than 20 metals and some specific metal species. A wealth of data in this field of science confirms the conclusions reached at that time. The following text summarizes present evidence, including a number of concepts and approaches introduced in the last decade. It cites recent reviews of presently available evidence.

This chapter introduces biomonitoring, both exposure biomonitoring and effects biomonitoring. It explains the importance of estimating the target dose, to define the mechanism or mode of action (MOA) of a toxic agent, and how the description of adverse outcome pathways (AOPs) is useful for risk and hazard assessment.

3.2 GENERAL CONSIDERATIONS ON EXPOSURE, ENVIRONMENTAL, AND BIOLOGICAL MONITORING

The target dose in the critical organ is of great importance for risk assessment. It determines when and how large a proportion of an exposed group of persons will suffer an adverse effect. The adverse effect that occurs at the lowest external exposure is the critical effect, and there is a corresponding target dose at the site of action. It is crucial for risk assessment and preventive action. Because the target dose (on a molecular level) is seldom possible to measure in vivo, the concentration of the substance under consideration in the critical organ is a useful surrogate measurement, often well correlated to the target dose. Although there are a few examples of direct measurements of the concentration in the critical organ (see Section 3.3.2), in many instances it is not possible to measure this concentration in vivo, and other measurements of the substance in media such as blood or urine forms the basis for estimating dose in the critical organ and target dose. Such *biomonitoring* or *biological monitoring* includes repeated measurement of substances or their metabolites in tissues, secreta, excreta, or expired air in order to evaluate occupational or environmental exposure and health risk (see also Appendix). *Biomarkers of exposure* relate external exposure to the levels of the substance under consideration (or its metabolites, or the product of interaction with target molecules) in a body tissue or fluid (see also Appendix). This concept includes interaction products between metallic species and target molecules, i.e., "target dose" (e g metal—enzyme complexes or metal-DNA adducts).

Fig. 3.1 starts with the classical identification of external exposure or dose by measurements in the external environment, i.e., environmental monitoring. External dose is composed of inhaled dose (airborne exposure) and daily intake (oral exposure) as discussed in Chapter 2. Fig. 3.1 also indicates that it is possible to perform direct studies of the relationship between these dose measurements and response in terms of occurrence of disease (and other less severe adverse health effects). However, such direct studies have to deal with several difficulties that are easier to handle when using biomonitoring instead of or as a complement to environmental monitoring. Fig. 3.1 indicates the connecting and transforming role of toxicokinetics between the external dose and internal dose (already dealt with in Chapter 2, Section 2.6). Toxicokinetics also explains and quantifies uptake in the critical organ and ideally the target dose for the critical effect. A lower target dose may be required in order to induce the critical effect in a susceptible subgroup of the exposed population compared to those with average susceptibility. Chapter 6 reviews examples of such differences in susceptibility. Neurotoxicity from methylmercury occurs in adults at approximately 10 times higher brain concentrations of the substance compared to fetuses and newborn infants. Another example: a relatively low blood and tissue concentration of methylmercury gives rise to cardiovascular toxicity (myocardial infarction) in a population with low intake of polyunsaturated fatty acids (PUFA).

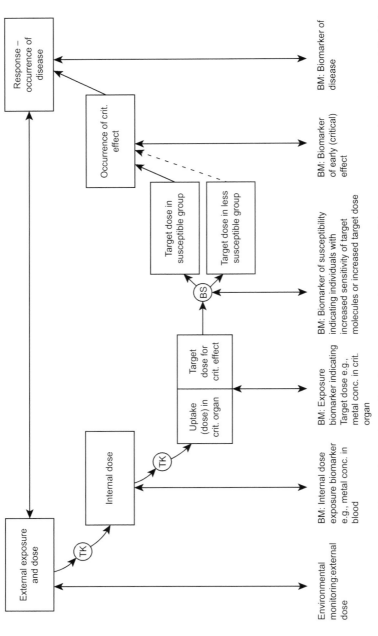

Figure 3.1 Biomonitoring and biomarkers. Relationships between external exposure and dose, environmental monitoring, biological monitoring (*BM*), and response. The importance of toxicokinetics (*TK*) and susceptibility (as shown by biomarkers of susceptibility [*BS*]) to adverse (critical [*crit.*]) effects is indicated.

Myocardial infarction thus emerges as the critical effect in a population group with such a pattern of risk factors. In groups with normal intakes of PUFA and less pronounced other cardiovascular risk factors, such toxicity does not occur. Chapter 6 also reviews other examples of susceptible groups. A subgroup accumulating higher target doses than the average individual provides another explanation on why a subgroup may suffer effects at lower external exposures than the average individual would do. In both instances, biomarkers of susceptibility indicate such differences in susceptibility. Biomarkers of effects indicate the occurrence of critical effects and/or disease. A general overview of biomonitoring (Fowler, 2016) provides further more detailed information. Santonen et al. (2015) focused their biomonitoring review on metallic compounds.

3.3 BIOMONITORING

3.3.1 Exposure Biomonitoring: Tissues and Fluids in Use

Biomonitoring of human exposures to metals and their compounds has utilized a number of tissues and fluids, most commonly blood and urine. Chemical analysis by inductively coupled plasma mass spectrometry in samples of these biomonitoring media is the most commonly used method at present for exposure monitoring. It is important to use adequate quality control in sampling and chemical analysis in order to avoid errors, often experienced in the past (Smith and Nordberg, 2015).

Blood: Blood is a mixture of blood cells and blood plasma. Blood cells are mainly erythrocytes, but a small proportion of blood cells are leukocytes and platelets. After clotting of blood, the remaining fluid is blood serum. Biomonitoring makes use of all of the mentioned blood components. However, for many metals and their compounds, plasma and serum concentrations are lower than those in blood cells. In the past, many chemical analytical methods were not sensitive enough for detection of the existing concentrations in plasma or serum; most biomonitoring programs for metals have used whole blood or packed blood cells. With the advent of more sensitive technology in recent years, this practice may change in the future. Presently available information is mostly about whole blood metal analyses. Adjustment for hemoglobin may be useful for metals with considerable higher concentrations in erythrocytes than in plasma, for example, when whole blood values of cadmium or lead are used, but only few investigators use such a correction (Santonen et al., 2015). Lead in whole blood is one of the most widely used measurements in occupational and environmental bio-monitoring. Lead concentrations in blood plasma are, as mentioned, much lower than whole blood concentrations. Measurements performed to date demonstrate no obvious advantages over whole blood values from a bio-monitoring perspective (Tian et al., 2013).

Urine: The kidney produces urine from blood plasma. Blood flows through the capillaries of the glomeruli in the kidney and fluid (primary urine) from blood plasma enters into the kidney tubules by filtration. Albumin in plasma and larger proteins remains in the blood compartment, but water, glucose, salts, amino acids, and small proteins in the urinary filtrate flow along the kidney tubules where a major proportion of these substances are reabsorbed into the tubular cells and further back into the blood stream. Some substances undergo tubular secretion by transfer from the blood through the tubular cells into urine. The body conserves water, salts, and other useful substances by tubular reabsorption while a small volume of water carries excretion products into urine. Because urine originates from blood plasma, there is in principle a relationship between plasma and urine values. However, this relationship varies depending on how the kidney handles the metal compound under consideration.

Each individual consumes a variable volume of water and drinks every day, and the body excretes all surplus water. Therefore, the urine volume each hour reflects the hydration state of the body. When using the concentration of a metal compound in urine as an index of body burden, concentration in critical organ, or external exposure, it is important to correct for urine flow/hydration status in order not to add this variation to other uncertainties that exist. There are two ways to correct for urine flow, either by urinary creatinine or by the relative density of urine. By dividing the observed urinary concentration of the metal compound in question with the measured creatinine concentration in the same sample, a mass fraction excretion in relation to creatinine is obtained, for example, nanomoles of metal/millimoles of creatinine. The amount of creatinine excreted in urine depends on muscular mass and is relatively constant in the same person. While it is a useful method in order to decrease the dependence on diuresis, it is not perfect because there is a remaining small dependence on diuresis because creatinine excretion increases a little with urine flow. Relative density of urine is another method used to adjust for diuresis. This correction only concerns differences in urine density (related to diuresis). It is performed by correcting the observed value (uncorrected value, C_0) based on the density of a reference value (RD_{ref}), usually 1.018 or 1.024, and the density of the sample under consideration (RD_0) according to the following equation: corrected value $C_c = C_0 \times (RD_{ref} - 1.000)/(RD_0 - 1.000)$. When urine is very dilute or very concentrated, i.e., outside of the range 1.010–1.030, corrected values are unreliable and a new urine sample should be obtained (see Santonen et al., 2015). Urinary cadmium is widely used because it reflects the body burden and the accumulation of cadmium in the kidney (the critical organ). However, correction by creatinine is not sufficient to compensate for diuresis. Further adjustment of the ratio of urinary cadmium to creatinine is required in epidemiological studies, based on the observed regression coefficient between the two variables (Barr et al., 2005). While urinary cadmium concentrations higher than 2 µmol/mmol creatinine are related to accumulation in the critical organ, the kidney cortex, and the occurrence of low-molecular-mass (LMM) proteinuria, lower values are difficult to evaluate, partly because most studies published at present did not compensate for the residual dependence on diuresis (further discussed in Chapter 8, Section 8.3).

Other tissues and fluids: For metal compounds accumulating in hair, metal concentration in hair may serve as a useful indicator of exposure and accumulation in critical organ. Because hair incorporates metals from the scalp, when formed, determinations of segments of hair can serve to describe past exposure history. Such data form an important basis for calculations of dose–response relationships between methylmercury exposure and neurological disease among farmers in Iraq exposed via contaminated grain (Chapter 8, Section 8.9). Other examples of media used are mercury determinations in saliva in monitoring of inorganic mercury exposures and cadmium in feces in monitoring of dietary cadmium exposure.

3.3.2 Biomonitoring as a Basis for Estimating Target Dose and Critical Organ Concentration

As noted in the statements in the introduction of this chapter, the toxic effects that occur at the lowest doses are those that occur in relation to the critical concentration in the critical organ or specifically at the lowest target dose. Direct biomonitoring of the concentration of the toxicant in the critical organ is possible for a few metallic compounds. The *critical concentration in the critical organ (also named the critical organ concentration)* is the mean concentration of a substance in the critical organ at the time the substance reaches its critical concentration in the most sensitive type of cell in the organ according to the International Union of Pure and Applied Chemistry (Duffus et al., 2007). It reflects, on the tissue level, the target dose at the molecular level.

In certain instances, it has been possible to measure the concentration of the substance in the critical organ. Cadmium is an example. Among workers occupationally exposed to cadmium, a noninvasive instrumental technology enabled measurements in vivo of the amount of cadmium in the critical organ (the kidney) and in an organ with high accumulation (the liver). Results of such measurements in combination with measurements of a biomarker of effect, i.e., urinary excretion of a LMM protein ($\beta2$-microglobulin), indicating the presence or absence of kidney dysfunction, form the basis for dose-—response relationships. A relationship between concentrations of cadmium in the critical organ and occurrence of an adverse (critical) effect in terms of kidney dysfunction was thus established (e.g., Roels et al., 1981; Roels et al., 1983; Ellis et al., 1984).

An S-shaped curve described the relationship between the total kidney cadmium burden and the percent probability of kidney dysfunction (Fig. 3.2). According to data displayed in Fig. 3.2, 22 mg of cadmium kidney burden corresponds to a 10% response (i.e., 90% of the workers are protected from developing LMM proteinuria). The corresponding cadmium concentration in the kidney cortex is 190 mg/kg according to the known relationships between whole kidney cadmium and kidney cortex cadmium (see Chapters 2 and 8). In this case, the critical organ concentration for each participant was determined, and the obtained data provided a basis for risk assessment and preventive action (see Chapters 8 and Appendix). These observations are from the 1980s, and they are still the best available example of in vivo measurements of critical organ concentrations for metals. Later contributions have tried to measure lower concentrations in groups from

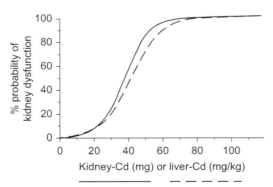

Figure 3.2 The percent probability of having kidney dysfunction in relation to kidney or liver cadmium burden determined by in vivo measurements of kidney cadmium in workers. *Modified from Ellis, K.J., et al., 1984. Environ. Res. 33, 216.*

the general population, but many of these measurements were below the detection limit of the method. Unfortunately, biomonitoring by in vivo measurements of substance concentrations in the critical organ is only possible for a few substances, but it is desirable to develop such in vivo measurements for other substances in order to enable similar measurements because they provide an excellent basis for dose—response assessment and related risk assessment (see further Chapter 8). For most substances including metals and their compounds, it is not possible to perform direct measurements of concentrations in the critical organ. Measurements of concentrations in blood or urine form a basis for indirect estimations of target dose (concentration in critical organ). It is possible and sometimes preferable to use other tissues and body fluids, but blood and urine are the most frequently used.

When the metal concentration in a tissue or biological fluid correlates accurately with the concentration in the critical organ, the target dose and, with the appearance of effects, biomonitoring provide a more accurate means of evaluating the risk of adverse effects compared to measurements of exposure. Often it is also easier and more convenient to perform such measurements than measurements of external exposure. In occupational lead exposure, for example, determination of lead in blood is less time consuming and gives information that is more accurate concerning risk of adverse effects compared to measurements of external exposure. This is true, also when monitoring inhalation exposure by personal sampling during a full working shift. The reason for this is that it integrates exposure during a longer time compared to air measurements during a single day. In addition, the blood lead concentration reflects the soft tissue pool of lead that correlates to the concentration in the critical organ. Measurements of the concentration of lead in bone tissue, a measurement that can be performed in vivo, provide an excellent estimate of the integrated exposure during a long period because of the long (years) half-life of lead in bone (Skerfving and Bergdahl, 2015). Interpretations of results obtained in biomonitoring programs, using exposure biomarkers, must take into account the toxicokinetics of the metal compound under consideration. For example, while mercury concentrations in urine are meaningful for a person exposed to inorganic mercury, such measurements are less valuable in methylmercury exposures. The explanation is that there is a good correlation between urinary concentrations of mercury and the concentration in the critical organ (the kidney) for inorganic mercury but a poor correlation for methylmercury because of the very limited excretion of this mercury species in urine. An accurate toxicokinetic model is the best way to describe the relationships between concentrations in biomonitoring media and concentration in the critical organ. Chapter 2 discussed such models and considerations given these are valid for the present discussion. Such toxicokinetic models provide an excellent quantitative description of the correlations mentioned in the forgoing text.

3.3.3 Use of Biomonitoring Data and Toxicokinetic Models to Estimate Dietary Intake

Biomonitoring data is sometimes a basis for estimating the corresponding external exposure. Toxicokinetic models (see Chapter 2) can support such conversion. Such models including the one-compartment model describe the uptake, distribution and elimination of drugs, and various organic chemicals as well as metallic compounds (WHO, 1978; Chapter 2). They provide relationships between exposure dose/daily intake, tissue concentrations, and excretion of the chemical compound studied. Ruiz et al. (2010) and Ruiz and Fowler (2015) described the extrapolation of external exposures from biomonitoring measurements as "reverse dosimetry". Amzal et al. (2009) and EFSA (2009) provide examples of the use of a one-compartment model to convert biomonitoring data. Based on data from an observational study of cadmium intake and determinations of urinary cadmium excretion in the same individuals, Amzal et al. (2009) developed a one-compartment model of cadmium toxicokinetics and derived the conversion factor between urinary cadmium and daily intake. The results of these calculations were used by the European Food Safety Authority (EFSA, 2009) when setting their recommendations of tolerable weekly intake (TWI) of cadmium (for further details of TWIs for cadmium recommended by various organizations, see Chapter 8). The International Commission for Radiological Protection used the one-compartment model extensively for calculating radiation doses to various body organs (see further Chapter 5).

3.3.4 Studying Health Outcomes by the Use of Biomarkers: Biomarkers of Effects

Biomarkers of effects are biochemical or biological changes indicating adverse functional change or disease detected in biomonitoring media such as blood or urine. Changes that are precursors to disease, but are reversible, are of particular value in order to prevent the occurrence of disease (Santonen et al., 2015).

A good example of such biomarkers are those indicating early stages of interference with heme synthesis, studied in lead-exposed groups of workers and members of the general population. These biomarkers, for example, lead-induced changes in the activity of δ-aminolevulinic acid dehydratase (ALAD) in erythrocytes, constitute early, reversible changes in the heme synthesis pathway. They constitute part of the biochemical mechanism of action of lead on heme synthesis. The decrease in ALAD activity by lead in combination with an effect by that metal on the enzyme ferrochelatase is an important event, ultimately leading to the development of anemia (see Section 3.4.1).

Other useful biomarkers indicate early stages of kidney dysfunction. Several proteins and enzymes determined in urine are useful for detection of changes in kidney function long before clinical kidney disease develops. Increased urinary albumin excretion is an indicator of increased permeability of the glomeruli in the kidney. Exposure to inorganic mercury or cadmium (see Chapter 8) causes such increased albumin excretion. Nephrotic syndrome with albumin excretion may occur after inorganic mercury exposure. Increased albumin excretion may also occur after exposure to other metallic compounds. Increased urinary concentrations of LMM proteins like β2-microglobulin, α1-microglobulin (protein HC), or retinol-binding protein indicate an impaired reabsorption capacity by the renal tubular cells. Determinations of these proteins in urine are useful biomarkers of renal tubular dysfunction. Exposure to inorganic mercury and cadmium causes accumulation of these metals in renal tubular cells and the mentioned biomarkers can detect early toxic lesions (see Section 3.4.2 and Chapter 8).

Exposure to metals and their compounds may cause neurotoxicity both in adults and in children (including fetuses). Minamata disease, caused by methylmercury exposure, is an example. This disease is a severe form of neurotoxicity first identified among fishermen and their families who ate methylmercury-contaminated fish caught in Minamata Bay, Japan. Severe poisoning, even fatalities, occurred among adults and women who gave birth to infants with cerebral palsy or severe neurodevelopmental deficits. This disease occurred also in other countries (see Chapter 5, Section 5.3.2 and Chapter 8). Neurotoxicity may also occur after exposure to metallic mercury vapor, lead and its compounds, manganese and manganese compounds, inorganic arsenic exposure, and thallium exposures. It is an important and challenging task to detect early stages of neurotoxicity in order to prevent the development of more severe forms of neurologic disease. Success until recently has been limited when trying to use, for example, serum prolactin or urinary homovanillic acid as indicators of changes in the dopaminergic system (de Burbure et al., 2006). Increasing evidence supports the potential utility of determinations in serum, plasma, urine, and cerebrospinal fluid of biomarkers of neurotoxicity such as microRNAs, F2-isoprostanes, translocator protein, glial fibrillary acidic protein, ubiquitin C-terminal hydrolase L1, myelin basic protein, microtubule-associated protein-2, and total tau (Roberts et al., 2015). Further research will determine the usefulness of these biomarkers for early detection of neurotoxicity by metals and their compounds.

Several metals and their compounds may give rise to toxic effects in the lungs, for example, beryllium, cobalt, cadmium, inorganic arsenic, and inorganic mercury. Impaired lung function is documented by tests measuring lung capacity and forced expiratory volume. X-ray examination, tomography, or MRI documents pathologic changes in the lung tissue, forming the basis for clinical diagnosis. Media used for biomonitoring of adverse effects on lungs are blood, serum, sputum, exhaled air, and exhaled breath condensate (EBC). Nitric oxide exhalation is a useful biomarker of inflammation in pulmonary tissues. It has a wide general use in diagnosis and follow-up of asthma, but so far only to a limited extent in metal-induced lung disease. Both FeNO (fraction of NO exhaled) in exhaled air and TNF-alpha (an inflammation biomarker) in EBC were measured in beryllium-exposed workers (Radauceanu et al., 2016), and the report pointed out the need for further studies. A biomarker of oxidative stress, malondialdehyde, was increased during the workweek in EBC from workers exposed to hexavalent chromium (Caglieri et al., 2005). Immunologic mechanisms are important for the development of some lung diseases. There are specific tests on blood cells, for example, for the evaluation of risks of berylliosis (also named chronic beryllium disease). The beryllium blood lymphocyte proliferation test identifies persons who are sensitized to beryllium, and these persons are those who are at risk of developing clinical or subclinical forms of berylliosis (Kreiss et al., 1997). Proteins specific to pulmonary tissues may serve as useful biomarkers of adverse effect. Hermans and Bernard (1999) launched analyses of such "pneumoproteins" in serum as an index of lung toxicity for air pollutants, and such measurements may be useful for metallic compounds affecting the lungs. CC16—Club cell protein 16—also named Clara cell protein 16 is such a protein. Its concentration in serum is a reflection of the number of Clara cells (Club cells) in the lung. So far, these biomarkers are research tools, mainly for other agents than metallic compounds.

Several other biomarkers are in use in studies of adverse effects of metals and their compounds on various tissues in the body. Circulating hormones indicate the functional integrity of endocrine organs. Bone-specific alkaline phosphatase, cross-linked N-telopeptide of collagen, osteocalcin, and urinary calcium may indicate bone effects by exposure to metallic compounds. Results from many studies of genotoxicity biomarkers in relation to exposures to metals and their compounds reflect a great interest that exists in possible relationships. As explained in the review by Davidson et al. (2015), most of the metals and metal compounds that are considered carcinogenic, with the exception of chromium, do not interact with DNA and are not mutagenic. Evidence from studies of relationships between metal exposure and genotoxicity biomarkers thus is mostly negative, except for chromium compounds. Gene—environment studies are epidemiological studies using biomarkers of genetic variation. The best example is that a specific leukocyte antigen (HLA) variant is involved in the presentation of beryllium to the immune system, giving rise to a high risk of berylliosis. Other examples of gene—environment interactions also exist, for example, the impact of polymorphisms in *AS3MT*, the gene that encodes arsenite methyltransferase, for arsenic metabolism (Broberg et al., 2015).

3.4 MECHANISM OF ACTION, MODE OF ACTION, AND ADVERSE OUTCOME PATHWAYS AS A BASIS FOR HAZARD AND RISK ASSESSMENT

MOA (mode of action) and *mechanism of action* are almost synonymous terms, but a somewhat different meaning is implicated in risk assessment (see further discussion in Section 3.4.2). MOA is a less detailed biochemical description of events than the mechanism of action, which usually implies exact knowledge of the biochemical event, for example, inhibition of a specific enzyme or alkylation of specific sites in DNA.

3.4.1 Mechanism of Action

When we know the molecular mechanism for an adverse effect and there is epidemiological evidence of dose—response relationships, such data provide strong support for causality and such evidence is a very useful basis for risk assessment. Such information that is generally accepted by the scientific community is, however, available only for few metallic compounds.

Many studies have investigated the effect of lead on heme metabolism. A considerable body of knowledge therefore exists concerning the molecular mechanisms leading to changes in heme metabolism in lead-exposed humans, and a summary is available on this extensive evidence (Skerfving and Bergdahl, 2015). This is probably the best example of well-documented quantitative relationships between metal exposure, molecular mechanisms, and adverse health effects. One of the salient features of classical occupational lead poisoning is anemia with basophilic stippling of erythrocytes. The mechanism behind this effect is a series of interactions by lead with enzymes in the heme synthesis pathway and, in addition, interference by lead on the enzyme pyrimidine $5'$nucleotidase ($5'$-NT/P5N).

In the bone marrow, the erythroid cells synthesize heme that constitutes an essential part of hemoglobin. Lead interacts with several enzymes in the heme synthesis pathway thus inhibiting heme synthesis. Fig. 3.3 shows known and suspected interactions between lead and the various enzymes in the heme synthesis pathway. One important enzyme affected by lead is ALAD catalyzing the conversion of delta-aminolevulinic acid into porphobilinogen. Another important step in heme synthesis affected by lead is the incorporation of iron into protoporphyrin IX by ferrochelatase, an

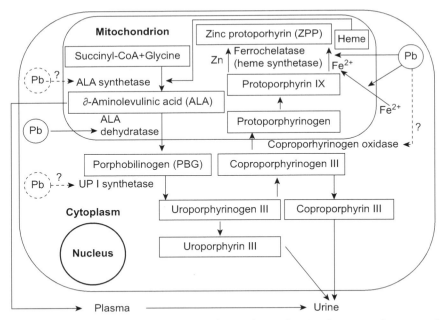

Figure 3.3 Lead interference with heme biosynthesis showing known and suspected interactions by lead (Pb). *From Skerfving, S., Bergdahl, I.A., 2015. Lead. In: Nordberg, G.F., Fowler, B.A., Nordberg, M. (Eds.), Handbook on the Toxicology of Metals, vol. 2. Academic Press, Elsevier, Amsterdam, Boston, pp. 911—967.*

enzyme also inhibited by lead. An additional effect of lead is that it decreases the availability of iron in mitochondria. These biochemical effects can be regarded as the molecular initiating events (MIEs) leading to decreased hemoglobin concentrations. Inhibition of ALAD and ferrochelatase cause an accumulation of delta-aminolevulinic acid and coproporphyrins in tissues with increased levels in serum/plasma and urine. In lead workers, such increases indicate lead exposure and interference with heme synthesis. Many studies in the past describe these relationships and the use of these measurements as tools in biomonitoring. Inhibition of ferrochelatase hampers the incorporation of iron into protoporphyrin IX. Zinc protoporphyrin (ZPP) is then formed instead of heme (iron protoporphyrin). Lead exposure increases ZPP in erythrocytes. A simple fluorimetric method can detect such accumulation in a blood sample for biomonitoring of lead exposure in workers. ALAD inhibition in erythrocytes occurs at very low lead exposures.

Table 3.1 illustrates how increasing lead exposure causes a cascade of events leading to successively more severe interference with heme biosynthesis and at higher exposures also with nucleotide metabolism causing clinically relevant anemia. Approximately 5% increase in the occurrence of ALAD-inhibition in erythrocytes occurs at a lead concentration in blood of 0.14 μmol/L. A similar increase of ZPP in erythrocytes occurs at 1 μmol/L and anemia with basophilic stippling of erythrocytes at >3.5 μmol/L. Higher blood lead levels result in a greater proportions of those exposed to be affected (Skerfving and Bergdahl, 2015; Murata et al., 2003). The formation of increased ZPP, also named free erythrocyte protoporphyrin (FEP), occurs in relation to biomarker concentrations of lead.

Table 3.1 Lowest concentrations of lead in blood (*Pb-B*) related to approximately 5% prevalence of indicated changes in heme synthesis or anemia

Heme biosynthesis biomarker	Pb-B μg/L (μmol/L)
ALAD inhibition in erythrocytes	27 (0.14)
Delta-aminolevulinic acid increase in plasma	33 (0.16)
ZPP increase in erythrocytes	200 (1.0)
Accumulation of pyrimidine nucleotides in erythrocytes	300 (1.5)
Decreased hemoglobin concentration	500 (2.5)
Anemia with basophilic stippling of erythrocytes	>700 (>3.5)

ALAD, δ-aminolevuinic acid dehydratase; *ZPP*, zinc-protoporphyrin.
Data from Skerfving, S., Bergdahl, I.A., 2015. Lead. In: Nordberg, G.F., Fowler, B.A., Nordberg, M. (Eds.), Handbook on the Toxicology of Metals, vol. 2. Academic Press, Elsevier, Amsterdam, Boston, pp. 911–967; Murata, K., et al., 2003. J. Occup. Health 45, 209.

Fig. 3.4 (from WHO, 1980) shows a clearly S-shaped relationship between blood lead levels and the percentage of a group of lead-exposed persons exceeding the cutoff limit for FEP. Lead in whole blood (Pb-B) is a biomarker of exposure and critical organ concentration/target dose. Because of the close correlation between lead concentrations in erythrocytes and the concentration in hematopoietic cells in the myeloid tissue in the bone marrow, whole-blood lead concentrations or erythrocyte lead concentrations are very good biomarkers of target dose related to hematological effects of lead. This is a valid assessment and the established relationships observed in humans between blood lead concentrations and appearance of adverse hematological effects fulfill the criteria of causality specified by Hill (Chapter 4, Section 4.4.2) and IPCS (The International Program on Chemical Safety) (Boobis et al., 2008; see below Section 3.4.2). It is at present not fully clarified to what extent the MIEs described here form the background for other effects of lead such as increased blood pressure, hypertension, and developmental toxicity to the brain, the latter effect presently considered to be the critical effect of lead from exposures in the general population. As mentioned, the molecular mechanisms explaining the

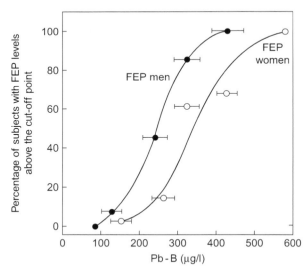

Figure 3.4 Relationship between blood lead (*Pb-B*, μg/L) and percentage of subjects with free erythrocyte protoporphyrin (FEP) above the cutoff point. *Modified from WHO, 1980. Recommended Health — Based Limits in Occupational Exposure to Heavy Metals. Tech. Rep. Ser. 647. WHO, Geneva.*

neurotoxic effects of lead are not scientifically established. Chapters 5 and 8 give further information on dose—response relationships for the various adverse effects of lead. It is interesting to note that polymorphism in the ALAD gene is associated with health outcomes in some epidemiological studies (Scinicariello et al., 2010; Tian et al., 2013), thus indicating a probable role of porphyrin metabolism for the studied health outcomes. Other cellular toxic mechanisms are reported after lead exposure, for example, perturbation of cellular calcium handling (Fullmer, 1992) and oxidative stress (Matovic et al., 2015), but their roles as MIEs are unclear. In general, the mechanism of action is of considerable importance for hazard assessment of carcinogenicity. For example, the International Agency for Research on Cancer (IARC, 2012) uses this criterion when classifying the carcinogenicity of various metals and metal compounds (Chapter 4, Sections 4.4.6 and 4.4.2.2). Although toxicokinetic data are valuable when comparing the target dose in animals and humans, according to IARC, there are no generally recognized quantitative toxicokinetic-toxicodynamic (TKTD) models for metallic compounds (or any other chemical substance) describing cancer risks. Chapter 5 discusses available quantitative models and extrapolation methods.

3.4.2 Mode of Action and the Human Relevance Framework

According to the US Environmental Protection Agency (Dellarco and Baetcke, 2005) and the IPCS (Sonich-Mullin et al., 2001; Boobis et al., 2008), the "Mode of Action" provides a less detailed description than the molecular mechanism of the events leading to an adverse effect. The MOA is sufficient to draw a reasonable working conclusion concerning a chemical's influence on the precursor events leading to an adverse effect. The IPCS has developed a structured framework (Boobis et al., 2008) for analysis of the MOA in animals to address human relevance—the Human Relevance Framework. The first step is to determine whether the weight of evidence based on experimental observations is sufficient to establish a hypothesized MOA. An adaptation of the considerations of causality in epidemiological studies by Sir Austin Bradford Hill (see Chapter 4, Section 4.4.2) to experimental data is used in this step. The method identifies key events. Subsequently, the MOA is compared qualitatively and quantitatively between animals and humans. Similar to the classical Hill considerations, IPCS (Boobis et al., 2008) lists the following criteria for human relevance:

- concordance of dose—response relationships;
- temporality of associations;

- strength, consistency, and specificity of toxicological response with key events;
- biological plausibility and coherence.

Such considerations result in a clear statement of conclusions concerning the applicability of the proposed MOA for humans. This framework intends to provide a transparent evaluation that is of value in further assessment of the compound, such as dose—response relationships.

For example, long-term exposure to cadmium compounds in animals or humans gives rise to accumulation of cadmium in kidney cells and impaired kidney function. The accumulation of cadmium occurs most prominently in tubular kidney cells. Cadmium accumulation in the kidneys of workers is possible to measure (Section 3.3.2 above). Such accumulation induces the synthesis of a metal-binding protein, metallothionein (MT). At low levels of exposure, the protective effects of MT dominate and no measurable cellular damage occurs. Accumulation of higher concentrations of cadmium leads to insufficient protection by MT, and cellular damage occurs. Several biochemical changes take place in tubular kidney cells when cadmium ions interact with cellular targets. Some studies report a decrease of zinc-dependent enzymes. Other studies report perturbations of cellular calcium transport and interaction by cadmium with cellular membrane targets (Nordberg et al., 1994). This is a probable MOA to induce the cellular changes leading to decreased reabsorption function by tubular cells in the kidney. He et al. (2009) presented data from animals indicating a role for zinc transporter ZIP 8 in relation to cadmium toxicity to the testicles and kidneys. Reactive oxygen species formation also takes place (Matovic et al., 2015), but we do not know the exact role of the various cellular changes for the functional impairments in renal tubular cells. Despite this uncertainty, dose—response relationships both at a tissue level (Section 3.3.2) and in relation to biomarkers of exposure in humans and animals are available based on extensive experimental and epidemiological studies (Nordberg et al., 2015). Based on such information, a TKTD model is available that allows calculation of relationships between external exposure, internal dose, accumulation in the critical organ, and the likelihood of kidney dysfunction. This model is a useful tool for comparison with epidemiological findings of renal tubular dysfunction in population groups with various levels of cadmium exposure in the occupational and general environments. Chapter 5 describes such comparisons. A good consistency exists between the TKTD modeled dose—response relationships and those observed in epidemiological studies of cadmium-exposed population groups. Because of that it seems reasonable to accept these sets of data as an example of the successful use of MOA–TKTD modeling despite the fact that there is no full understanding of the detailed sequence of biochemical and cellular events leading to the adverse effect.

In addition to the TKTD model for cadmium, Chapter 5 summarizes other available TKTD models for metallic compounds. At present, only few well-established quantitative MOA–TKTD models exist for metals and their compounds, but further work in this area may result in useful models for additional metal compounds in the future.

3.4.3 Adverse Outcome Pathways

In the last decades, increasing research efforts have dealt with molecular mechanisms of toxicity. Davidson et al. (2015) gave an overview of a number of such mechanisms of metal toxicity and carcinogenicity. As mentioned in the foregoing text, the MOA concept, relates a series of key events along a biological pathway from the initial chemical interaction to the adverse outcome (AO) (see Section 3.4.2.). These toxicity pathways can lead to adverse health effects (OECD, 2012a). According to Vinken (2013), toxicity pathways align with AOPs, which have their roots in the area of ecotoxicology. An AOP refers to a conceptual construct that portrays existing knowledge concerning the linkage between a direct MIE and an AO at a biological level of organization relevant to risk assessment (Ankley et al., 2010; OECD, 2012a). In comparison with the MOA, the scope of an AOP is much broader, as it starts with the exposure and can go up to the population level. It thus includes some of the components of the concept MOA–TKTD. AOPs for a number of different human-relevant toxicological endpoints are available or underway. In response to the increasing use of the AOP tool, the OECD has published a draft guidance document for the development and assessment of the completeness of AOPs (OECD, 2012a). The following text summarizes a few of these considerations.

AOP development identifies the main information blocks and subsequently summarizes data and then evaluates them (OECD, 2012a). An AOP typically relies on three information blocks, namely the MIE, intermediate step(s), and the AO. An in-depth literature survey or data from experimental studies including "omics-based" data, in vitro data, and in vivo data is the basis for these building blocks (OECD, 2012a). The first anchor of an AOP is the MIE and refers to the interaction of a chemical with a biological system at the molecular level, such as ligand—receptor interactions or binding to proteins and nucleic acids. The second AOP anchor is the AO describing the actual apical toxicological endpoint. The AO may be located at different levels of biological organization, ranging from the cellular to the population level, and can relate to either a chronic or a systemic toxicological outcome, or an acute or local adverse effect. An AOP only has one MIE and one AO, but may involve an unlimited number of intermediate steps.

A graphical presentation of the different AOP information blocks is the most common way of data summation. According to OECD (OECD, 2012a), the evaluation of a newly developed AOP includes two steps: (1) a weight-of-evidence assessment according to specified criteria similar to those developed by Bradford Hill (see Chapter 4, Section 4.4.2). This evaluation step establishes or rejects a causal link between the blocks of the AOP. (2) The second evaluation step is a confidence assessment, answering the following five questions: how well characterized is the AOP? How well are the initiating and other key events causally linked to the outcome? What are the limitations in the evidence in support of the AOP? Is the AOP specific to certain tissues, life stages, or age classes? Are the initiating and key events expected to be conserved across taxa?

An AOP described by Vinken (2013) and OECD (2012b) is the one for skin sensitization (Fig. 3.5). Allergic contact dermatitis is a delayed type of

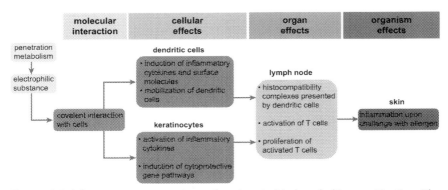

Figure 3.5 Adverse outcome pathway for chemical-induced skin sensitization. The initial step (*left*) includes the penetration of the chemical into the skin, sometimes accompanied by local metabolism, yielding an electrophilic substance. The latter serves as a hapten and covalently binds to skin proteins, which defines the molecular initiating event. The haptenized chemical induces an inflammatory reaction in keratinocytes and simultaneously activates dendritic cells. Activated dendritic cells then move to lymph nodes, where T lymphocytes (*T cells*) are activated and proliferate. Subsequent contact with the chemical causes an allergen challenge that induces clinical effects. This is the adverse outcome in the skin. *Adapted from Vinken, M., 2013. Toxicology 312, 158; OECD, 2012b. The Adverse Outcome Pathway for Skin Sensitization Initiated by Covalent Binding to Proteins. Part I: Scientific Evidence. OECD. www.oecd.org.*

hypersensitivity reaction caused by many chemicals, for example, nickel and nickel compounds. This hypersensitivity reaction consists of two phases: induction and elicitation. In the induction phase, the chemical generates an immunological memory, and in the elicitation phase, subsequent exposures give rise to clinical effects (Maxwell et al., 2011).

Penetration into the outer epidermis layer of the skin is the first event in the induction phase. A covalent interaction occurs between the chemical or its metabolite (acting as a hapten) and skin proteins, an event called haptenization. This is the MIE. The haptenized chemical (i.e., the hapten—protein complex) then triggers an inflammatory response in keratinocytes with expression of proinflammatory interleukin-1 beta. In dendritic cells and epidermal Langerhans cells, similar actions take place, and these cells become activated. In fact, activated dendritic cells migrate to local lymph nodes, where they present parts of the haptenized chemical to naive T lymphocytes that differentiate and proliferate into chemical-specific memory T lymphocytes, which circulate freely in the body. The next contact with the chemical initiates the elicitation phase. The chemical penetrates the skin and is haptenized. The haptenized chemical enters into dendritic cells, and they recruit the chemical-specific memory T lymphocytes to the epidermis. The memory T lymphocytes secrete proinflammatory cytokines and mobilize cytotoxic T lymphocytes. This leads to clinical symptoms and signs such as skin rash, blisters, and pruritus (itchy skin) constituting the AO. The OECD (2012b) established this AOP framework (Fig. 3.5) after a favorable evaluation by the above-mentioned (see Section 3.4.2) weight-of-evidence criteria and confidence questions. Discussions at a symposium in 2015 (Wittwehr et al., 2017) considered that the systematic organization of knowledge into AOP frameworks can inform and help direct the design and development of computational prediction models that can further enhance the utility of mechanistic and in silico data for chemical safety assessment. This publication (Wittwehr et al., 2017) suggested TKTD models presenting computer calculations of predicted risks for skin sensitization based on in vitro testing of chemicals. Chapter 4, Section 4.5.1, presents an in vitro method (OECD 442E) based on the AOP in Fig. 3.5. This method is considered to support discrimination between sensitizers and nonsensitizers. Chapter 5 discusses quantitative AOP models. No published information seems to be available comparing model-generated data to actual observational data from humans concerning dose—response relationships for dermal exposure to nickel and its compounds and related occurrence of dermatitis. Chapter 8, Section 8.10, summarizes available information about allergic contact dermatitis induced by nickel.

3.4.4 Biomonitoring Equivalents

In recent years, extensive biomonitoring programs have provided information on existing concentrations of metallic compounds in blood or urine of the general population. Examples are the NHANES studies in the United States and various national and international biomonitoring programs in Europe. For several of the studied compounds, there is a lack of information on risks of adverse health effects at the concentrations detected. There is a need to address the question of what these levels mean in terms of potential public health risks. These considerations lead to the development of the Biomonitoring Equivalents (BEs) concept (Meek et al., 2008). Hays et al. (2008) summarized guidelines for derivation of BEs. These methods make use of established limits in exposure media (air, drinking water, and food), representing acceptable risks and converting them into corresponding levels in biomonitoring media such as blood or urine. Chapter 7, Section 7.3.3, gives further information about BE.

3.5 SUMMARY

It is clear from the above discussion that there are a number of recent technical and conceptual advances in risk assessments for metals that make use of evolving approaches in toxicology and risk assessment. These approaches involve incorporation of modern tools of molecular and computational biology that have the potential to develop more sensitive and accurate risk assessments for metals on an individual or mixture exposure basis. Validation studies, which link these modern approaches and understanding of initial molecular events to the onset of clinical outcomes, are now essential to permit complete acceptance of tools for risk assessment practice. Fortunately, thanks to the human relevance framework based on the considerations by Bradford Hill, noted above, we have a conceptual framework for conducting such validation studies.

REFERENCES

Amzal, B., et al., 2009. Environ. Health Perspect. 117, 1293.
Ankley, G.T., et al., 2010. Environ. Toxicol. Chem. 29 (3), 730.
Barr, D.B., et al., 2005. Environ. Health Perspect. 113, 192.
Boobis, A.R., et al., 2008. Crit. Rev. Toxicol. 38, 87.

Broberg, K., Engström, K., Ameer, S., 2015. Gene-environment interactions for metals. In: Fowler, B.A., Nordberg, G.F., Nordberg, M. (Eds.), Handbook on the Toxicology of Metals, fourth ed. Academic Press, Elsevier, Amsterdam, Boston, pp. 239–264.

Caglieri, A., et al., 2005. Environ. Health Perspect. 114, 542.

Clarkson, T.W., Friberg, L., Nordberg, G.F., Sager, P.A. (Eds.), 1988. Biological Monitoring of Toxic Metals. Plenum Press, New York, pp. 1–686.

Davidson, T., Ke, Q., Costa, M., 2015. Selected molecular mechanisms of metal toxicity and carcinogenicity. In: Nordberg, G.F., Fowler, B.A., Nordberg, M. (Eds.), Handbook on the Toxicology of Metals, fourth ed. Academic Press, Elsevier, Amsterdam, Boston, pp. 173–196.

de Burbure, C., et al., 2006. Environ. Health Perspect. 114 (4), 584–590.

Dellarco, V.L., Baetcke, K., 2005. Toxicol. Sci. 86, 1.

Duffus, J.H., et al., 2007. Pure Appl. Chem. 79 (7).

EFSA, 2009. EFSA J. 980, 1.

Ellis, K.J., et al., 1984. Environ. Res. 33, 216.

Fowler, B.A. (Ed.), 1979. Environ. Health Perspect. 28, 1.

Fowler, B.A., 2016. Molecular Biological Markers for Toxicology and Risk Assessment. Elsevier Publishers, Amsterdam, p. 153.

Fullmer, C.S., 1992. Neurotoxicology 13, 799–807.

Hays, S.M., et al., 2008. Reg. Toxicol. Pharmacol. 51, S4.

He, L., et al., 2009. Toxicol. Appl. Pharmacol. 238, 250.

Hermans, C., Bernard, A., 1999. Am. J. Respir. Crit. Care Med. 159, 646.

IARC, 2012. Arsenic, metals, fibres and dusts. In: IARC (Ed.), IARC Monographs, vol. 100C. IARC, Lyons France.

Kreiss, K., et al., 1997. Occup. Environ. Med. 54, 605.

Matovic, V., et al., 2015. Food Chem. Toxicol. 78, 130.

Maxwell, G., et al., 2011. ALTEX 28, 50.

Meek, M.E., et al., 2008. Reg. Toxicol. Pharmacol. 52, S3.

Murata, K., et al., 2003. J. Occup. Health 45, 209.

Nordberg, G.F., 1976. Scand. J. Work Environ. Health 2, 37.

Nordberg, G.F., et al., 1994. Environ. Health Perspect. 102 (Suppl. 3), 191.

Nordberg, G.F., Nogawa, K., Nordberg, M., 2015. Cadmium. In: Nordberg, G.F., Fowler, B.A., Nordberg, M. (Eds.), Handbook on the Toxicology of Metals, fourth ed. Academic Press, Elsevier, Amsterdam, Boston, pp. 667–742 (Chapter 32).

OECD, 2012a. Proposal for a Template and Guidance on Developing and Assessing the Completeness of Adverse Outcome Pathways.

OECD, 2012b. The Adverse Outcome Pathway for Skin Sensitization Initiated by Covalent Binding to Proteins. Part I: Scientific Evidence. OECD. www.oecd.org.

Radauceanu, A., et al., 2016. Toxicol. Lett. 263, 26.

Roberts, R.A., et al., 2015. Toxicol. Sci. 148, 332.

Roels, H., et al., 1981. Environ. Res. 26, 217.

Roels, H., et al., 1983. Toxicol. Lett. 15 (4), 357.

Ruiz, P., et al., 2010. Environ. Res. 198, 44.

Ruiz, P., Fowler, B.A., 2015. Exposure assessment, forward and reverse dosimetry. In: Nordberg, G.F., et al. (Eds.), Handbook on the Toxicology of Metals. Academic Press, Elsevier, Amsterdam, Boston.

Santonen, T., et al., 2015. Biological monitoring and biomarkers. In: Nordberg, G.F., Fowler, B.A., Nordberg, M. (Eds.), Handbook on the Toxicology of Metals, fourth ed., vol. 1. Academic Press, Elsevier, Amsterdam, Boston, pp. 155–171.

Scinicariello, F., et al., 2010. Environ. Health Perspect. 118, 259.

Skerfving, S., Bergdahl, I.A., 2015. Lead. In: Nordberg, G.F., Fowler, B.A., Nordberg, M. (Eds.), Handbook on the Toxicology of Metals, vol. 2. Academic Press, Elsevier, Amsterdam, Boston, pp. 911—967.

Smith, D.R., Nordberg, M., 2015. General chemistry, sapling, analytical methods, and speciation. In: Nordberg, G.F., Fowler, B.A., Nordberg, M. (Eds.), Handbook on the Toxicology of Metals, fourth ed., vol. 1. Academic Press, Elsevier, Amsterdam, Boston, pp. 15—44 (Chapter 2).

Sonich-Mullin, C., et al., 2001. Regul. Toxicol. Pharmacol. 34, 146.

TGMA, Task Group on Metal Accumulation, 1973. Environ. Physiol. Biochem. 3, 65.

TGMI, Task Group on Metal Interaction, 1978. Environ. Health Perspect. 25, 3.

TGMT, Task Group on Metal Toxicity, 1976. A consensus report from an international meeting organized by the Subcommittee on the Toxicology of Metals of the Permanent Commission and International Association on Occupational Health. In: Nordberg, G.F. (Ed.), Effects and Dose-Response Relationships of Toxic Metals. Elsevier, Amsterdam, pp. 1—111.

Tian, L., et al., 2013. Toxicol. Lett. 221, 102.

Vinken, M., 2013. Toxicology 312, 158.

WHO, 1978. Environmental Health Criteria No. 6. In: WHO (Ed.), Principles and Methods for Evaluating the Toxicity of Chemicals. WHO, Geneva.

WHO, 1980. Recommended Health — Based Limits in Occupational Exposure to Heavy Metals. Tech. Rep. Ser. 647. WHO, Geneva.

Wittwehr, C., et al., 2017. Toxicol. Sci. 155, 326.

CHAPTER FOUR

Hazard Identification and Assessment

Abstract

Hazard identification is a central part in the process of evaluating the safety of a metallic or any other chemical compound. Such identification evaluates the totality of information about chemical and toxicological properties. It is important to consider different metal compounds (species) separately when evaluating metabolism, toxicokinetics, and effects. The basis for classifying toxicological properties are adverse effects observed in humans, in animals, in in vitro systems, and as modeled by computational tools. Information about chemical and toxicological properties allows the classification of substances as persistent, bioaccumulative, toxic, corrosive or irritating to the skin or mucous membranes of the respiratory or gastrointestinal tract; sensitizing to the skin or respiratory tract; toxic to reproduction and development; and mutagenic or carcinogenic. The hazard identification process characterizes the weight of evidence for causation of specific adverse effects as sufficient, limited, or insufficient. Concerning induction of effects in humans, human data are of great importance and data from animals or in vitro systems are also valuable. The mechanism of action or the mode of action, when known, provides additional support. Sometimes it is possible to describe an adverse outcome pathway. Based on all available information, a systematic analysis leads to a grading of the weight of evidence supporting that the chemical compound causes the adverse effect under consideration. Human exposures known or predicted to occur form the basis for the assessments. It is important to follow applicable ethical and legal rules when performing studies involving human subjects or animals.

4.1 INTRODUCTION

Human exposure to metallic chemical species occurs both because of their natural occurrence in the environment and because of mining, refining, and their use for various purposes in society, as indicated in Chapters 1 and 2. Regardless of the framework in which human metal exposures occur, hazard identification and assessment is a central point in the overall evaluation to be used when regulating processes or uses causing human exposure. When identifying the hazards caused by exposure to a specific metal or metal compound, it is necessary to have access to a minimum set of toxicological information. The availability of more abundant data,

Risk Assessment for Human Metal Exposures
ISBN: 978-0-12-804227-4
https://doi.org/10.1016/B978-0-12-804227-4.00004-2

99

perhaps also including adverse effects observed in humans, improves the quality of the identification process. The hazard identification process classifies the weight of evidence for causation of specific adverse effects as sufficient, limited, or insufficient. Such evaluations use in vivo (humans, experimental animals) and in vitro evidence (tests in cell culture and biochemical systems) as well as computational tools. Primary considerations for metals and their compounds are the existing or expected human exposures for specific chemical species of the metal.

For some metallic compounds, extensive toxicological and epidemiological information exists. Some metals/metalloids and their compounds are very toxic, and they have therefore been studied and regulated for a long time, long before the present legal framework was established. The restrictions in the use of some metals/metalloids and their compounds that has been in effect previously under specific legal rules in European countries are now included in the Registration, Evaluation, Authorization and Restriction of Chemicals (REACH) legislation implemented in the European Union (EU) countries. The European Chemicals Agency (ECHA) supervises this legislation. Hazard identification and assessment is a central point in the overall evaluation used when regulating chemicals and is crucial for the classification, labeling, and packaging (CLP) regulation in the EU and the Lautenberg Chemical Safety Act (Public Law 114—182 114th Congress, 2016) in the United States. The CLP regulation in the EU is in concordance with the Globally Harmonized System of Classification and Labelling of Chemicals (GHS) set up by the United Nations (UN) (see also Chapter 7).

When identifying hazards from a chemical compound, we use all possible adverse effects of that compound as a basis for the evaluation. The weight of evidence is the basis for statements about specific hazards identified for a specific chemical substance. Physicochemical properties in combination with biological data are important for classification (REACH and CLP) of substances as persistent, bioaccumulative, and toxic. ECHA (2017a,b) gives detailed criteria for such classification. The classification may specify various categories of danger (for example, very toxic, toxic, harmful, and corrosive) depending on the hazards identified for human health and the environment.

Special considerations are applicable for nanomaterials. The fact that the same properties of nanomaterials that are desirable in some applications, such as the ability to cross biological barriers and the manifestation of high surface reactivity, may also give rise to toxicity is referred to as the "nanomaterials paradox." Karlsson et al. (2015) reviewed available evidence on toxic effects observed for different metallic nanoparticles. The amount of information on specific metallic nanoparticles are highly variable. Some have already been used for a long time (e.g., TiO_2) without evidence of high toxicity, but for other materials, not widely used in the past, much more work is needed to provide reliable hazard assessments.

Another important consideration in hazard identification is whether a specific mode of action (MOA) or adverse outcome pathway (AOP) can explain an adverse effect or outcome (AO) caused by exposure to a specific metal compound. When there is a sufficient database for assessment, the weight of evidence is determined and if a specific effect is likely to be caused by the chemical in question, the judgment is that there is sufficient evidence that the chemical causes a specific type of toxicity/adverse effect. The assessment is made in relation to exposures known to occur in the working environment, general environment, or special circumstances. Quantitative information concerning both exposure/dose and the occurrence of effects makes it possible to describe dose—response relationships (see Chapter 5). The following text will first point out some fundamentally important considerations such as chemical speciation, knowledge about mechanism, or MOA and, when available, AOPs. Considering such information is crucial to a successful and scientifically valid hazard assessment.

4.2 SPECIATION

The publication "Elemental Speciation in Human Health Risk Assessment" (IPCS, 2007) emphasizes the fundamental importance of speciation in risk assessment. The need to consider different metal compounds (species) separately when evaluating metabolism, toxicokinetics, and effects is well recognized for some metals and was reviewed by Yokel et al. (2006) (see also Chapter 8). Mercury is a classic example; for this metal, it is not only necessary to separate organic from inorganic mercury compounds but also metallic mercury from inorganic mercury salts. For example, the long-term toxicity of methylmercury for humans considerably exceeds that of phenylmercury or divalent inorganic mercury. Inhalation of mercury vapor causes neurotoxicity while exposure to divalent inorganic mercury gives rise to adverse kidney effects (see further description in Chapter 8).

Arsenic occurs as inorganic, as well as organic, compounds. Exposure to high doses of organic arsenic occurs in fish-eating human populations. The stable organic arsenic compounds in fish and crustaceans are of low toxicity and are quickly excreted in urine. Exposure to inorganic arsenic through drinking water occurs in some segments of the human population, particularly in Bangladesh, causing increased risks of skin diseases, cancer, and other diseases (see Chapter 8). Usually, trivalent inorganic arsenic compounds are considered more toxic than pentavalent ones. Evidence for carcinogenicity is mostly available for the trivalent form or for a mixture of trivalent and pentavalent forms because they occur in groundwater used as drinking water (IARC, 2012).

It is fundamentally important to recognize the different kinetics, metabolism, and toxicity of different species of metals. Hazard and risk assessments must consider such basic information. It is therefore increasingly important to analyze not only the metals as such but also the different forms in which they occur. Reliable methods are available for the analysis of different compounds of arsenic, mercury, and other metals/metalloids (see IPCS, 2007) (see also Chapters 2, 3, and 8). Because it was difficult in the past to determine the various chemical species in exposure media and in media used for biological monitoring, most evaluations in the past only considered total metal content. Speciation has not been a part of hazard and risk assessment of metals, except for mercury, where early chromatographic methods identified methylmercury in fish. These findings were the basis for early risk assessments of human exposures to this very toxic compound. At present, chemical analytical methods allow the determination of specific species of metals/metalloids in exposure media and media used for biological monitoring. Thus, it is possible at present to employ elemental speciation and speciation analysis for several metals/metalloids in human health hazard and risk assessment. Risk assessors and regulators should consider such information in their daily work (IPCS, 2007).

4.3 MECHANISM OF ACTION, MODE OF ACTION, AND ADVERSE OUTCOME PATHWAYS

Although *MOA (mode of action)* and *mechanism of action* are synonymous in common language, in hazard and risk assessment a somewhat different meaning is understood, as discussed in Chapter 3, Sections 3.4.1 and 3.4.2. The US Environmental Protection Agency (USEPA) recognizes such a difference (see Dellarco and Baetcke, 2005) as do other risk assessment organizations like International Program on Chemical Safety (IPCS) (Sonich-Mullin et al., 2001; Boobis et al., 2008). The "mode of action" represents a less detailed biochemical description of events than is meant by the "mechanism of action," as will be discussed in the following text. Chapter 3 gave an introduction to the use of biomonitoring for estimating the target dose causing a toxic effect. The adverse/toxic effect that occurs at the lowest exposure is the critical effect that is crucial for preventive action. The critical effect is often a different effect at single or short-term exposure than at long-term exposure, to be discussed in the following text and in Chapter 5. This chapter will consider the use of information on mechanism of action, MOA, and AOPs for identifying hazards. It will thus consider if the weight of evidence is sufficient to declare that the chemical compound in question can cause a specific adverse effect under the exposure conditions that prevail, e.g., cancer, reproductive and developmental effects, immunotoxicity or allergic sensitization, and related diseases.

4.3.1 Mechanism of Action

When there is knowledge about the molecular mechanism explaining an adverse effect of exposure to a chemical compound, particularly if there is also epidemiological evidence on dose–response relationships, such information provides strong evidence supporting causality. Chapter 3 gives an example of such an effect (anemia) caused by lead exposure. Lead interferes with enzymes in the heme synthesis pathway inhibiting the formation of heme (Section 3.4.1).

Davidson et al. (2015) reviewed selected molecular mechanisms of metal toxicity and carcinogenicity. Carcinogenic metals/metalloids, with the exception of chromium, do not interact with DNA and are not mutagenic. Other mechanisms explain the carcinogenicity of these chemical species such as modification of gene expression and epigenetic effects, for example, DNA methylation. Interference with cell signaling by metallic compounds and intracellular formation of reactive oxygen species may cause cellular lesions. Extensive research identified many such mechanisms in cells in vitro as well as in vivo in experimental animals, but there are only few examples where sufficient knowledge is available to consider the molecular mechanism fully known and applicable to dose–response relationships of adverse effects observed in humans.

Since the mid-1990s, the International Agency for Research on Cancer (IARC) has used data on mechanisms of carcinogenesis in hazard assessments for cancer (see preface in IARC, 2012, 2018). IARC lists the following changes in organs, tissues, or cells as being of importance, for their evaluations:

1. *Physiological changes* related to exposure, e.g., mitogenesis, compensatory cell division, escape from apoptosis and/or senescence, the presence of inflammation, hyperplasia, metaplasia and angiogenesis, alterations in cellular adhesion, changes in steroidal hormones, and changes in immune surveillance.

2. *Functional changes at the cellular level related to exposure*: alterations in cell signaling pathways, changed activities of enzymes, alterations in DNA repair, alterations in kinases that govern cell cycle progression, changes in apoptotic rates, changes in DNA replication and transcription, and intercellular communication, e.g., changes in gap junction processes.

3. *Changes at the molecular level related to exposure*: the formation of DNA adducts and DNA strand breaks, mutations in genes, chromosomal aberrations, aneuploidy, and changes in DNA methylation patterns.

The IARC also takes into consideration other data influencing mechanisms, e.g., structure—activity relationships (SARs) and physical and chemical properties. However, according to the IARC, high-output data (such as those derived from gene expression microarrays and from testing hundreds of agents for a single endpoint) pose a problem for use in the evaluation of carcinogenic hazard. For high-output data, there is a possibility of over interpretation of changes in individual endpoints (e.g., changes in the expression of a single gene) when the finding cannot be considered in a broader context.

4.3.2 Mode of Action

The foregoing section pointed out that the USEPA (see Dellarco and Baetcke, 2005) and the IPCS (Sonich-Mullin et al., 2001; Boobis et al., 2008) consider that the MOA provides a less detailed description than the "mechanism of action" of the molecular events leading to an adverse effect. However, the MOA provides a sufficient basis for practical conclusions concerning a chemical's influence on the precursor events leading to an adverse effect. Boobis et al. (2008) described a structured framework developed by IPCS for analysis of the MOA in animals to address human relevance—the Human Relevance Framework (see also Chapter 3, Section 3.4.2). The first step is to determine whether the weight of evidence based on experimental observations is sufficient to establish a hypothesized MOA. This first step uses an adaptation of Hill's considerations (see the following Section 4.4.2) to experimental data for such evaluation. A comparison of the MOA, qualitatively and quantitatively, between animals and humans strives to derive clear conclusions concerning the applicability of the proposed MOA for humans. This human relevance framework intends to provide a transparent evaluation that is of value in further evaluation of the chemical compound, such as estimation of dose—response relationships. On a scientific basis, this is justifiable based on the conservation of biological systems between experimental animals and humans.

4.3.3 Adverse Outcome Pathways

The AOP concept, introduced in Chapter 3, Section 3.4.3, is an extension of the MOA concept. An AOP is a conceptual construct describing existing knowledge concerning the linkage between a molecular initiating event and an AO at a biological level of organization such as a clinical symptom or a disease. Further, an AOP can start with exposure and include toxicokinetic modeling. Chapter 3 describes an AOP for skin sensitization, further considered and used in hazard identification in the following text (Section 4.5.1). Organization for Economic Co-operation and Development (OECD) has developed and published a number of AOPs for various adverse effects of importance in safety evaluations (OECD, 2012, 2017).

4.4 HUMAN DATA

4.4.1 General Considerations on Human Data

Obviously, the best basis for risk or hazard assessment of human exposures are data from humans. General medical knowledge about human diseases, pathology, physiology, and biochemistry furnishes an important background, complemented by specific knowledge about adverse effects observed in humans as a result of exposure to the metallic species under consideration. Case reports may be available and detailed clinical studies of a limited number of similarly exposed persons with a specific disease may exist. *Toxicovigilance* is a term used to encompass the active detection, validation, and follow-up of clinical adverse events related to toxic exposures in humans (Descotes and Tesud, 2005). Case studies can seldom establish causality but can generate hypotheses for further studies. In exceptional cases, when there are unique features such as association with a rare disease, e.g., Minamata disease from methylmercury exposures, causality may be indicated even in a limited number of cases.

If ethical considerations according to the Declaration of Helsinki are observed, experimental *studies in human volunteers* can be performed (see Section 4.8.1 for further ethical aspects). Possible studies include the kinetics of metal compounds at low doses, and studies of mild, reversible effects of low doses. In the scientific literature, however, there are only few reports of such studies for metallic compounds.

Studies of groups of exposed and unexposed persons concerning the occurrence of disease or other adverse health effects (i.e., cohort-type *epidemiological studies*) often provide useful information if well performed.

For uncommon diseases, case—control studies may be more feasible (Grandjean and Budtz-Jorgensen, 2015). Such analytical epidemiological studies can contribute to the establishment of causal connections between exposure and effect. When interpreting such studies, one must consider the possible influence of confounding and other weaknesses inherent in epidemiological studies. Descriptive epidemiological studies and correlation studies (also named *ecological studies*) may be valuable as a complement to other observations. They are mainly hypothesis generating and can seldom establish causality by themselves. Considerations for causality in epidemiological studies are the subject of the subsequent section.

4.4.2 Causality in Epidemiological Studies: Hill's Considerations

Epidemiological studies often establish statistically significant associations between exposures to chemical agents and occurrence of disease or other adverse health effects. Such associations are not always descriptions of cause and effect but may be due to confounding factors. Sir Austin Bradford Hill (1965) published nine considerations to take into account when establishing causality in epidemiological studies. These, now classical considerations, are still valid:

1. *Strength of association*, meaning that it is more likely that an association with a large relative risk is causal than one with a small relative risk.
2. *Consistency*, meaning that if association can be found in several studies by different investigations, causality is supported.
3. *Specificity*, meaning that the effect is specific to the exposure. In metal toxicology, this is rarely the case. Although the presence of specificity implies causality (e.g., for asbestos exposure and mesothelioma), its absence does not exclude it.
4. *Temporality*, meaning that exposure must precede effects.
5. *Biological gradient*, meaning that an association for which a dose—response relationship has been demonstrated is likely to be causal unless there is confounding.
6. *Biological plausibility*. If the mechanism of injury is known from animal experiments, this supports causality. However, if the mechanism is not known, or if there are no animal experiments reproducing the same effect of a specific exposure that, in itself, is not sufficient reason to reject causality.
7. *Coherence* between the observed association and other observations. Hill (1965) used the example of the association between cigarette smoking and lung cancer. It is coherent with the temporal rise in lung cancer with increased smoking in the population in the 1940s—1960s.

8. *Experiment.* Removal of a suspected agent gives rise to a decrease in disease occurrence or the disappearance of the disease.

9. *Analogy.* Similarity of exposure may indicate a causal relationship to disease. Hill (1965) mentions thalidomide and if a similar drug would be used and malformations were observed, causality would be supported by analogy.

According to Hill (1965), these are nine viewpoints from which we should study associations before we designate causation. They are not rules of evidence that must be obeyed before we accept cause and effect. What they can do is to help us make up our minds—is there any other answer equally or more likely than cause and effect?

Neutra et al. (2018) noted that the publication by Hill (1965) has been very important and still is important for rulings by judges in the United States. However, the original intention by Sir Austin Bradford Hill should be upheld, i.e., these considerations are not compulsory criteria for causality, but viewpoints from which we should study causality.

4.4.3 Requirements for Data and Sources of Human Data

The Food and Agriculture Organization/World Health Organization (WHO) Joint Expert Committee on Food Additives and Contaminants performs evaluations based on available data in humans and, traditionally, data from long-term studies in animals to derive recommendations (see Chapter 5, Section 5.2.1).

In the EU, the REACH regulation, and the CLP regulation require that producers and importers of chemical substances register the substances. In the registration process, the applicant must supply the required information to the ECHA in order for the substances to be used (see Chapter 7, Section 7.2.5, for further description of the general structure and implementation of these regulations). Many thousand chemical compounds are registered. Metals, metalloids, and their compounds represent only a small proportion of the registered compounds. Depending on the amount handled, the regulation requires submission of more or less detailed information. In addition to information about a number of physicochemical properties, there are requirements information about skin and respiratory irritation and sensitization, acute toxicity, and other toxicological properties (ECHA, 2017a). These properties are all important for the labeling of chemicals.

For metallic compounds used for a long time in society, information is available from the scientific literature on local effects and acute toxicity (see Section 4.4.4 below), but there are many new uses of metallic compounds for which information is lacking. According to the mentioned regulations, new tests for health or environmental hazards of substances and mixtures may only be performed when the manufacturer, importer, or downstream user has exhausted all other means of generating information. Such methods recommended in REACH include alternative methods/ approaches to animal testing of a substance, e.g., the use of existing data, quantitiative SARs (QSARs), and read–across methods, provided they are considered adequate.

In addition to the human data on local effects and acute toxicity mentioned above, human data are available on adverse effects of long-term exposures. Because of its serious nature, induction of cancer by chemical substances attracts special attention. Evaluations of carcinogenicity by IARC (see below) uses data published in the international scientific literature and publicly available documents from government agencies. In addition to human data of the various categories mentioned in the previous Section 4.4.1, IARC uses other types of data, for example, in vivo, ex vivo, and in vitro data on biochemical mechanisms of toxicity (see Section 4.5.2 below).

4.4.4 Availability of Human Data and Considerations of Causality for Local Irritation Effects, Skin and Respiratory Sensitization, and Acute Toxicity

4.4.4.1 Human Data on Local Corrosive/Irritation Effects on Skin and Mucous Membranes; Skin and Respiratory Sensitization

A considerable amount of human data is available from the scientific literature on *local corrosion/irritation on skin and mucous membranes* by metals/ metalloids and their compounds. For example, a number of such compounds cause corrosive/irritant dermatitis. Arsenic compounds, beryllium compounds, trimethyl bismuth compounds, hexavalent chromium compounds, cobalt compounds, nickel compounds, platinum coordination complexes such as hexachloroplatinates, acidic inorganic tin compounds, organic tin compounds such as tributyl tin all cause such adverse effects in humans. Inhalation of aerosols of nickel compounds, hexavalent chromium compounds, and arsenic compounds may cause ulceration of mucous membranes in the airways and subsequent perforation of the nasal septum (Nordberg et al., 2015). Because the dermal manifestations in terms of skin rash and eczematous changes occur soon after exposure and subside after a relatively short period of nonexposure, the causality of such changes is possible to determine with reasonable certainty. Ulcerations of the nasal epithelium and perforation of the nasal septum are rare clinical signs in nonexposed persons and the relation to exposure to the mentioned agents are therefore possible to determine, provided the physician investigates and records the presence of such exposures. The CLP regulation makes a distinction between corrosion and irritation, the former causing destruction of living tissue with ulceration and necrosis, while irritation causes inflammation. The regulation also gives specific considerations of "serious eye damage" (ECHA, 2017a).

Exposure to a number of metals and metallic compounds may cause *dermal sensitization and allergic dermatitis*, for example, beryllium and beryllium compounds, hexavalent chromium compounds, cobalt compounds, nickel and nickel compounds, and platinum coordination complexes such as tetra- and hexachloroplatinates (Nordberg et al., 2015). As an example, the present book describes human data for the sensitizing effect and subsequent elicitation of dermatitis by nickel and nickel compounds. Chapter 3, Section 3.4.3, describes the AOP for dermal sensitization by allergens and mechanisms for subsequent AO in terms of dermatitis. Chapter 8, Section 8.10, describes epidemiological evidence on dose—response relationships in humans for dermal nickel exposure and adverse effects in the form of dermatitis. Such information is used in the EU for prevention of nickel-related allergic dermatitis (see Chapter 8, Section 8.10). In the present chapter, Section 4.5.1 discusses possibilities to predict skin sensitization based on in vivo data from animal experiments and by in vitro tests.

Several metals and metal compounds give rise to *respiratory sensitization and related lung diseases* in humans. The most serious one is probably chronic beryllium disease; severe cases may have a fatal outcome. Occupational exposure to cobalt or cobalt compounds are related to an increased occurrence of cobalt asthma or hard metals asthma. Respiratory sensitization to other metals and metal compounds may lead to asthma, for example, in relatively rare cases after sensitization to hexavalent chromium or nickel compounds (Chapter 8, Section 8.10). Platinum salt sensitivity with asthma-like symptoms occurs in workers exposed to tetra- and hexachloroplatinates, a condition also named "Platinosis" (Nordberg et al., 2015). When good exposure assessments are available and temporal relationships as well as dose—response relationships to the occurrence of lung diseases can be established, the causal nature of epidemiological associations between exposure and disease occurrence can be established. These diseases sometimes are identified as critical effects, and observed dose—response relationships determine occupational exposure levels.

4.4.4.2 Acute Toxicity—Human Data

Like with other toxicological data, acute toxicity data on humans are very useful when available; they have considerable weight in hazard assessments used for CLP regulation. Possible sources of data are those already mentioned—epidemiological data, data from toxicovigilance at poisoning centers, and biomonitoring data, for example, in industrial workers. The short time interval between exposure and the appearance of symptoms of acute toxicity makes it reasonable in many cases to consider a causal relationship. The acute toxicity in humans of several metals/metalloids after a single high oral dose or short-term high-dose inhalation is well known. Examples include arsenic trioxide, cadmium and its compounds, inorganic copper compounds, mercury vapor, vanadium pentoxide, and zinc chloride (Chapter 8 and/or Nordberg et al., 2015). The acute toxicity in humans is not known for a number of metallic compounds, not previously extensively used in commerce. Because experimental exposure studies are not possible in humans, an obstacle to the use of human data is the limited availability and the limited information on levels of exposure in many accidental poisoning cases. For chemical compounds in general, most of the information that is available on acute toxicity is from animal studies and other sources (see Section 4.5.1 below).

4.4.5 Reproductive and Developmental Toxicity—Human Data

Lead may cause decreased male fertility in humans and decreases of certain parameters of semen quality (Skerfving and Bergdahl, 2015). An association between cadmium in urine and the occurrence of increased levels of prostate-specific antigen was found in a cadmium-polluted area in China (Zeng et al., 2004). There are studies of uncertain relevance reporting adverse effects on male reproductive parameters in humans for mercury, manganese, chromium, nickel, and arsenic (Apostoli et al., 2007). Elevated blood lead levels in the general population occurred during the latter part of last century (until around 1990 in Sweden) in many western industrialized countries. A main reason was the use of lead-containing additives in petrol and related emissions of lead into air from motor vehicles. Several epidemiological studies (review Landrigan et al., 2007) demonstrated developmental effects of lead on the brain function of children at low exposure levels. Such effects are partly due to exposure of the fetus through the mother in utero and partly due to exposure during childhood. These effects are considered as the critical effect when general population groups are exposed (Skerfving and Bergdahl, 2015). Methylmercury is a neurotoxic metallic compound present in several species of fish. Consumption of fish containing methylmercury by pregnant women may cause exposure to the fetus and cause neurodevelopmental deficits in their children after birth. This is the critical effect in such exposures (Chapter 8, Section 8.9).

4.4.6 Classification of Carcinogenicity Using Human Data; International Agency for Research on Cancer Group 1

Evaluations of available human and other relevant information in order to establish whether a chemical compound may cause cancer in humans, i.e., the classification of chemical compounds as carcinogens for humans is of great importance for prevention of cancer. Human data relevant for classification of carcinogenicity may range from case reports to extensive epidemiological studies (see Section 4.4.1 above). The IARC organizes meetings of Task Groups performing such evaluations of the causality for cancer. The resulting documents are published by the IARC (e.g., IARC, 2006a,b, 2012). The IARC has selected and developed their criteria for causality for cancer in epidemiological studies during the history of this organization, see preamble in IARC (2006a,b, 2012, 2018). Classification of an agent as "carcinogenic to humans" (IARC Group 1) usually requires that there is sufficient evidence of carcinogenicity in humans. Such evidence is based on epidemiological studies of good quality showing a statistically significant association between exposure to the agent and the occurrence of cancer; in addition, the IARC working group should be convinced that bias and confounding could be ruled out with reasonable confidence. Since the mid-1990s, classification in Group 1 can be supported by a combination of limited evidence of carcinogenicity in humans, sufficient evidence of carcinogenicity in experimental animals, and strong evidence in exposed humans that the agent acts through a relevant mechanism of carcinogenicity. Some of IARC's criteria for causality thus are similar to the considerations by Hill, for example, consistency and biological plausibility. Other criteria are unique for IARC, for example, the mechanistic criteria, but they have a certain similarity to Hill's considerations of biological plausibility.

Other classification categories in the IARC system, for example, Group 2A "Probably carcinogenic to humans" also requires some human evidence (see Section 4.5.2.2 below). However, classification in IARC Group 2 mainly uses nonhuman data (see Section 4.5.2.2). Other organizations use similar criteria when classifying chemical substances and other exposures as human carcinogens (see Section 4.7).

4.5 DATA FROM STUDIES ON ACUTE AND CHRONIC TOXICITY IN ANIMALS, CELLS, AND MOLECULAR SYSTEMS IN VITRO; COMPUTATIONAL SYSTEMS

4.5.1 In Vivo and In Vitro Data: Relevance for Humans—Noncancer Effects

As mentioned in the foregoing section, human data on skin irritation, skin sensitization, and acute toxicity are available for those metallic compounds which have been widely used in society. However, there is a lack of such data for metal compounds newly introduced or not yet used extensively. Information concerning local effects and acute and chronic systemic toxicity in experimental animals provides useful information on potential effects in humans. Although similar considerations might be applied, as those in the human relevance framework used for evaluation of MOA (Section 4.3.2 above), effects observed in animals usually are considered of relevance for humans, even if quantitative dose—response relationships may differ between animals and humans (see further Chapter 5). Achievement of a reasonable degree of safety for humans is only possible when the nonhuman data are of good quality. Even limited human data, complementing good nonhuman data, improves the risk assessment considerably both from a qualitative (hazard identification) and a quantitative (dose—response analysis) point of view (see also Chapter 5). As illustrated by the AOP for skin sensitization (see Chapter 3 and below), in vitro data on cells and molecular systems provide very useful information when the MOA for toxic metals can be described. In situations in which such mechanisms can be shown to be valid at dose levels occurring in human tissues at realistic exposures for humans and animals, such in vitro data are extremely valuable for the extrapolation of observations in animals to humans, and it is sometimes possible to use in vitro data for hazard identification and classification (see below).

Suitably designed animal studies performed according to accepted guidelines provide relevant information. The OECD (website: www.oecd.org) publishes test guidelines for the various specific animal bioassays for local effects like skin irritation and skin sensitization, acute, subchronic, and chronic systemic toxicity; developmental and reproductive toxicity; immunotoxicity; and carcinogenicity. Tests in experimental animals performed to satisfy regulatory requirements and published in recent years usually fulfill the OECD requirements or similar guidelines, but experiments performed to answer other research questions and older data may not. Even if the size of groups does not meet the requirements of the guidelines, positive findings may still be useful. Such incomplete data, does not allow assessment of the absence of observed effects.

In the past, when human data were absent or incomplete, a complete set of data on *local corrosive effects on the skin, eyes, and respiratory tract, as well as acute toxicity from animal experiments* was required for toxicological evaluation. However, ethical considerations (see Section 4.8.2) make it desirable to limit the use of animals to a minimum, particularly when tests are related to animal discomfort and/or pain. As mentioned above, this is also an explicit policy in the REACH legislation in EU. A number of validated in vitro test systems for skin corrosion/irritation are listed by ECHA (2017a). The EU Reference Laboratory for Alternatives to Animal Testing (EURL ECVAM; http://ihcp.jrc.ec.europa.eu/) provides information on validation and regulatory acceptance of available tests.

Adequate information on skin corrosion/irritation based on nontesting extrapolation or from in vitro tests, sometimes makes it possible to omit tests in animals (see ECHA, 2017b) and still meet the requirements in the REACH framework. Skin corrosion/irritation and acute toxicity following high-dose exposures are important for labeling of chemicals, for example, in the EU (CLP regulation). Successful results from evaluations of in vitro systems for the effects mentioned provide an important background for the ban in the EU on the animal testing of cosmetic products.

Very low doses of metallic and other chemicals may sometimes induce *skin and respiratory sensitization and related allergic dermatitis or respiratory disease*, and such adverse effects can be critical effects in the safety assessment. Hultman and Pollard (2015) described general features of the immunotoxicology of metals and their compounds and reviewed available evidence in the scientific literature in humans, animals, and in vitro systems. Their review included skin sensitization and allergic dermatitis induced by metallic species. Because sensitization effects occur at very low doses, it is important to find adequate test systems for such effects. Since the turn of the century (2000), there is extensive use of animal tests such as the guinea pig maximization test and local lymph node assay (LLNA) in order to predict the risk for skin sensitization in humans (cf. OECD, see www.oecd.org). In the last decade, our understanding has increased concerning the molecular and cellular mechanism behind skin sensitization and allergic dermatitis (Wittwehr et al., 2017). There is now international agreement about what is meant by skin sensitization. Skin sensitization refers to an allergic response following skin contact with the tested chemical, as defined by the UN GHS

(UN, 2017) and the present text uses this definition. According to Wittwehr et al. (2017), there are a number of in vitro tests for predicting skin sensitization in humans. Jaworska et al. (2013) presented an integrated strategy using a number of in vitro assays. These authors predicted 95% of chemicals for sensitization hazard and 86% for LLNA potency class. Ahmed et al. (2016) identified a number of human sensitizers including nickel in a test using skin explants in vitro. Nickel sensitization is difficult to predict in other assays. Chapter 3 presented an AOP for skin sensitization (Fig. 3.5). OECD recently published an in vitro test method (OECD, 2017) based on such an AOP (test 442E). This method combines three in vitro tests to predict sensitization in humans. The three in vitro test methods address a Key Event on the AOP: (1) the human Cell Line Activation Test or h-CLAT method, (2) the U937 Cell Line Activation Test or U-SENS, and (3) the Interleukin-8 Reporter Gene Assay or IL-8 Luc assay. All three tests support the discrimination between skin sensitizers and nonsensitizers in accordance with the UN GHS.

Animal experiments can reproduce several features of *respiratory sensitization* in humans and related lung diseases for many of the metallic species mentioned in Section 4.4.4 on human evidence. However, the chronic and progressive nature of chronic beryllium disease in humans has been difficult to reproduce in animals (Jakubowski and Palczynski, 2015). Induction of respiratory sensitization in animals can occur via inhalation or dermal exposure. Respiratory sensitization mechanisms not only have some similarities with those for skin sensitization but also some differences. Respiratory sensitization usually favors Th2 response with induction of IL4, IL5, and IgE antibodies. Animal tests examining local lymph nodes after inhalation are used to some extent, but no validated in vitro tests are available (ECHA, 2017a,b).

Experiments in animals are the basis of *repeated dose toxicity*. Such experiments concerning general systemic toxicity include subacute, medium term, and chronic toxicity studies. OECD (www.oecd.org) provides detailed information on methods. Hazard evaluation uses a weight-of-evidence approach when identifying specific hazards from repeated dose toxicity studies. Although considerable efforts are made to find alternatives to animal testing, no validated in vitro systems are recognized at present for use in chemical safety assessments as replacements for repeated dose toxicity studies in animals. Correlations between changes in several parameters, e.g., between clinical or biochemical measurements, organ weights, and histopathological findings, are considered in the evaluation. Publications by ECHA (2017a) and the IPCS (2009) and WHO (2016) give further guidance. A project aiming at the development of in vitro methods to replace animal tests for repeated dose toxicity is "Safety Evaluation Ultimately Replacing Animal Testing" (SEURAT 1), conducted in Europe. It was finalized in 2016, and the results formed the basis for continuation of this important research in the EU–ToxRisk program.

The long-term toxicity of relatively low daily doses often is more important than acute toxicity for the overall risk and hazard assessment used for preventive action in the work environment and in the general environment because it determines the lowest acceptable long-term exposure. Thus, this assessment influences the acceptable exposure limits for protection of workers and the public from adverse effects from chemicals. Chapter 3 (Section 3.3.2; see also Chapter 5, Section 5.1.3) pointed out the crucial role of the critical effect in toxicological evaluations aiming at such protection. Because some effects are known to occur also at very low-level exposures (e.g., cancer, reproductive and developmental effects and immune–related effects including allergy), these effects are often identified as the critical effect. Identification of such effects is particularly important and is crucial in hazard identification and assessment. The foregoing paragraph considered dermal and respiratory sensitization. The following text will deal with systemic toxic effect such as reproductive and developmental effects and cancer.

Apostoli and Catalani (2015) reviewed mechanisms for induction of *reproductive and developmental effects* and reviewed available information in this field for metals and their compounds. As mentioned in Section 4.4.5, neurodevelopmental toxicity is the critical effect of both environmental lead exposure and environmental methylmercury exposure in humans. It is therefore very important to make an evaluation of such effects for new metallic compounds that are introduced and used for various purposes in society. According to the REACH and CLP regulations in EU, *reproductive toxicity* information must be provided (ECHA, 2017a,b). It is important to consider available information on genotoxicity, carcinogenicity, germ cell mutagenicity, and reproductive toxicity (CMR properties) before deciding whether any testing for reproductive toxicity potential is required. If, for example, data from the scientific literature can be used for CMR classification, testing is not necessary. Depending on the usage volume, more or less detailed tests are prescribed, for example, reproductive/developmental toxicity screening (see OECD). Validated in vitro tests replacing animal tests are not available, but complementary data can be provided, for example, in the form of in vitro embryotoxicity test and tests in vitro of estrogen receptor transactivation (see OECD).

4.5.2 In Vitro and In Vivo Data—Mutagenicity and Carcinogenicity

4.5.2.1 Mutagenicity

There is a testing strategy according to the REACH legislation for this adverse effect (ECHA, 2017a,b). Like the situation for other toxicological properties of chemicals, the requirements for data on mutagenicity are related to the amount of substance used or imported. Before in vivo testing, existing data has to be assembled and evaluated to see if criteria for CMR classification are already fulfilled based on such existing data. Mutagenicity is important for labeling according to the CLP regulation. According to ECHA (2017a), however, officially adopted methods are not available for estimating health risks associated with (low) exposures of humans to mutagens. In fact, most—if not all tests used today—are developed and applied to identify mutagenic properties of the substance, i.e., identification of the mutagenic hazard per se. In today's regulatory practice, the assessment of human health risks from exposure to mutagenic substances is covered by assessing and regulating the carcinogenic risks of these agents. The reason for this is that, according to ECHA, mutagenic events underlie these carcinogenic effects. Therefore, mutagenicity data are not used for deriving dose descriptors for risk assessment purposes. Mutagenicity information is thus used in combination with carcinogenicity for guidance according to REACH on how to assess the chemical safety for mutagenic substances. Laulicht et al. (2015) reviewed published data on cancer induction by metallic chemical species and Davidson et al. (2015) reviewed molecular mechanisms considered to be of importance in such cancer induction. It is of interest to note that the carcinogenicity of metallic compounds, with the exception of chromium compounds, is not considered related to genotoxicity or mutagenicity.

4.5.2.2 Carcinogenicity

The following sections of the present chapter reviews hazard identification for *carcinogenicity* according to IARC based mainly on in vivo and in vitro data. The foregoing Section 4.4.6 described the criteria for classification of a chemical as carcinogenic to humans (IARC Group 1). For such classification, human data are required.

4.5.2.2.1 International Agency for Research on Cancer Classification of Carcinogenicity—Groups 2 and 3

Classification of substances in Group 2 is done when, at one extreme, the degree of evidence of carcinogenicity in humans is almost sufficient, as well as, at the other extreme, when there are no human data but there is evidence of carcinogenicity in experimental animals. Agents are assigned to either Group 2A, "probably carcinogenic to humans," or Group 2B, "possibly carcinogenic to humans," based on epidemiological and experimental evidence of carcinogenicity and mechanistic and other relevant data. The terms *probably carcinogenic* and *possibly carcinogenic* describe different levels of evidence of human carcinogenicity and have no quantitative significance, with *probably carcinogenic* signifying a higher level of evidence than *possibly carcinogenic*.

IARC Group 2A—The Agent is Probably Carcinogenic to Humans: this is the usual classification when there is limited evidence of carcinogenicity in humans and sufficient evidence of carcinogenicity in experimental animals. In some cases, an agent is classified in this category when there is inadequate evidence of carcinogenicity in humans and sufficient evidence of carcinogenicity in experimental animals, with strong evidence that such carcinogenesis is mediated by a mechanism that also operates in humans. Exceptionally, an agent may be classified in this category solely on the basis of limited evidence of carcinogenicity in humans. An agent may be assigned to this category if it clearly belongs, based on mechanistic considerations, to a class of agents for which one or more members have been classified in Group 1 or Group 2A.

IARC Group 2B—The Agent is Possibly Carcinogenic to Humans: agents for which there is limited evidence of carcinogenicity in humans and less-than-sufficient evidence of carcinogenicity in experimental animals are assigned to this category. When there is inadequate evidence of carcinogenicity in humans but sufficient evidence of carcinogenicity in experimental animals, this classification category may also be used. In some instances, an agent for which there is inadequate evidence of carcinogenicity in humans and less-than-sufficient evidence of carcinogenicity in experimental animals may be placed in this group if there is supporting evidence from mechanistic and other relevant data. An agent may be classified in this category solely on the basis of strong evidence from mechanistic and other relevant data.

IARC Group 3: agents for which there is inadequate evidence in both humans and animals and in vitro are classified into Group 3, "not classifiable as to its carcinogenicity in humans," as stated in the preamble of the IARC monographs (IARC, 2006a,b, 2012, 2018). A discussion about the interpretation of long-term carcinogenicity assays and other methods for hazard classification of carcinogens is ongoing (see Boobis et al., 2016; Loomis et al., 2017). Loomis et al. (2017) pointed out the importance of taking into account available epidemiological evidence and evidence on mechanism of action when known. Section 4.6 gives a historical overview of carcinogenicity classification of metallic compounds including current classifications.

In addition to the classifications by IARC, other frequently cited carcinogenicity classifications are those made by authorities in the EU, USEPA, and American Conference of Industrial Hygienists (ACGIH) (see Section 4.7.3).

4.5.3 Computerized Systems Supporting Hazard Identification and Assessment

Computerized systems, also called in silico *methods*, are available for extrapolations of toxicological properties of chemical substances. Read–across systems estimate an unknown chemical or toxicological property from adjacent chemical substances in a chemical series. SARs (structure–activity relationships) allow estimates of the toxicological properties of a chemical compound with unknown toxicological properties from the known toxicity of other chemical compounds with similar chemical structure. For quantitative estimates based on structure similarities, the term *quantitative SAR* (or QSAR) is used. Fowler (2013) presented a number of methods including SAR and QSAR in a series of chapters on the use of computerized models in regulatory toxicology. In the implementation of REACH and CLP, ECHA recommends the use of SAR and QSAR as tools for estimating various properties of chemical substances. ECHA (2017a) lists a number of computational tools, for example, OECD QSAR toolbox that is freely available on the Internet.

Most frequently, analysis by the computerized systems allies to organic substances and only to a limited extent for inorganic metallic compounds. For many of the metals included in this book, all soluble inorganic compounds of the metal, for example, cadmium, are considered to have the same systemic toxicological properties because the toxicity is due to the metal ion formed when the compound is dissolved in water or biological fluids. This kind of simple "read across" extrapolation is widely used in this book. The following section summarizes some observations on the historical development of observations of carcinogenicity in humans and animals.

4.6 OBSERVATIONS OF CARCINOGENICITY OF METALLIC COMPOUNDS DURING 40 YEARS

Data from animal experiments are important in classification of carcinogenicity. Such evaluations have a history of more than 40 years. In 1980, an international workshop/conference (Belman and Nordberg, 1981) discussed the role of metals and their compounds in carcinogenesis. The scientists participating in this workshop were not able to reach any firm conclusions concerning the use of so-called *short-term* tests in predicting the carcinogenicity of chemical compounds. On the other hand, the meeting in 1980 concluded that results from lifetime studies on animals are predictive of probable carcinogenicity in humans, especially when the routes of exposure and sites of the tumors are the same. Joint WHO/IARC working groups that had met in 1977 and 1978 (see preamble of IARC volume 23; IARC, 1980) came to similar conclusions. IARC adopted these principles, and they are still widely used in their documents on carcinogenicity of chemicals for humans. The preamble to IARC's recent publications related to metallic and other compounds state that agents for which there is sufficient evidence of carcinogenicity in experimental animals also present a carcinogenic hazard to humans. In the absence of additional scientific information, IARC considers that such agents pose a carcinogenic hazard to humans (IARC, 2012, 2018).

Exposure to several metals/metalloids (arsenic, beryllium, cadmium, chromium, and nickel) are proven to be carcinogenic both in humans and animals. Chronological observations on the carcinogenicity of metallic compounds at the international meeting in 1980 (Belman and Nordberg, 1981) was the starting point, as depicted in Fig. 4.1. These chronological observations were made as judged by case reports, animal experiments, and epidemiological studies. This evaluation has been updated by us, and all metals/metalloids whose compounds are classified by the IARC as human carcinogens or probable human carcinogens (IARC, 2006a,b, 2010, 2012) are included (shown in Fig. 4.1). Data by Takenaka et al. (1983) and Pershagen et al. (1984) are used as a basis for the indication in Fig. 4.1, that there is good evidence in animals for carcinogenicity of trivalent inorganic arsenic. Before this evidence was available (1984) arsenic was considered as an exception from the rule that substances giving rise to cancer in humans also give rise to cancer in animals. The carcinogenicity of the first five metallic elements listed in Fig. 4.1 (As, Cr, Ni, Be, and Cd)

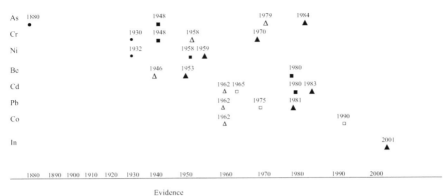

Figure 4.1 *Chronology of observation on carcinogenicity of metallic compounds.* At an international meeting in 1980 (Belman and Nordberg, 1981), the first five elements listed in the figure were judged as contributing to human cancer. The suspected metallic compounds are not listed in the figure but, as pointed out in the review, specific metallic compounds usually constitute the carcinogenic entity. Data by Takenaka et al. (1983) and Pershagen et al. (1984) have been added, providing evidence for carcinogenicity of As in animals. The carcinogenicity of these first five metallic elements and/or their compounds has been confirmed by the IARC (2012) and includes GaAs. Data on inorganic Pb compounds, Co with W-carbide, and In as InP were reviewed by the IARC (2006a,b); TiO$_2$ by IARC (2010); and welding, molybdenum trioxide (MoO$_3$) and indium tin oxide by IARC (in preparation) and Guha et al. (2017). Pb, Co with W-carbide, and InP are considered by the IARC to be probable human carcinogens (group 2A) and the respective metals are indicated in the figure; welding with UV radiation is carcinogenic (group 1), indium tin oxide (In$_2$O$_3$; SnO$_2$) is possibly carcinogenic to humans (2B). For other exposures to metallic compounds, which have been classified by IARC, see text, Section 4.6. *Updated and redrawn from Belman and Nordberg (1981).*

and/or their compounds has been confirmed by the IARC (2012) and includes GaAs. Data on inorganic Pb compounds, Co with W–carbide, and In as InP were reviewed by the IARC (2006a,b). Pb, Co with W-carbide, and InP are considered by the IARC to be probable human carcinogens (group 2A), and the respective metals are indicated in Fig. 4.1. TiO$_2$ was reviewed by IARC (2010); molybdenum trioxide (MoO$_3$) and indium tin oxide by IARC (2018) (Guha et al., 2017). According to the evaluations published by IARC, these agents are possibly carcinogenic to humans (2B). Antimony trioxide, indium tin oxide (In$_2$O$_3$; SnO$_2$), methylmercury compounds, titanium dioxide, vanadium pentoxide, molybdenum trioxide, and iron–dextran complex are also possible human carcinogens (Group 2B) but are not listed in the figure. Cisplatin, occupational exposure to welding fume with UV radiation, occupational exposure in iron and steel founding, and aluminum production are carcinogenic to humans (Group 1) but are not listed in Fig. 4.1. The reason why we have not listed these carcinogenic exposures is that, for cisplatin, exposure is almost entirely to patients in treatment for cancer; welding fume is a very complex mixture; and it is difficult to identify a single metal or a fixed set of metals responsible for the effect. In occupational exposures in iron and steel founding and in aluminum production, the suspected carcinogens are nonmetals and that is the reason why these exposures are not included in the figure.

It is important to be cautious when extrapolating data from nonhuman studies to humans, not only because of possible differences in metabolism and toxicokinetics among species but also because exposure situations will differ. Exposure doses that occur in real life are often lower than those used in animal experiments. Most animal studies use only single substance exposures and such studies do not reproduce the complex exposure situation that often occurs for humans. Furthermore, the number of animals exposed is usually small compared with the number of people who may be exposed, particularly when environmental exposures occur. The classical long-term animal tests did not include the very young, very old, and other risk groups, such as people with deficient or suboptimal nutritional intakes and people who already suffer from preexisting diseases. Some presently used testing protocols in animals include exposure from gestation (cf. OECD). At present, epidemiological studies, when available, and animal tests in combination with (limited) human data and complemented by information about toxicokinetics and mechanism of action (or MOA) in vitro, in animals and in humans, are the major information sources for risk assessment of metal compounds. As mentioned previously (Section 4.4.6), the IARC classification system for carcinogenicity in humans uses the specified principles for classification into Group 1 (carcinogenic in humans). As mentioned in Section 4.5, experimental data in animals and in vitro systems form the main basis for classification of exposures into Group 2 although epidemiological data are also required for classification in Group 2A (probably carcinogenic in humans). Agents for which there is inadequate evidence in both humans and animals and in vitro are classified into Group 3, "not classifiable as to its carcinogenicity in humans," as stated in the preamble of the IARC monographs (IARC, 2006a,b, 2012, 2018).

4.7 CARCINOGENICITY CLASSIFICATION BY NATIONAL/UNION AUTHORITIES AND BY OTHER ORGANIZATIONS

4.7.1 Carcinogenicity Classification in the European Union

Three agencies/committees in the EU publish classifications of carcinogenicity of chemical substances: ECHA, EFSA (European Food Safety Authority), and SCOEL (Scientific Committe on Occupational Exposure Levels). ECHA and EFSA often use the carcinogenicity classification according to REACH and CLP, described below as classification according to ECHA.

4.7.1.1 Classification According to SCOEL

SCOEL have their own classification system with classification in categories A—D. A are nonthreshold carcinogens, while B and C are genotoxic carcinogens without and with a threshold, respectively. Group D is for nongenotoxic carcinogens.

4.7.1.2 Carcinogenicity Classification According to ECHA (REACH and CLP Regulations)

Carcinogens are classified into one of two main categories based on strength of evidence and additional considerations. In certain instances, route-specific classification may be warranted if it can be conclusively proved that no other route of exposure can cause the hazard.

4.7.1.2.1 Category 1: Known or Presumed Human Carcinogens

Classification into Category 1 is based on epidemiological and/or animal data. A substance may be further distinguished as:

Category 1A, known to have carcinogenic potential for humans, classification is largely based on human evidence.

Category 1B, presumed to have carcinogenic potential for humans, classification is largely based on animal evidence.

The strength of evidence mainly determines classification into Category 1A and 1B.

Evidence considered human studies, establishing a causal relationship between exposure and the development of cancer (known human carcinogen), or animal experiments providing sufficient evidence of animal carcinogenicity (presumed human carcinogen). In addition, on a case-by-case basis, scientific judgment may warrant a decision of presumed human carcinogenicity derived from studies showing limited evidence of carcinogenicity in humans together with limited evidence of carcinogenicity in experimental animals.

4.7.1.2.2 Category 2: Suspected Human Carcinogens

When the evidence from humans, animals, and additional considerations is not sufficiently convincing to place the substance in Category 1A or 1B, the substance may be placed in Category 2 (suspected human carcinogen).

The evidence supporting placement into this category may be derived either from limited evidence of carcinogenicity in human studies or from limited evidence of carcinogenicity in animal studies. The ECHA (ECHA, 2017b) refers to the IARC (see Preamble to IARC Monographs, IARC, 2012, 2018) concerning what is considered limited and sufficient evidence for carcinogenicity. Further, ECHA points out the need for expert judgment in carcinogenicity classification.

4.7.2 Classification According to the USEPA (2017)

According to information available from USEPA (2017), the agency gradually (from 1996) shifted its methodology for carcinogenicity to the new 2005 guidelines. These new guidelines reflect EPA's accumulated experience and advances in our knowledge on cancer assessment. Assessments prepared under the 1986 guidelines continue to be valid. Therefore, the dose—response assessments of carcinogens reflect a mixture of the application of 1986 guidelines and the more recent guidelines.

4.7.2.1 Hazard Identification for Carcinogenic Effects (USEPA)

2005 (current) guidelines: EPA's guidelines recognize three broad categories of data: (1) human data (primarily epidemiological), (2) results of long-term experimental animal bioassays, and (3) supporting data, including a variety of short-term tests for genotoxicity and other relevant properties, pharmacokinetic and metabolic studies, and SARs. In hazard identification, the three categories of data are combined to characterize the weight of evidence regarding the agent's potential as a human carcinogen. The current, 2005 guidelines express the weight of evidence by narrative statements and express them separately for the oral and inhalation routes. The general categories recognized are:

- carcinogenic to humans
- likely to be carcinogenic to humans

- suggestive evidence of carcinogenic potential
- inadequate information to assess carcinogenic potential
- not likely to be carcinogenic to humans

    The 1986 guidelines use the following categories:

    Group A—carcinogenic to humans: agents with adequate human data to demonstrate the causal association of the agent with human cancer (typically epidemiologic data).

    Group B—probably carcinogenic to humans: agents with sufficient evidence (i.e., indicative of a causal relationship) from animal bioassay data, but with either limited human evidence (i.e., indicative of a possible causal relationship, but not exclusive of alternative explanations; Group B1) or little or no human data (Group B2).

    Group C—possibly carcinogenic to humans: agents with limited animal evidence and little or no human data.

    Group D—not classifiable as to human carcinogenicity: agents without adequate data either to support or refute human carcinogenicity.

    Group E—evidence of noncarcinogenicity for humans: agents that show no evidence for carcinogenicity in at least two adequate animal tests in different species or in both adequate epidemiologic and animal studies.

The current carcinogenicity classification by USEPA may be via the 1986 or the current guideline. A table gives this information for metallic compounds and other substances on the USEPA website. In the future, the table may also include excerpts of narrative weight of evidence and dose—response assessments for carcinogens. Since the publication of EPA's original cancer guidelines in 1986, new knowledge is available. The 2005 guidelines recognize both linear and nonlinear dose—response models. Nonlinear methods are to be used if there is sufficient evidence to support them. Chapter 5 further describes quantitative models for dose—response extrapolation of cancer effects.

4.7.3 Classification According to the American Conference of Governmental Industrial Hygienists

The American Conference of Government Industrial Hygienists (ACGIH, 2016) has different classifications based on the concept that MOAs, and dose—response relationships in animals have implications for human safety:

    A1—confirmed human carcinogen

    A2—suspected human carcinogen

    A3—animal carcinogen. The agent is not likely to cause cancer in humans except under uncommon routes or levels of exposure. The agent is carcinogenic in animals at a relatively high dose, by route(s) of administration, at site(s), histologic type(s), or by mechanism(s) that may not be relevant to worker exposure.

A4—not classifiable as a human carcinogen

A5—not suspected as a human carcinogen.

4.8 ETHICAL CONSIDERATIONS FOR STUDIES OF EFFECTS OF CHEMICAL COMPOUNDS WITH HUMANS OR ANIMALS

4.8.1 Studies With Humans

Information based on observations in humans is crucial in risk assessment of human exposures to metals and their compounds. Information in humans may come from a number of sources as mentioned in Section 4.4.1. Clinical observations of cases of poisoning is one example. Detailed clinical studies of a limited number of similarly exposed persons with a specific disease may result from toxicovigilance. Case studies, except in exceptional situations, cannot establish causality but can generate hypotheses for further studies.

If ethical considerations according to the Declaration of Helsinki (see below) are observed, experimental studies in human volunteers can be performed. Possible studies include the kinetics of metal compounds at low doses and studies of mild, reversible effects of low doses. For metals, however, there are few examples of the latter type. Epidemiological studies using a cohort or case—control approach (see Section 4.4.1) often provide useful information. Such analytical epidemiological studies can contribute to the establishment of causal connections between exposure and effect, after due consideration of possible influence of confounding and other weaknesses (see Section 4.4.2). Descriptive epidemiological studies, correlation studies, and ecological studies may provide a complement, but they are mainly hypothesis generating and cannot in themselves establish causality. Section 4.4.2 dealt with additional considerations in relation to causality in epidemiological studies.

Ethical considerations are of paramount importance when research involves human subjects. The appropriateness of a particular behavior can be evaluated by applying a set of generally acceptable governing principles (WHO, 2009). The most commonly identified principles in bioethics are:

1. individual autonomy (the ability to make decisions for oneself)
2. beneficence (the obligation to "do good" for others)

3. nonmaleficence (the obligation to avoid causing harm to others)
4. justice (the value of distributing benefits and burdens fairly).

These principles provide a general framework for analysis, which can then be applied to the facts of a particular ethical dilemma to reach a resolution. The WHO document (WHO, 2009) discusses these and other methods for ethical considerations of practical research questions.

The European Commission published a "European Textbook on Ethics in Research" (Hughes, 2010). The authors introduce the subject by descriptions of abuses of human subjects that have occurred in the past. The book discusses the value of research versus the justification of involving human subjects. It lists a number of reports and documents that are available in the area including the Helsinki declaration (see below) and the Oviedo convention on Human Rights and Biomedicine. The intention of this textbook is to introduce the subject to members of research ethics committees established in most European countries.

The Helsinki declaration: in 1964, the World Medical Association established recommendations guiding medical doctors in biomedical research involving human subjects. This "Declaration of Helsinki" governs international research ethics with human subjects. It was revised a number of times, with the latest in 2013. It is the basis for Good Clinical Practices used today.

The declaration of Helsinki first states general principles regarding how physicians should promote and safeguard the health of patients and those who participate in medical research and the importance to follow ethical, legal, and regulatory norms and standards. It further points out that when involving human subjects:

- Medically/scientifically qualified individuals with appropriate education in ethics should perform the research.
- The importance of the objective of the research must outweigh the risks to the research subjects.
- If risks turn out to outweigh benefits, physicians/investigators must assess whether to stop the study.
- Research with vulnerable groups is only justified if the research is responsive to the health needs of this group. This group should stand the benefits from the knowledge from the research.
- Research must be based on knowledge in the scientific literature, laboratory and as appropriate, animal experimentation.
- Design and performance of research must be described in a protocol including ethical considerations, funding and potential conflicts of interest.

- The research protocol must be submitted to and reviewed by an independent research ethics committee before the study begins. The researcher must provide monitoring information to the committee, especially about any serious adverse event, and submit a final report of the study's findings.
- Informed consent from research participants is necessary. Participants have the right to withdraw their consent at any time without reprisal.
- For research based on material contained in a biobank, physicians must seek informed consent for its collection, storage and use. In exceptional situations where consent would be impossible or impracticable to obtain, the research may be done after approval of a research ethics committee.
- The research project must be registered in a publicly accessible database before its start. Researchers have a duty to make publicly available the results of their research and to adhere to guidelines for ethical reporting.

Legislation applying the principles of the Helsinki declaration exists in many European countries, but only in relation to clinical trials, there is an EU Directive: European Clinical Trials Directive 2001/20/EC. In Sweden, the law on ethical review of research involving humans (SFS 2003:460) conforms to the rules in the Helsinki Declaration.

In the United States, there are multiple pieces of legislation at both the state and national levels. These are also administered by a number of agencies such as the National Institutes of Health (NIH) and the US Food and Drug Administration under the Department of Health and Human Services. A core set of regulations governing research on humans is embedded in the Code of Federal Regulations—Title 45 of the CFR part 46, which establishes rules governing institutional review boards (IRBs) at institutions conducting research on human subjects. For a more complete discussion of these rules and other related pieces of legislation see www.medschool.duke.edu, where the recent (January 25th 2018) NIH rules are included.

4.8.2 Studies With Animals

4.8.2.1 Rules in the European Union

The EU aims at a complete replacement of experiments on living animals by other research methods. At present, it is not yet possible to reach this goal. The European Directive 2010/63/EU on the protection of animals used for scientific purposes describes the rules for animal experiments in the Union.

In this EU Directive, "procedure" means any use, invasive or noninvasive, of an animal for experimental or other scientific purposes.

A "project" is a program of work having a defined scientific objective and including one or more procedures.

The Directive states the principle of replacement, restriction, and refinement of animal experiments (3R principle). Wherever possible, a scientifically satisfactory method or testing strategy, not entailing the use of live animals, shall be used instead of a procedure. The number of animals used in projects should be reduced to a minimum without compromising the objectives of the project. "Member States shall ensure refinement of breeding, accommodation and care and of methods used in procedures, eliminating or reducing to the minimum any possible pain, suffering, distress or lasting harm to the animals."

Subsequently, the Directive lists the recognized *purposes* of research: basic research; applied research for prevention; diagnosis or treatment of disease in humans, animals, or plants, as well as studies of physiological conditions and welfare in animals, safety of drugs, foodstuffs, and other substances or products and a few other types of research. Although, not mentioned in the Directive, it is notable that there is a ban on animal testing of cosmetic products in the EU according to EU regulation 1223/2009, fully implemented 2013.

The methods of killing animals shall ensure a minimum of pain. Special rules apply to the use of endangered species, nonhuman primates, and animals taken from the wild, and stray and feral animals of domestic species. The common species of animals used are animals bred for use in procedures.

Choice of methods: a procedure should not be used if another method for obtaining the result sought, not using animals, is recognized under the legislation of the Union. The procedure should be chosen, which uses the minimum number of animals, causes the least pain and suffering, and uses animals with the lowest capacity to experience pain.

Local or generalized anesthesia should be used except when it is judged to be more traumatic to the animal than the procedure itself.

All procedures are *classified* as "nonrecovery," "mild," "moderate," or "severe." Nonrecovery means that the procedure is performed on an animal in general anesthesia, and the animal is killed subsequent to the procedure without regaining consciousness.

There are rules for reuse of surviving animals and rehoming of domestic species.

A competent authority should authorize breeders, suppliers, and users of animals. They must have sufficient staff with adequate competence and a designated veterinarian with expertise in laboratory animal medicine.

They should set up an animal welfare body advising the staff on the welfare of the animals. They should keep records of relevant information such as the number and the species of animals bred, acquired, supplied, and used in procedures and the dates for procedures. There are rules for marking and information records for dogs, cats, and nonhuman primates. The care and accommodation of animals must be adequate. The competent authority should perform inspections to ensure that rules are followed. The commission shall undertake controls of the infrastructure and operation in the member states.

Project evaluation: the purpose of the project must justify the use of animals, and the project must comply with the 3R principle. The competent body takes a decision and communicates it to the applicant within 40 days after submission of a complete application. The competent body makes a retrospective assessment in certain cases. All projects using nonhuman primates and projects involving procedures classified as "severe" shall undergo a retrospective assessment.

Member states should publish *nontechnical summaries* of authorized projects. These summaries do not specify the names of users and personnel involved. Each member state shall set up a *National Committee for the Protection of Animals used for scientific purposes*.

There are rules for avoidance of duplication of procedures, and member states are required to accept data from other member states. The commission and the member states shall contribute to the development and validation of alternative approaches to procedures using animals. A Union Reference Laboratory has roles specified in an annex.

The EU member states are required to translate the rules in the EU Directive to national legislation. Here we take Sweden as an example. The Animal Welfare Act and the Swedish Board of Agriculture's Regulation and General Advice on Laboratory Animals (SJVFS 2015:24) are applicable. This legislation prescribes detailed rules for research with animals and for animal husbandry and authorization of experiments in accordance with the EU Directive (see above). The competent body authorizing animal experiments in Sweden is the regional Animal Ethics Committees. Decisions by the regional committees can be appealed to the central animal ethics committee at the Swedish Board of Agriculture (Jordbruksverket).

4.8.2.2 Rules in the United States

In the United States, the US Department of Agriculture (USDA) plays a central role in overseeing the ethical treatment of animals in research.

The USDA Animal Plant Health Inspection Service administers the Animal Welfare Act and the Horse Protection Act, which establishes rules for the ethical and humane treatment of animals in research. As with human subjects, institutions conducting research on animals must establish an approved IRB usually designated as an Institutional Animal Care and Use Committee to oversee animal research in that institution. For a more complete discussion regulations, please see www.aphis.usda.gov.

REFERENCES

ACGIH (American Conference of Governmental Industrial Hygienists), 2016. American Conference of Governmental Industrial Hygienists TLVs and BEIs. ACGIH, Cincinnati, OH.

Ahmed, S.S., et al., 2016. J. Appl. Toxicol. 36, 669.

Apostoli, P., Telisman, S., Sager, P., 2007. Reproductive and developmental toxicity of metals. In: Nordberg, G.F., et al. (Eds.), Handbook on the Tooxicology of Metals, third ed. Academic Press, Elsevier, pp. 214–250.

Apostoli, P., Catalani, S., 2015. Effects of metallic elements on reproduction and development. In: Nordberg, G.F., et al. (Eds.), Handbook on the Toxicology of Metals, fourth ed. Academic Press, Elsevier, Boston, Amsterdam, pp. 399–423.

Belman, S., Nordberg, G.F. (Eds.), 1981. Environ. Health Perspect. 40, 1.

Boobis, A.R., et al., 2008. Crit. Rev. Toxicol. 38, 87.

Boobis, A., et al., 2016. Regul. Toxicol. Pharmacol. 82, 158.

Davidson, T., Ke, Q., Costa, M., 2015. Selected molecular mechanisms of metal toxicity and carcinogenicity. In: Nordberg, G.F., Fowler, B.A., Nordberg, M. (Eds.), Handbook on the Toxicology of Metals, fourth ed., vol. 1. Academic Press, Elsevier, Amsterdam, Boston, pp. 173–196.

Dellarco, V.L., Baetcke, K., 2005. Toxicol. Sci. 86 (1), 1–3.

Descotes, J., Tesud, F., 2005. Toxicol. Appl. Pharmacol. 207, 599.

ECHA, 2017a. In: ECHA (Ed.), Guidance on Information Requirements and Chemical Safety Assessment Chapter R7b: Endpoint Specific Guidance. ECHA, Helsinki, Finland.

ECHA, 2017b. Guidance on the Application of the CLP Criteria, Version 5.0 ed. ECHA.

Fowler, B.A. (Ed.), 2013. Computational Toxicology: Applications for Risk Assessment. Elsevier, Amsterdam.

Grandjean, P., Budtz-Jorgensen, E., 2015. Epidemiological approaches to metal toxicology. In: Nordberg, G.F., Fowler, B.A., Nordberg, M. (Eds.), Handbook on the Toxicology of Metals, vol. 1. Academic Press, Elsevier, Amsterdam, Boston, pp. 265–279.

Guha, N., et al., 2017. Lancet Oncol. 18, 581.

Hill, A.B., 1965. Proc. R. Soc. Med. 58, 295–300.

Hughes, J., 2010. European Textbook on Ethics in Research. EUR24452EN (EU).

Hultman, P., Pollard, K.M., 2015. Immunotoxicology of metals. In: Nordberg, G.F., et al. (Eds.), Handbook on the Toxicology of Metals, fourth ed. Academic Press, Elsevier, Boston, Amsterdam, pp. 379–398.

IARC, 1980. Some Metals and Metallic Compounds. In: IARC Mongraphs, vol. 23. Lyon, France.

IARC, 2006a. Cobalt in Hard Metals and Cobalt Sulfate, Gallium Arsenide, Indium Phosphide and Vanadium Pentoxide. In: IARC Monographs on the Evaluation of Carcinogenic Risks to Humans, vol. 86. Lyon, France.

IARC, 2006b. Inorganic and Organic Lead Compounds. In: IARC Monographs, vol. 87. Lyon, France.

IARC, 2010. Carbon Black, Titanium Dioxide, and Talc. In: IARC Monographs, vol. 93. Lyon, France.

IARC, 2012. Arsenic, metals, fibres and dusts. In: IARC (Ed.), IARC Monographs, vol. 100C. IARC, Lyons, France.

IARC, 2018. Welding, Welding Fumes, and Some Related Chemicals. In: IARC Monographs, vol. 118. Lyon, France (in preparation).

IPCS, 2007. Elemental Speciation in Human Health Risk Assessment. EHC 234.

IPCS, 2009. Principles and Methods for the Risk Assessment of Chemicals in Food. World Health Organization, International Programme on Chemical Safety, Geneva. Environmental Health Criteria, 240.

Jakubowski, M., Palczynski, C., 2015. Beryllium. In: fourth ed.Nordberg, G.F., et al. (Eds.), Handbook on the Toxicology of Metals, pp. 635—666.

Jaworska, J., et al., 2013. J. Appl. Toxicol. 33, 1353.

Karlsson, H.L., Toprak, M.S., Fadeel, B., 2015. Toxicity of metal and metal oxide nanoparticles. In: Nordberg, G.F., Fowler, B.A., Nordberg, M. (Eds.), Handbook on the Toxicology of Metals, fourth ed. Academic Press, Elsevier, Amsterdam, Boston.

Landrigan, P., et al., 2007. Am. J. Ind. Med. 50, 709.

Laulicht, F., et al., 2015. Carcinogenicity of metal compounds. In: Nordberg, G.F., et al. (Eds.), Handbook on the Toxicology of Metals. Academic Press, Elsevier, Boston, Amsterdam, pp. 351—378.

Loomis, D., et al., 2017. Regul. Toxicol. Pharmacol. 88, 356.

Neutra, R.R., et al., 2018. Jurimetr. J. 58, 127.

Nordberg, G.F., Fowler, B.A., Nordberg, M., 2015. In: Handbook on the Toxicology of Metals, fourth ed. Academic Press, Elsevier, Amsterdam, Boston, New York.

OECD, 2012. Proposal for a Template and Guidance on Developing and Assessing the Completeness of Adverse Outcome Pathways.

OECD, 2017. Skin Sensitization Test 442E. www.oecd.org.

Pershagen, G., et al., 1984. Environ. Res. 34, 227.

Skerfving, S., Bergdahl, I.A., 2015. Lead. In: Nordberg, G.F., Fowler, B.A., Nordberg, M. (Eds.), Handbook on the Toxicology of Metals, vol. 2. Academic Press, Elsevier, Amsterdam, Boston, pp. 911—967.

Sonich-Mullin, C., et al., 2001. Regul. Toxicol. Pharmacol. 34 (2), 146—152.

Takenaka, S., et al., 1983. J. Natl. Cancer Inst. 70, 367.

UN, 2017. Globally Harmonized System of Classification and Labelling of Chemicals, seventh ed. UN, ECE, New York, Geneva. http://www.unece.org/trans/danger/publi/ghs/ghs_rev07/07files_e0.html#c61353

USEPA, March 2017. Risk Assessment for Carcinogenic Effects.

WHO, 2009. Research Ethics Committees Basic Concepts for Capacity Building.

WHO, 2016. Guidance Document for WHO Monographers and Reviewers. Available at: http://www.who.int/foodsafety/chem/jecfa/guidelines/en/.

Wittwehr, C., et al., 2017. Toxicol. Sci. 155 (2), 326—336.

Yokel, R.A., et al., 2006. Toxicol. Environ. Health Part B 9, 63.

Zeng, X., et al., 2004. Environ. Res. 96, 338.

CHAPTER FIVE

Dose—Effect and Dose—Response Assessment

Abstract

Dose—effect and dose—response assessments are important to the overall risk assessment process by providing a quantitative estimation of the relationship between dose/exposure and the occurrence of adverse effects from human exposure to metallic species. This chapter defines the concepts of dose—effect and dose—response relationships, discusses the importance of identifying the critical effect and estimates the critical concentration for toxicity in the critical organ. It further describes how to use these concepts in quantitation of the overall relationship between external exposure, internal exposure/dose, and the likelihood of occurrence of adverse effects in groups or populations. This chapter gives definitions of the no-observed-adverse-effect level, benchmark dose, and its lower confidence limit, which are important concepts in risk assessment. It further describes various approaches to estimate a low (acceptable) risk to humans, based on experimental and epidemiological data. The chapter gives special emphasis on quantitative estimation of dose—response relationships based on the mechanism of action and toxicokinetic and toxicodynamic modeling and describes results of such modeling in terms of dose—response curves. It includes discussions of the use of adverse outcome pathways.

5.1 CONCEPTS IN QUANTITATIVE TOXICOLOGICAL ANALYSIS

5.1.1 Dose—Effect and Dose—Response

Terminology to distinguish different dimensions of the relationship between dose/exposure and effect/response was introduced by the Task Group on Metal Toxicity (1976) (see also Task Group of Metal Interactions, 1978). Since its introduction, this terminology has been used in metal toxicology and sometimes even more widely. The term "effect" means a biological change caused by exposure to a toxic substance. Sometimes this effect can be measured on a graded scale of severity, although at other times, one may only be able to describe a qualitative effect. When data are available for a graded effect, one may establish a relationship between dose/exposure and the gradation of the effect in the population; this is

Risk Assessment for Human Metal Exposures
ISBN: 978-0-12-804227-4
https://doi.org/10.1016/B978-0-12-804227-4.00005-4

the *dose—effect* relationship. An example may be inhalation exposure to lead (Pb) by workers and the amount or concentration of δ-aminolevulinic acid (ALA) excreted in urine, an indicator of adverse changes in porphyrin metabolism (see Chapter 3). The term *response* is used to mean the proportion of a population that demonstrates a specific effect. Its correlation with estimations of dose/exposure provides the *dose—response* relationship. An example may be the relationship between different lead concentrations in industrial air and the percent of industrial workers with more than 5 mg/L of ALA in urine. Chapter 2 described the similar meaning of the terms *dose* and *exposure*. Although the presentation in this chapter mostly uses the term *dose*, it is good to remember the similarity with the term *exposure*. The International Union of Pure and Applied Chemistry (IUPAC) (Nordberg et al., 2004; Duffus et al., 2007, 2009) has recommended the following:

Dose—effect relationship: association between dose and the resulting magnitude of a continuously graded change, either in an individual or a population.

Dose—response relationship: association between dose and the (cumulative) incidence of a defined biological effect in an exposed population, usually expressed as percentage.

This terminology, clarifies the difference between these concepts. This chapter and other chapters of this book use this terminology. Because the words "effect" and "response" are synonyms in common language, this use of these terms is, however, not self-evident. In epidemiology, the terms "prevalence" and "incidence" are well established. One may consider a replacement of the term "dose—response" by more precise terms such as "dose—prevalence" and "dose—incidence." Prevalence means the number of existing cases of disease or persons with an adverse effect at a defined point in time. Incidence is the number of new cases occurring during a defined period. However, up to the present, such terms have not been much used outside the field of epidemiology; they are seldom used in toxicology. Therefore, the definitions of "dose—effect" and "dose—response," as traditionally used in metal toxicology (and by the IUPAC), will be used in this book because these concepts facilitate distinction between two dimensions of relationships. The dose—effect concept describes the relationship with the severity of effect, and the dose—response concept describes the distribution of a specific effect in the population. The use of these concepts supports clear descriptions and discussions on these relationships that are of great importance in risk assessment.

5.1.2 The S-Shaped or Sigmoid Curve

Dose—response data often display an S-shaped or sigmoid curve. For dose—effect relationships, similar curves may occur, but other shapes are also possible. The S-shaped curve in Fig. 5.1 describes dose—response in terms of percentage of an exposed group displaying an adverse effect in relation to dose/exposure. This is explained by the fact that the value on the response scale (%) includes the summation of all responders at dose levels up to and including that dose, i.e., a summation of the frequency distribution as shown in Fig. 5.1. Mofett et al. (2015) give further considerations concerning dose—effect and dose—response curves.

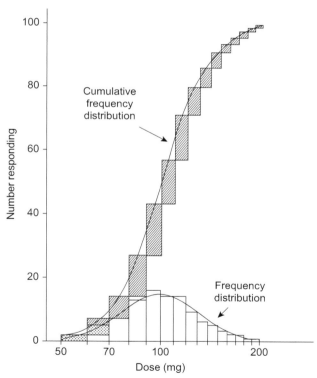

Figure 5.1 Relationship between dose (mg) and percent (0—100) response. The figure displays the frequency distribution curve showing percent responders in specific narrow dose intervals and the S-shaped (cumulative) percent response (number responding) in relation to dose (mg). *Reproduced with permission from McGraw Hill, Brunton et al., Goodman and Gilman's. The Pharmacological Basis of Therapeutics, twelveth edition, 2011.*

5.1.3 Critical Organ, Critical Concentration, Critical Effect, and No-Observed-Effect Level

A major issue in health effects evaluation is to identify adverse effects and to establish exposures or doses at which the adverse effects occur. At high doses, severe effects occur, even death of the exposed individual; low doses give rise to less-severe effects. Laboratory methods can sometimes detect effects at exposure levels without evident symptoms or signs of disease, i.e., subclinical effects. Such effects can still be adverse effects if they impair the function of organs or other physiological systems. In occupational and environmental health, this type of effect is of great importance because these professions deal with the prevention of adverse effects and the promotion of health for the population. Prevention of mild and early adverse effects automatically prevents more severe effects, which are pathophysiological consequences of the early effects. Mild and early adverse effects are in focus in these professions and such effects are fundamentally important in guiding the related risk assessments.

The *critical effect* is the effect used as a basis for setting exposure recommendations and for risk management. Depending on the exposure scenario, exposure duration can be short- or long-term. In short-term/acute exposures, there are often different adverse effects (acute toxic effects) than in long-term exposures. The critical effect, thus, often is a different one in acute/short-term exposures than in long-term exposures. The critical effect, particularly in long-term exposures, is often subclinical. The organ (or tissue), which suffers functional impairment in relation to the critical effect, is named the *critical organ*. In some instances, there is a direct relationship between the tissue concentration of a toxicant in an organ and the appearance of effects. The lowest tissue concentration giving rise to an effect in an organ of a particular individual is the *critical concentration* in that individual. The toxic effect that occurs at the lowest dose is the one that corresponds to the critical concentration in the critical organ (biomonitoring of metallic compounds in critical organs is discussed in Chapter 3). The concept of a critical concentration is applicable only to effects that occur at a specific threshold concentration in tissues/organs named *deterministic effects* or *threshold effects*. Appendix gives formal definitions (by the Task Group on Metal Toxicity or IUPAC) of the concepts mentioned.

Exposure of a group or population to a toxic agent with observation of several effects generates a set of dose—response curves, displayed in Fig. 5.2.

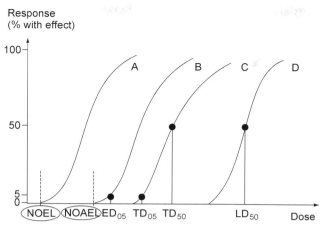

Figure 5.2 Spectrum of dose–response curves for deterministic (threshold-type) effects of a metal compound. No-observed-effect level (*NOEL*), no-observed-adverse-effect level (*NOAEL*), effect dose 5% (*ED$_{05}$*), toxic dose 5% (*TD$_{05}$*), toxic dose 50% (*TD$_{50}$*), and lethal dose 50% (*LD$_{50}$*) are indicated. *From Nordberg and Fowler (2015), with permission.*

Severe and lethal effects occur at high doses (curve D, Fig. 5.2). The median lethal dose (LD$_{50}$) is a well-known concept. In the past, animal experiments determining the dose–response curve for lethality were common, but such experiments are of very limited value in environmental and occupational health, and they should also be limited based on ethical considerations. At lower doses (curve C, Fig. 5.2), there will be toxic effects leading to disease. In the middle of curve C (Fig. 5.2), the median toxic dose (TD$_{50}$) is displayed for a specific toxic effect that may represent a clinical disease not leading to death. At slightly lower doses, TD$_{05}$ (the toxic dose for 5% of the exposed group) may be identified. Even lower doses (curve B, Fig. 5.2) may produce adverse functional changes without clinical effects identified by biomonitoring. When such subclinical changes are precursors to clinical disease, they are useful as critical effects. The part of this curve representing relatively low doses and low response levels (e.g., the level when 5% of the exposed group displays this effect, i.e., the effect dose for 5% [ED$_{05}$]) is of interest in occupational and environmental health. At lower doses, when there are no observable adverse (critical) effects, the no–observed–adverse–effect level (NOAEL) is reached (Fig. 5.2). The curves in Fig. 5.2 are the result of observations in specific dose groups forming the curve. The NOAEL is the highest dose level at which a group of individuals have been exposed without any statistically significant adverse effects being demonstrated. At even lower doses (curve A, Fig. 5.2), there may be a dose—response curve describing slight, but statistically significant, changes in enzymes for which there is a high reserve capacity; a small decrease does not imply any decrease in organ function—so called *subcritical effects*. Doses below this curve, at which no effects whatsoever occur represent the no-observed-effect level (NOEL), which is the highest dose without effects (Fig. 5.2). The European Chemicals Agency (ECHA) uses the term *no-adverse-effect level* (or NAEL) instead of NOAEL. The concept used by ECHA is "dose descriptor," i.e., NAEL is a "dose descriptor" when implementing the Registration, Evaluation, Authorisation and Restriction of Chemicals (REACH) regulation (see further Chapter 7). The *derived no-effect level* (DNEL) corresponds approximately to the NOEL (ECHA, 2012). A Gaussian distribution in sensitivity among persons making up the group studied explains the S-shaped dose—response curves for threshold type effects (Fig. 5.2). Fig. 5.1 displays the relationship between this Gaussian frequency distribution and the cumulative dose—response curve. Dose—response curves of this classical shape occur in healthy laboratory animals exposed to various doses of a single toxicant. Exposure to more than one chemical agent modifies these curves (see Chapter 6 about mixed exposures). In Fig. 5.2, the dose—response curves are roughly parallel and relatively steep; they represent well-defined adverse effects in terms of clinical disease or adverse functional changes such as inhibition of a specific enzyme. Effects resulting from more complex, multitarget events display dose—response curves that may be shallower, thus extending over a larger range of doses and down to very low dose levels. Such effects are similar to stochastic/nonthreshold effects (see Section 5.2.2). It is of particular importance in preventive medicine, to identify mild and early effects. Prevention of such effects may result in prevention also of later, perhaps more severe effects, particularly when the early effects are precursors of the later more severe effects. Published discussions are available for dose—response relationships and the *critical concentrations*, *critical organs*, and *critical effects* for human exposures to the metals mercury, lead, and cadmium and their compounds (Nordberg, 1992; Task Group on Metal Accumulation, 1973; Task Group on Metal Interactions, 1978; Task Group on Metal Toxicity, 1976, Nordberg et al., 2018, Chapter 8). Some of these concepts are mainly applicable to deterministic/threshold-type effect, but the critical effect concept may also be used when stochastic/nonthreshold effects are considered. These concepts are further described and examples given of their use by Friberg and Kjellstrom

(1981), Kjellstrom et al. (1984), Nordberg (1992), WHO/IPCS (1992), Järup et al. (1998), and Nordberg et al., 2018, and definitions are given by the IUPAC (Duffus et al., 2007, see also Appendix).

When a random interaction of the metal compound with DNA occurs or when a series of events such as in multistage carcinogenesis constitutes the background for the effect, such effects are *stochastic effects* or *nonthreshold effects*. Assumptions are common that such effects display a linear component of the dose—response curve at low doses (see further discussion in Section 5.2.2). Cancer and some reproductive and developmental effects belong to this category of effects (Section 5.2.2).

5.1.4 The Lower Confidence Limit of the Benchmark Dose

In toxicology and risk assessment, the concept of benchmark dose in its original form (BMD_{or}) was introduced by Crump (1984) as the statistical lower confidence limit on the dose producing a predetermined level of change in adverse response (the benchmark response [BMR]) compared with the response in untreated animals. Using this concept instead of the NOAEL in risk assessment has several advantages, because this concept considers the variance in observations in a more systematic way. When there is a larger number of observations and less variance, BMD_{or} values are higher, and data sets with more variance generate lower BMD_{or} values for the same BMR. The BMD_{or} approach thus makes more use of available data and provides more safety.

A different definition by Gaylor et al. (1998) of the benchmark dose (BMD_{Ga}), stated that the benchmark dose (BMD) is the point estimate of the dose corresponding to a specified low level of risk. For example, the dose giving rise to a 10% increase in adverse response BMD-10_{Ga} is the same point in the dose—response curve as ED-10 or TD-10 (see Section 5.1.2) or PCC-10 (see Section 5.1.4). These authors suggested the use of the lower confidence limit (LBMD) of the BMD_{Ga} instead of a NOAEL in risk assessments. The LBMD (lower confidence limit of BMD) as defined by Gaylor et al. is the same concept as the lower confidence limit of the BMD (BMDL) used by the USEPA (United States Environmental Protection Agency) (2017a) and identical to the original BMD_{or}, BMD in the form originally defined by Crump (1984). The benchmark concept as it was originally defined by Crump (BMD_{or}) was promoted by the IUPAC (see Duffus et al., 2007, 2009, 2017). The different definitions of BMD are not always noted, but it is important to be aware of them. It is interesting to note that Crump, in his more recent publications, has changed his terminology to the one used by USEPA (see, for example, Crump, 2002).

WHO/IPCS (2009) and USEPA (2017a) describe mathematical models for use in dose—response modeling and the calculation of BMD and BMDL. Software for calculating BMD and BMDL are available from USEPA (2017a). Publications presenting calculations of the BMD and BMDL often use the mentioned methods. The present book uses the terminology by USEPA and WHO/IPCS (2009). The software available from USEPA provides various mathematical models. They differ in some details from those used by Gaylor et al. (1998). When reporting BMD and BMDL values, it is important to indicate which definition of BMD is used and to specify the exact mathematical models that are applied. The first use of the BMD concept was with dose—response data in experimental animals. The available information on the background response is an important consideration when calculating the BMD/BMDL. If the "control" group is small with a large variance, it will cause difficulties when calculating BMDL regardless of whether experimental data in animals or epidemiological data are considered. Sand et al. (2003) advanced the "hybrid" approach and extrapolation of epidemiological data to the zero dose in order to overcome some of these problems. Metals, however, are elements, always present in a variable level in the earth's crust, and zero exposure is not possible. The issues of causality and confounding factors are important considerations in animal experiments, and they are even more important in epidemiology (see Section 5.4.2). Such considerations are important when calculating the BMD and BMDL based on epidemiological data. Recent studies show that diuresis can be a confounding factor for tubular effects of cadmium. Creatinine-adjusted urinary cadmium excretion introduces an error and influences dose—response relationships of cadmium-induced low-molecular-mass proteinuria (Akerstrom et al., 2014; Chaumont et al., 2013; Nordberg et al., 2018, Chapter 8, Section 8.3). Interactions are also important. An example is renal dysfunction in population groups exposed to cadmium in China. The BMDL for Cd was considerably lower in the presence of concomitant exposure to arsenic than in the absence of such exposure (Jin et al., 2004; Hong et al., 2004; Nordberg et al., 2005; Chapter 6 on mixed exposures). Probabilistic risk assessment approaches can take into account variability within exposed populations; this is a further refinement to these statistical methods. The BMD based on dose—response relationships, discussed in the foregoing text, is a point on the dose scale. The dose—response relationship, as defined in this book, uses so-called *quantal data* and such use of the BMD concept is common. Conversion of dose—effect data (continuous data) to dose—response data can have advantages, for example, in order to use observations considered "abnormal" from a clinical chemistry point of view—usually those deviating by more than two times the standard deviation from the mean among healthy persons. For cadmium, adverse long-term health outcomes in terms of low-molecular-mass proteinuria (β2-microglobulin) occur in relation to biomarkers of exposure in population groups (see Chapter 8, Section 8.3), and the BMD and BMDL are meaningful points in the dose scale that can be used for risk assessment.

Sand et al., 2003 and WHO/IPCS, 2009 provided models to extend the BMD concept for use with dose—effect data (continuous data). They discussed the use of data obtained in epidemiological studies and emphasized the importance of confounder adjustment (Budtz-Jørgensen et al., 2001; Crump, 1995, 2002; Grandjean and Budtz-Jorgensen, 2015; Kalliomaa et al., 1998). BMD calculations based on dose—effect are useful in risk assessments, but it is important to define the implications in terms of health risk. Both dose—effect and dose—response models are sometimes combined in a hybrid approach (WHO/IPCS, 2009; Sand et al., 2003). It is important to specify whether dose—response (quantal or dichotomous) data or dose—effect data (continuous data) are used when presenting BMD and BMDL values in risk assessments, for example, in risk assessment of the adverse effects of cadmium in general population groups (Suwazono et al., 2010; Akesson et al., 2014). BMD based on dose—response should specify the BMR. Methods used to define the magnitude of effect are of interest when considering dose—effect data. Grandjean and Budtz Jorgensen (2015) pointed out that measurement imprecision in the dose scale (e.g., in epidemiological studies) will also affect the BMD and BMDL. When taking all the considerations discussed in this section into account, then BMD/BMDL calculations are very useful and provide numbers that can be efficiently utilized in risk assessments.

5.1.5 Population Critical Concentration

The Task Group on Metal Toxicity (1976), like IUPAC (Duffus et al., 2007, 2017, see also Appendix), defined the critical concentration on an individual basis as it varies among individuals. The dose—response relationship expressing the occurrence of a particular effect as a function of metal concentration in the critical organ thus displays the frequency distribution of individual critical concentrations. A single critical concentration for a group of individuals thus does not exist even for a specified effect. Presentation of such misleading information sometimes appears and causes problems. Friberg and Kjellstrom (1981) therefore suggested the introduction of a *population critical concentration* (PCC) instead of an unspecified *critical concentration* when assessing data based on a population. To the PCC should be appended a number indicating the response rate expected at this PCC: PCC-50 would be the concentration in the critical organ at which 50% of a population has the critical effect and PCC-20 is the concentration at which 20% has the critical effect and thus has exceeded their individual critical concentrations. The PCC concept is similar to the use of LD_{50} and ED_{50} in toxicology and is similar to the presently most-often-used BMD concept (see Section 5.1.3).

Decisions of importance in risk assessment and risk management of chemicals often concerns maximum acceptable response rate for a given effect based on risk estimation. If 5% is the maximum, then PCC-5 has to be established. If 0.1% is the maximum, then it is important to establish PCC-0.1 with sufficient precision. Exposure standards are often required, and it is therefore necessary to define the exposure that gives rise to 5% response. To arrive at this exposure, the impact of interindividual parameters has to be taken into consideration. Variations in metabolism/toxicokinetics and sensitivity to a toxic substance will be parameters of importance. High fractional absorption, unfavorable interactions with other substances, high retention, and low excretion together with high tissue sensitivity within the critical organ may favor an effect even at low exposure levels. Knowledge of the PCC in combination with toxicokinetic (TK) information makes it possible to estimate exposure levels related to a specific risk of an adverse effect. The proportion of a population with concentrations above the critical concentration is equal to the probability of adverse effect in that population. For cadmium, this proportion has been estimated by Kjellstrom (1985a,b), Järup et al. (1998), and Nordberg et al., 2018 (see also Chapter 8, Section 8.3). Jin et al. (2004) estimated the PCC in terms of urinary cadmium (UCd; a biomarker of the Cd level in the kidney cortex) related to adverse kidney effects in terms of PCCUCd-05 (i.e., PCC of urinary cadmium for 5% of the studied group). These authors also reported the lower confidence limit of this value (i.e., LPCCUCd-05), which is identical to the BMDL-05 in the *benchmark dose* terminology (see Section 5.1.3).

The combined impact of distributions of exposure, toxicokinetics, metabolism, and effects are discussed in Chapters 2, 3, and 8, as well as in papers by Nordberg and Strangert (1976, 1978, 1985), Kjellstrom (1985b), Sakurai et al. (1982), Järup et al. (1998), Diamond et al. (2003), Ruiz et al. (2010), and Nordberg et al. (2018) and in Chapter 8.

5.2 ESTIMATING ACCEPTABLE OR RECOMMENDED EXPOSURE LEVELS IN HUMANS BASED ON DOSE—RESPONSE STUDIES IN ANIMALS

Good data from epidemiological studies in humans are available only for a limited number of metals and their compounds (see Section 5.4). For other metals and their compounds, mainly data from studies in animals and in vitro systems are available. This section describes the use of data from animal experiments and combined studies in humans and animals for quantitative risk analysis to arrive at recommended safe exposures for humans.

5.2.1 Threshold-Type Critical Effects

This section summarizes a set of principles used for chemical substances giving rise to threshold-type (deterministic) critical effects. For substances with genotoxic or carcinogenic effects or other nonthreshold effects, Section 5.2.2 gives a summary of relevant principles.

There is a long tradition in food toxicology (see IPCS, 2009) of using animal data as a basis for recommended acceptable daily human intakes (ADIs) of food additives. The FAO/WHO have traditionally based their recommendations on long-term and chronic toxicity studies in animals and have derived NOAEL from such data. In previous assessments, NOAEL was the point of departure (POD) for deriving intake recommendations.

Since 2000, these organizations sometimes used the BMDL as the POD for the derivation of health-based guidance values such as ADI. The usual procedure is to divide the NOAEL in animals by a safety factor of 100 in order to arrive at an ADI. This method was widely used in the past; it has lately been developed by the use of additional data, when available (see later). In principle, the method is applicable also for metals and their compounds, but only few metals or their compounds have been used as food additives, the most common one being iron. An ADI or recommended daily allowance (RDA) for iron used human data as a basis for assessment (see Chapter 6 on essential metals and interactions).

For contaminants in food and metal compounds occurring in food and drinking water as natural components of the environment, the FAO/WHO sets a provisional tolerable weekly intake (PTWI) or monthly intake (PTMI). Sometimes the organizations recommend a provisional tolerable daily intake (see IPCS, 2009). They use similar evaluation principles as for ADI when establishing these recommendations. Instead of using a safety factor of 100, the margin of exposure (MOE), also named margin of safety

(MOS) may be used. This is a comparison between the POD and the actual or estimated human exposure. Acceptable safety corresponds to an MOE of 100 or more, meaning that the estimated human exposure is 100 times lower than the NOAEL or BMDL in animals. The method used to arrive at an ADI (or PTWI, i.e., dividing the NOAEL in animals by 100) is only applicable for substances that are not carcinogenic. For stochastic effects like carcinogenesis and other nonthreshold effects, the FAO/WHO recommend linear extrapolation to low doses and risks (see Section 5.2.2). The safety factor (or uncertainty factor [UF] or assessment factor) of 100 consists of a factor of 10 to account for extrapolation from animals to humans and another factor of 10 to account for variability in the human population. Using safety factors does not allow the incorporation of actual data on toxicokinetics and toxicodynamics into the evaluation, even if such data are available in animals and in humans. Renwick (1993) and WHO/IPCS (1999; see also IPCS, 2009) suggested that (in the absence of actual data) the safety factor (UF or assessment factor) of 10 for interspecies differences can be subdivided into two factors: a factor of 4 for interspecies differences in toxicokinetics and another factor of 2.5 representing interspecies differences in toxicodynamics. The factor of 10 for variability in the human population can be subdivided into a factor of 3.2 for variability in toxicodynamics and another factor of 3.2 for variability in toxicokinetics (Table 5.1).

Table 5.1 shows default factors based on experience that there are considerable differences between animals and humans concerning the toxicity of metallic compounds as well as other substances. Differences are due to a combination of differences in tissue sensitivity to a particular substance (i.e., a toxicodynamic difference) in combination with differences in toxicokinetics and metabolism. Instead of the factor indicated in Table 5.1 for extrapolation between animals and humans, the ECHA uses assessment factors modified for different animal species by allometric scaling. According to ECHA (2012), for doses given to various animal species, the interspecies assessment factor varies and is 4×2.5 for rats, 7×2.5 for mice, and 4×1.4

Table 5.1 Default factors in risk assessment[a]

Interspecies = 10	Interindividual = 10
TK = 4; TD = 2.5	TK = 3.2; TD = 3.2

TD, toxicodynamics; TK, toxicokinetics.
[a]According to WHO/IPCS (1999).

for dogs. If inhaled concentration of a toxicant is considered, no allometric scaling is required because the inhaled volume of air (respiratory rate and volume) is proportional to the metabolic rate of various animal species.

Certain types of toxic effects are difficult to detect in general tests in animals, for example, neuropsychiatric disorders. Many specific and specialized tests are available, and it is important to look for adequate animal models when there is reason to suspect effects, not picked up by conventional tests.

The following text gives a few examples of differences influencing risk extrapolation between animals and humans. The default factors (Table 5.1) are intended to compensate for such differences when they are unknown. When we know these differences and can quantitatively estimate them, they can form a basis for chemical-specific assessment adjustment factors (see below, this section). The organic compound methylmercury is very toxic to humans. It is highly stable, has a long half-life, and accumulates in the human body as methylmercury. In rats, methylmercury is much more readily transformed into inorganic mercury than in humans, it has a shorter half-life and the effects are less severe (Chapter 8). Rats, therefore, tolerate higher doses per kilogram body weight compared to humans. Methylation of arsenic occurs to a considerable degree in humans as well as in many animal species. The trivalent monomethylarsenic acid [MMA(III)] is a highly toxic species that may play a role in arsenic-induced carcinogenesis. In the marmoset monkey, however, there seems to be no methylation at all (Chapter 8). Another monkey, the rhesus monkey, seems to be more resistant than humans and other animal species to cadmium-induced kidney dysfunction (Chapter 8). When there are such known differences between humans and animals and an adequate animal model exists for extrapolation to humans, it is, of course, important to use such a model to obtain data relevant for humans.

Extrapolation from animals to humans is improved if the specific observed differences in toxicokinetics can be used in the extrapolation, i.e., the chemical-specific assessment factor (CSAF; this is the same as the adjustment factor used by the WHO/IPCS). It is the case, however, that in many instances such differences are unknown and extrapolation has to rely on the default factors (e.g., those listed in Table 5.1). Chapter 8 summarizes data on selected individual metals. There are only few examples of the use of default factors in deriving recommended safe levels of exposure for humans. Instead, metals-specific information is available or the use of some metals is so limited that no recommendations are considered necessary. When human epidemiological data are available, an evaluation of the adequacy of the "factor" method is possible by comparison with actual human dose—response data observed for the metal species in question. An attractive and useful alternative to the use of safety factors (UFs, assessment factors, or CSAF) is the calculation of risks based on estimates of variability in toxicokinetics and toxicodynamics in humans. Section 5.3 describes probabilistic approaches to calculating risks for adverse effects based on such actual data and estimates.

5.2.2 Carcinogenesis and Other Stochastic/Nonthreshold Effects

The International Agency for Research on Cancer (IARC, Chapter 4; IARC, 2006a,b; 2012, 2017) publishes hazard assessments focusing on the weight of evidence for carcinogenicity. Although the preface of the most recent publications states that consideration of quantitative dose—response information is possible if there are adequate epidemiologic data (IARC, 2017), currently available IARC publications present no quantitative risk estimation. Other scientific bodies have long since developed quantitative estimations of cancer risks to humans based on combined animal and (limited) human data. The International Commission for Radiological Protection (ICRP) has a long history of successful estimations of importance for health protection in the field of radiation protection. The ICRP rules for protection against the carcinogenic effects of ionizing radiation (ICRP, 1977, 2016) assume that thresholds do not exist and that any exposure involves an increased risk.

For the carcinogenic effects of chemical substances, including metals, this philosophy has been adopted in many quarters. Several international symposia discussed the dose—response curve for carcinogenic substances. The one held by the Task Group on Air Pollution and Cancer (1978) was one of the earliest. Conclusions stated "in considering protection of human populations, and in the absence of firm evidence to the contrary, it is not justified to assume a 'threshold,' i.e., that there is a dose below which no response is obtained." The Task Group also considered that "in the absence of relevant dose—response data, the most appropriate way to estimate the risk of lung cancer is to assume that it will be directly proportional to the increase in dose. For small added doses, a simple linear dose—response curve, as used in radiation carcinogenesis, is appropriate." Thus, this Task Group, like several other scientific bodies, adopted the same philosophy as that long used in radiation protection, namely that thresholds do not exist and that any exposure may involve some risk. Similarities with ionizing radiation were considered as best founded in regard to (ultimate) carcinogens (i.e., not requiring metabolic activation) acting on directly exposed tissues. Cancer risks from ionizing radiation were initially modeled based on these principles. Later, the models were applied to chemicals that are relatively freely distributed among human tissues such as acrylamide. Published estimates are based on extrapolations from animal experiments to humans (e.g., Törnkvist et al., 2008), as well as direct risk estimates for humans. Similar extrapolations and calculations may be possible for some metals and metalloids. For extrapolation of cancer risks from high to low doses, a number of mathematical models have been proposed. These are discussed by Moffett et al., (2015) and by an Interdisciplinary Panel on Carcinogenicity (1984) and the WHO/IPCS (1999); see also USEPA (2017b). The dose—response models are quantitatively similar to one another at statistical response rates of 10%—100%, but yield substantially different estimates at lower response rates, where estimates may differ by orders of magnitude (see Fig. 5.3).

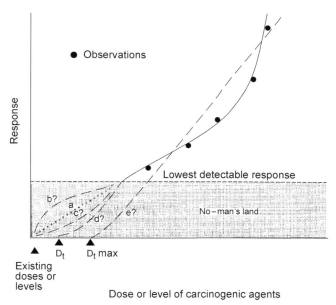

Figure 5.3 Illustration of traditional detection limits for epidemiological and experimental observations of cancer incidence (mortality) as a function of dose (exposure level) of a carcinogenic agent. Lower detection limits are, at present (2017), sometimes achieved in epidemiological studies (see Figure 5.4). "Response" indicates the response caused by the agent (i.e., the difference between incidence in exposed groups and incidence in the control group). For discussion of curves "a," "b," "c," and "d" and "e," see text. D_t, threshold dose. *Modified from the Swedish Governmental Cancer Committee, 1984. Cancer, Causes, Prevention. SOU 1984:64 (In Swedish with English Summary). Ministry of Health and Social Affairs, Stockholm.*

Epidemiological and experimental data from traditionally relatively small observation groups, including certain genetic data, led to the conclusion that a linear extrapolation to low doses in "no man's land" was best in agreement with available mechanistic knowledge for initiators. Even today, experimental observations, as well as epidemiological data, are often based on doses that are much higher than those considered as acceptable exposure levels. There- fore, there is a need for a rationale in support of extrapolation to low dose/ exposure levels. The situation is further complicated by the fact that observa- tions are often within an area of relatively high doses, and it is impossible to draw statistically valid conclusions concerning dose—response relationships at low doses. Fig. 5.3 illustrates this situation. A linear extrapolation according to curve "a" would lead to underestimation or overestimation of the risk if curve "b" or "c," respectively, was true. Exposures within the dose interval that occur in practice would wrongly be considered "dangerous" if the true relationship showed a threshold dose (Dt) according to curve "d" or "e."

Epidemiological studies in the 2010s included large population groups exposed to inorganic arsenic in drinking water (see also Chapter 8, Section 8.2). Chen et al. (2010) performed a prospective cohort study providing a basis for estimates of risks for bladder cancer in the range 0.2%—5%, as will be discussed in Section 5.4.4 (Fig. 5.6). Although in the very low dose range <1 μg/kg body weight per day, uncertainties still exist, these actual observations in the low dose and incidence range support the notion that dose—response curves for cancer extend into the low-dose range in a nearly linear manner. As shown in Fig. 5.6, this seems to be the case for inorganic arsenic exposure through drinking water, and it is probable that the situation may be similar for many other agents. The dose—response curve for bladder cancer described in Section 5.4.4 (Fig. 5.6) is most similar to curve "a" in Fig. 5.3.

There is reason to believe that for cancer promoters, a certain exposure (dose in target organs) is necessary for an effect to develop at all. Under such circumstances, a linear extrapolation from high to low doses may lead to overestimation of risks. Models based on initiation, promotion, and, when available, toxicokinetics have been presented (WHO/IPCS, 1999; Moffett et al., 2015). Regulatory agencies in countries around the world use such models to a variable extent for the extrapolation of observed relationships to specific response levels such as the 5% or 1% level. Below this level, a linear dose—response extrapolation is often used for further extrapolation into the low-dose range to establish regulations or recommendations of acceptable exposures.

In the United States, the EPA (USEPA, 2018) uses the "unit risk estimate" for inhalation and the "carcinogenic potency slope" for ingestion. The unit risk estimate represents the upper-bound excess lifetime cancer risk estimated to result from continuous exposure to an agent over a lifetime at a concentration of 1 $\mu g/m^3$ in air. The carcinogenicity potency slope is upper bound, usually approximating a 95% confidence limit, on the increased cancer risk from a lifetime oral exposure to an agent. This estimate, usually expressed in units of proportion (of a population) affected per mg/kg/day, is used in the low-dose region, i.e., corresponding to risks less than 1 in 100. These estimates are plausible upper-bound estimates of the risk (i.e., the actual risk is likely to be lower).

The linear dose—response relationship is often used for cancer, but it may also be considered for other effects. An example is the neurodevelopmental toxicity of lead (Skerfving and Bergdahl, 2015) or methylmercury (see Chapter 8, Section 8.9), giving rise to an impact on the intelligence quotient (IQ) in children. Such effects occur even at very low exposures. For lead, such effects occur in the most sensitive subsection of the population at exposures corresponding to a blood lead level of 0.25 $\mu mol/L$ (50 $\mu g/L$) and even lower in some studies. In the general population of industrialized countries such blood lead levels were common in the past and may still occur in limited subpopulations today. The linear dose—response relationship means that one may apply the concept of collective dose in risk assessment. This concept thus is applicable to carcinogenic substances that are persistent in the environment and that—as may be the case for metals—are ultimate carcinogens. It may also be applicable for other effects mentioned in the foregoing text. The collective dose is defined as the product of the average dose given to an individual in a defined exposure group and the number of individuals in that group (ICRP, 1977). The unit risk concept developed by the USEPA (2017b) is based on a linear extrapolation of observational data (see also Chapter 7).

5.3 DOSE—RESPONSE RELATIONSHIPS BASED ON MECHANISM OF ACTION, TOXICOKINETIC AND TOXICODYNAMIC MODELING, AND ADVERSE OUTCOME PATHWAYS

Local effects often occur at high-dose exposure in the skin after dermal exposure, mucous membranes in the oral cavity or gastrointestinal tract after oral intake, or the respiratory tract after inhalation. Such effects reflect a direct corrosive action. They usually are of the threshold type and can be prevented by avoiding the high exposures required for their elicitation. Other types of local effects are those occurring after sensitization, i.e., allergic reactions to metallic compounds causing dermatitis, eczema, gastrointestinal effects, and asthma. Nickel and chromium metals and their compounds are examples of metallic species with sensitizing properties. Chapter 3, Section 3.4.3, describes events of importance for the development of allergic contact dermatitis from such sensitizing agents. The information is structured in the form of an adverse outcome pathway (AOP; Chapter 3, Section 3.4.3).

When the mechanism of action is known for a *systemic toxic effect* caused by a metallic substance, and when relevant biomarkers of exposure and response are available, conditions are very favorable for defining safe exposure levels. An example of such circumstances is the induction of anemia by lead exposure described in Chapter 3 and below (Section 5.3.1.1).

When the mode of action is not known in detail, but when the levels of toxicant giving rise to impaired organ function are known or possible to estimate, dose—response relationships can be estimated. Nordberg and Strangert (1978) advanced methods, using estimated variability in toxicokinetics and toxicodynamics as a basis for risk estimation and estimation of the uncertainty in risk estimates. These models were later developed by the inclusion of mathematical simulation and consideration of the physiologically based TK models described in detail in Chapter 2. Models are available based on our knowledge of the particle size and solubility of metals or metal compounds that occur as air pollutants in particle form, their deposition in the lungs can be predicted and their uptake modeled. For metals taken up through the gastrointestinal tract, general knowledge about mechanisms are not so well developed, and observational data are required to estimate uptake into the blood. The same is true for transport and distribution to various organs in the body and for excretion (see Chapters 2 and 8). The transformation of metal ions into a bound state (e.g., DMT-1, MT for Cd) or oxidation/reduction reactions (e.g., Cr, Hg) influences their distribution and toxicity.

5.3.1 Systemic Effects that are Deterministic/Threshold-Type Effects

When a sufficiently high concentration is reached in the cells of the critical organ, some metal compounds (or species) elicit systemic effects with tissue damage/adverse changes in organ function. Such effects occur at a critical concentration determined by the sensitivity of the target molecules and the status of defense systems in a particular individual. *Threshold effects* is another term used to characterize such deterministic effects because there is a threshold concentration for each individual in the group or population. Organ sensitivity varies among individuals within a population. For example, adverse effects caused by cadmium in the kidney cortex is determined by sensitivity and the binding of Cd to target molecules in the renal cell membranes on one hand and the binding of Cd to intracellular metallothionein and other antioxidant defense systems on the other (see discussion below and cadmium section in Chapter 8). A relationship between tissue levels and occurrence of adverse effect can be established by the simultaneous measurement of (1) metal concentration in a critical organ either directly or indirectly through biomarkers and (2) of the occurrence of the adverse effects in a large number of individuals in a population.

When mathematical models of the toxicokinetics and toxicodynamics of the metal compound can be obtained, calculations of expected dose—response relationships can be performed (see subsequent Sections 5.3.2 and 5.3.3.)

5.3.1.1 Dose—Response Relationships Based on Known Mechanism of Action And/Or Observations in Humans

An example of an adverse effect, for which the mechanism of action is known, is lead-induced anemia. Dose—response relationships, based on observations in humans of biomarkers, reflecting this known mechanism of action, provide a very reliable basis for preventive action (see Fowler, 2016). Unfortunately, information on the mechanism of action in humans is available only for a few adverse effects of metallic substances. Chapter 3 described the mechanism of action for lead in causing anemia. Lead interferes with specific enzymes in the heme synthesis pathway. Table 3.1 of Chapter 3 describes dose—effect and dose—response relationships, i.e., lead levels in blood (Pb-B) and related changes in the heme synthesis pathway. Mild/early effects such as ALAD (delta-aminolevulinic acid dehydratase) inhibition in erythrocytes occur among 5% of an exposed group of persons at 0.14 μmol/L of Pb-B. Other more severe changes in the heme synthesis pathway occur at higher Pb-B levels and clinical anemia occurs at >3.5 μmol/L.

When there are limited data on humans, but an understanding of threshold-type relationships from animal data, rough estimates of relationships between tissue concentrations and the occurrence of effects can be obtained. In such situations, data are often limited to a small number of persons (e.g., workers) who have suffered the adverse effect because of high exposure. Experience from such calculations, performed more than 30 years ago for cadmium (Kjellstrom, 1985b; Friberg et al., 1986), can now be evaluated in relation to epidemiological data from exposed groups in the general population (Nordberg et al., 2018, Chapter 8, Section 8.3). There is relatively good agreement with epidemiological data, but the variance of critical concentration in the kidney cortex, as estimated from studies carried out in the 1970s and 1980s based on data from small groups of exposed workers, has turned out to be somewhat smaller than the variation observed in later epidemiological studies of the general population. The reason is that workers are a more homogenous group than the general population. The estimated PCC (e.g., PCC10) was adequate for workers but gave a somewhat higher than actual value for the general population.

Further understanding of the toxicokinetics of a metal compound (species) and a further developed quantitative TK model can be established. Concentrations in critical organs and tissues can be calculated for various exposure scenarios, as described in Chapter 2. Toxicodynamics describe the mechanisms of action of toxicants, how they can cause tissue damage, and under what conditions in terms of tissue concentrations and time of tissue exposure/dose that adverse effects on tissue structure and function occur. Calculations based on updated information complemented by Monte-Carlo simulated variation for cadmium will be described in the following Section 5.3.3. Similar models may be used in AOP approaches of risk assessment (see Section 5.3.4).

5.3.2 Toxicokinetic-Toxicodynamic Modeling of Dose—Response or Dose—Effect Relationships Based on the One-Compartment Model

The one-compartment model for elimination of a chemical substance from the body and/or a specific organ is described in Chapter 2. This model is the basis of the concept of biological half-life. The ICRP successfully used the one-compartment model for estimating body tissue radiation doses that are used to recommend maximum permissible exposure levels for radiation protection (ICRP, 1968, 1971, 1979, 1982). Radiation protection calculations by ICRP used a "standard man". This "standard man" and "reference man" were specified by the ICRP (1975). Interindividual variations in intake, absorption, distribution, and excretion may greatly influence metal accumulation in critical organs and are therefore important for correct predictions (Nordberg and Strangert, 1985). Systematic changes in organ weight and daily intake should be considered when estimating accumulation. Kjellstrom and Nordberg (1978, 1985) considered such factors in calculations regarding cadmium accumulation in the kidney. Also the Task Group on Reference Man (ICRP, 1975) and Choudhury et al. (2001) used such information. Age-dependent changes in organ composition and function need be taken into account when they are important to the modeling process. An example is provided by renal changes, identified as important in modeling the kinetics of cadmium (Kjellström and Nordberg, 1978; Travis and Haddock, 1980; Choudhury et al., 2001). Berglund et al. (1971) used the one-compartment model successfully for calculations of accumulation of methylmercury in the central nervous system and estimated dose–effect relationships of the neurological effects of this toxic mercury compound. This model was further used to calculate the variable brain and body burdens of methylmercury expected to occur as a result of different biological half-lives for methylmercury among persons exposed in the 1970s in Iraq. As explained in Chapter 2 and shown in that chapter in Figure 2.7 (from Shahristani and Shihab, 1974), half-lives were estimated to vary from 30 to 120 days. Other observations in persons exposed to methylmercury in Iraq showed that there was a large variation in the body burden, giving rise to clinical symptoms of poisoning among these persons.

Fig. 5.4 (from Bakir et al., 1973) shows the relationship between body burden and the percentage of persons displaying various symptoms. Curves are presented for relatively mild symptoms like paresthesia and more severe neurological symptoms as well as for lethal outcomes. Based on this information, Nordberg and Strangert (1976) calculated the risk of poisoning in adults in relation to the long-term daily intake of methylmercury (see Fig. 5.5), i.e., when a steady-state maximum body burden is reached. The lower part of the curve in Fig. 5.5 can be compared with clinical and epidemiological observations of the daily intake related to poisoning. Although information is limited, a reasonable fit seems to exist.

Recently, Rand et al. (2016) reported results from studies of the half-lives of methylmercury in human volunteers consuming considerably lower doses of methylmercury than the doses of this chemical compound that was consumed by the poisoning cases in Iraq. They found shorter half-lives (average 44 days, range 28–62 days). The reason for the different half-lives is not known—technical differences in measurement methodology or dose-related differences are possible.

Nordberg and Strangert (1978, 1985) developed and further discussed the principles of risk estimation by the use of interindividual variation of

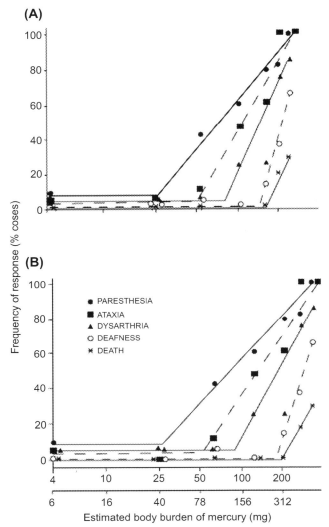

Figure 5.4 The relationship between frequency of signs and symptoms and the estimated body burden of mercury (A) at the time of onset of symptoms and (B) at the
time of cessation of ingestion of methylmercury in bread. Both scales on the abscissa
are for body burden of methylmercury and were calculated in different ways as
described by Bakir et al. (1973). For the top scale, use was made of the observed relationship between the blood mercury concentration and the ingested dose. The bottom
scale was estimated from the relationship between the blood mercury concentration
and the ingested dose, as reported by Miettinen (1972).

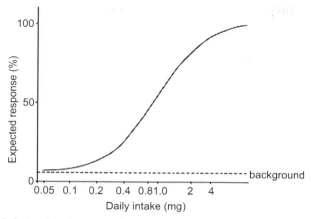

Figure 5.5 Relationship between long-term intake of methylmercury and risk of poisoning in adult persons. Based on information concerning interindividual variation in biological half-time and interindividual sensitivity to development of neurological effects (see text). *From Nordberg, G.F., Strangert, P., 1976. Effects and dose—response relationships of toxic metals. In: Nordberg, G.F. (Ed.), Elsevier, Amsterdam, pp. 273—282.*

toxicokinetics and toxicodynamics, i.e., organ sensitivity parameters. While these principles of dose—response estimation remain valid, epidemiological studies published more recently (cf. Chapter 8, Section 8.9) demonstrated that the critical effect of methylmercury is the induction of neurodevelopmental changes in the fetus of pregnant women. Epidemiological studies of dose—response relationships for this effect are available (see Berlin et al., 2015; Grandjean and Budtz-Jorgensen, 2015 and Chapter 8, Section 8.9). However, for the neurodevelopmental effects, toxicokinetic-toxicodynamic (TKTD) modeling is not available for comparison with the epidemiological findings.

5.3.3 Quantitative Toxicokinetic-Toxicodynamic Modeling of Systemic Effects Based on Multicompartment and Physiologically Based Kinetic Models

The foregoing section described toxicokinetic-toxicodynamic (TKTD) modeling with quantitative estimations of expected dose—response relationships for systemic effects of metallic toxicants using the one-compartment model. This section will deal with similar calculations using multicompartment and physiologically based models. Nordberg and Strangert (1985) published an early contribution to this field, using a multicompartment model for cadmium (Kjellstrom and Nordberg, 1978, described in detail in Chapter 2). Also, Thun et al. (1991) used the Kjellström–Nordberg model in calculations of airborne occupational exposures expected to give rise to kidney dysfunction after 45 years of exposure. Their calculations predicted that such long-term exposures at cadmium concentrations of 5–10 $\mu g/m^3$ in workroom air would cause such effects in a small proportion of workers. Choudhury et al. (2001) further developed the Kjellstrom– Nordberg model of cadmium kinetics by inclusion of Monte-Carlo simulation and other improvements mentioned in Chapter 2 (Section 2.6.2.1). Ruiz et al. (2010) used similar improvements and compared Berkeley Madonna model-generated urinary excretion estimations with measured urinary excretion data from the National Health and Nutrition Examination Survey (NHANES) data set of the general US population. Good concordance was observed between the model-generated and NHANES laboratory analytical data. Fransson et al. (2014) presented an updated version of the Kjellstrom–Nordberg model considering the data on kidney cadmium published by Akerstrom et al. (2013).

Diamond et al. (2003) used the modified model according to Choudhury et al. (2001) to calculate the long-term intake, giving rise to a kidney cortex concentration of 84 mg/kg. This value in the kidney cortex corresponds to the lower confidence level of a 10% response in terms of low-molecular-mass proteinuria—i.e. the lower confidence limit of PCC-10—in the US population (estimated by Diamond et al., 2003). At higher cadmium values in the kidney cortex, a higher proportion of the population will display changes in the excretion of such low-molecular-mass urinary proteins indicating tubular kidney dysfunction.

The urinary cadmium level and the daily long-term intake level corresponding to 84 mg/kg in the kidney cortex was calculated (Diamond et al., 2003; Nordberg et al., 2018) as 1.4 nmol/nmol creatinine (urinary Cd) and a long-term dietary intake of 1 $\mu g/kg$ body weight in women (2.2 $\mu g/kg$ body weight in men). Long-term intakes were calculated for 55 years (from birth). These estimates fit fairly well with the lowest observed adverse effect observed in epidemiological studies in the form of low-molecular-mass proteinuria. The cadmium section of Chapter 8, gives further description and discussion of these comparisons.

Chapter 2, Section 2.6.2, reviewed a number of multicompartment and physiologically based models. Several of these models, for example, multicompartment (e.g., the integrated exposure uptake biokinetic model) and physiologically based models developed by O'Flaherty (1993,1995), O'Flaherty et al. (2001) have been used to assist in risk assessment of metal exposures in humans, but published estimates of expected dose—response relationships are not available.

5.3.4 Adverse Outcome Pathways

An evolving area of risk assessment is the incorporation of basic molecular information on the mechanisms (mode of action) by which metals produce cell injury/cell death into the risk assessment process. This frequently involves measurement of molecular biomarkers which reflect deleterious effects. As pointed out in Chapter 3, AOPs describe existing linkage between molecular initiating events and adverse outcomes at a biological level of organization that is relevant to risk assessment. Important events are those playing central roles in cellular toxicity or cancer development (Fowler, 2016; Jennings, 2013; OECD, 2012; Vinken, 2013). The value of incorporating these tools into a risk assessment paradigm is that they may provide a direct linkage between exposure and effect in the target cell population when matched with chemical measurements of the metal or chemical of interest in the same cell population or organ. This information can hence greatly improve the precision of dose—response estimations and help provide adequate risk assessment for a given health outcome such as target organ toxicity or cancer. This information may be of particular value for risk assessments of sensitive subpopulations at special risk of toxicity.

Discussions at a symposium held in 2015 (Wittwehr et al., 2017) considered that the systematic organization of knowledge into AOP frameworks can inform and help direct the design and development of computational prediction models that can further enhance the utility of mechanistic and in silico data for chemical safety assessment. This publication (Wittwehr et al., 2017) suggested semiquantitative TKTD models described in Chapter 3, Section 3.4.3 and Chapter 4, Section 4.5.1 of predicted semiquantitative risks for skin sensitization based on in vitro testing of chemicals.

An example of an AOP is the detailed description of the molecular mechanisms for nickel-induced allergic dermatitis given in Chapter 3, Section 3.4.3. OECD (2012) and Vinken (2013) described an AOP for nickel-induced allergic contact dematitis that involves two components. One component termed "induction" is linked to the entrance of nickel into the skin and generation of haptens via binding with proteins in the skin cells. This process is designated the molecular initiating event (MIE). The haptenized proteins, in turn, generate an inflammatory response termed "elicitation component" as they are recognized and "remembered" by

T-lymphocytes of the cellular immune system as being foreign in nature. Subsequent exposure activates the elicitation response resulting in clinical dermatitis as the adverse outcome event. In principle, this AOP should provide a basis for prediction of the occurrence of the adverse outcome (dermatitis) in sensitized persons when they are subject to exposure at various levels in terms of dermal exposures. However, we, the authors of this book, have not been able to find any published quantitative predictions of expected outcomes. It would be of great interest if such predictive calculations could be presented so that a judgment can be made concerning the precision of such predictions based on comparisons with actual dose—response data observed in humans (see Section 5.4 and Chapter 8, Section 8.10).

Although a detailed description of the AOP for allergic nickel dermatitis is available, its use as a predictive tool in quantitative risk modeling and risk assessment is unclear. Preventive action for nickel is based on epidemiological observation of exposure and response (please see Chapters 3, 4, and 8 and OECD, 2012 for a more complete discussion).

5.3.5 Stochastic or Nonthreshold Effects

Although not widely applied, TKTD modeling is also useful for modeling dose—response relationships in carcinogenesis. When combined with an understanding of the mechanisms of action and quantitative relationships between tissue levels of carcinogenic metals and the appearance of tumors, such models should be of great value in risk assessment. Unfortunately, such data are not widely available. It is hoped that these methods may be used on a wider scale in the future. For metals, examples of such calculations in risk assessment are not currently available, but they have been used for other classes of chemical compounds (WHO/IPCS, 1999).

5.4 DOSE—RESPONSE ASSESSMENT BASED ON EPIDEMIOLOGICAL STUDIES

5.4.1 Local effects

Effects that occur as a result of direct corrosive action of the metallic compound on tissues exposed at the site of exposure or intake, i.e., the skin for dermal exposure, the oral cavity and the gastrointestinal tract for oral intake, and the respiratory tract for exposure by inhalation, invariably occur at high doses. Local effects that occur after sensitization may occur at very much lower doses and may be critical effects in environmental exposures.

5.4.1.1 Nickel

Patch tests detect *sensitization to nickel*. Menné (1994) summarized dose—response relationships in terms of exposure levels in patch tests and skin reactions in humans. He concluded that trace amounts of nickel present in the general environment do not induce nickel sensitization. Elicitation of nickel dermatitis is unlikely for concentrations $<0.1-1$ $\mu g/cm^2$ in contact with skin during occluded exposure and 15 $\mu g/cm^2$ when nonoccluded. He suggested a nonsensitizing nickel concentration of 0.5 $\mu g/cm^2/week$ for consumer items made of nickel alloys (see also Chapter 8, Section 8.10.6.1). Denmark implemented legislation to limit the dermal exposure to nickel in 1992, i.e., earlier than in the European Union as a whole. Jensen et al. (2002) found that the odds ratio for nickel sensitization was 3.34 ($P = .004$) for girls who had their ears pierced before 1992 when compared to girls without ear piercing. For girls who had their ears pierced after 1992, there was no statistically significant difference in comparison with girls without ear piercing.

5.4.2 Systemic, Noncarcinogenic Effects

Because of long-term interest and many studies performed during many years, there is presently a wide recognition of the adverse systemic effects of arsenic, cadmium, lead, manganese, mercury, and their compounds. A considerable amount of epidemiological data are available on human health effects. Chapter 4 discussed causality in epidemiological studies; such considerations are very important in quantitative risk assessment. It is a fundamental requirement to be reasonably sure that relationships are causal before a quantitative assessment is made. Sometimes, human data are available only on a limited number of exposed persons (e.g., in some occupational studies), and it may not be possible to calculate the BMDL. It may still be possible to estimate the NOAEL for use in risk assessment. Early application of the principles of TKTD modeling used limited observations in humans as a basis for calculating predicted risk levels and for estimation of the NOAEL. In the past, such calculations formed the basis for estimates of acceptable exposures before epidemiological data were available (Berglund et al., 1971, Chapter 8, Section 8.9). Recently published lower confidence limits of BMD levels, i.e., BMDL estimates, are based on epidemiological data with a larger number of observations. Chapter 8, section on cadmium, presents published calculations for exposures to cadmium. When using the reported numbers, consideration of possible confounding factors is important. Chapter 8, section on cadmium, describes recently identified problems with confounding by creatinine correction of urinary cadmium values when describing the dose—response relationship between urinary cadmium and low-molecular-mass proteinuria, an established adverse effect of cadmium exposure. Comparisons of the results of TKTD modeling with epidemiological findings provide perspectives on the causality of reported statistical associations. When there is no confounding or effect modification, or when such modifications are compensated, BMDL values are useful in risk assessment and risk management.

When identifying the critical effect, to be used in risk assessment, one must consider the effect in the most sensitive subsection of the population (e.g., the fetus of the pregnant mother when the exposure causes adverse effects on the fetus). Methylmercury is a metallic compound causing neurodevelopmental effects, and these effects are recognized as critical effects (see Chapter 8, Section 8.9). This effect results from a complex pattern of events (see Lucchini et al., 2015 "Neurotoxicity of Metals"). The dose—response curve for an impact on IQ in children born by mothers exposed to methylmercury extends to very low doses (see Chapter 8, Section 8.9).

5.4.3 Adverse Outcome Pathways and Identification of Sensitive Subpopulations at Risk

5.4.3.1 Genetic Variation in the Binding of Lead to ALA-Dehydratase and Susceptibility to Lead-Induced Hypertension

ALA-dehydratase (ALAD) is the primary binding protein for lead in blood (Skerfving and Bergdahl, 2015) and exists as two alleles (ALAD 1 and ALAD2) which vary in their affinity for this element (Scinicariello et al., 2010) and influence susceptibility to lead-induced hypertension as the adverse outcome measure on a genetic basis (Scinicariello et al., 2007). The binding of lead to the ALAD alleles is the MIE, which is controlled by genetic variation in the affinity of the ALAD alleles for lead, in turn regulates the bioavailability of lead to produce hypertension as the adverse outcome clinical measure (Scinicariello et al., 2007, 2010). This AOP is of clearly major importance for improving risk assessments by more precisely relating lead exposure levels to a major human health endpoint and helping to identify which individuals in the general population are at the greatest risk for lead-induced hypertension based upon genetic inheritance.

5.4.4 Carcinogenic Effects

Section 5.2.2 discussed how to estimate a safe level of exposure to a carcinogenic metal compound. The definition of such a level usually involves extrapolation from higher to lower exposures. It is still true that such extrapolation is necessary for many compounds even if current epidemiological studies of sufficient size can detect incidence in terms of 1/1000 in some studies. However, even modern epidemiological studies are unable to demonstrate such low response levels that are aimed at as acceptable in the general environment (i.e., lower than 1:100,000 in a lifetime). Observations on cancer outcome in exposed groups in epidemiological studies still are of great value as a starting point for extrapolations to low–risk values in quantitative risk assessment. A good example of a useful epidemiological study involving a metal/metalloid is the studies of relationships between exposure to inorganic arsenic in drinking water (see Fig. 5.6 and Chapter 8, Section 8.2). Fig. 5.6 displays a near–linear dose—response curve for bladder cancer extending down to low exposure levels in terms of intake of inorganic arsenic. In recent years, an increasing number of epidemiological observations have been reported on skin, lung, bladder, kidney, and other cancer types among subpopulation groups in a number of countries exposed to elevated levels of arsenic in drinking water. Dose—response relationships for these effects are also available (Chapter 8, Section 8.2). There are widespread arsenic exposures in drinking water in some parts of

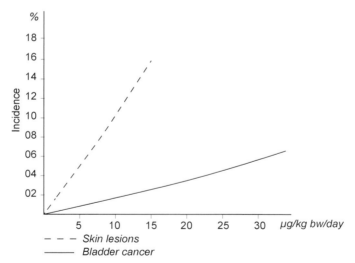

Figure 5.6 Incidence of skin lesions (*dotted line*) and bladder cancer (*unbroken line*) in relation to exposure to arsenic in drinking water. Incidence (above-background incidence) of skin lesions (keratosis and melanosis) per 9 years of exposure is estimated from Argos et al. (2011). Incidence of bladder cancer in life-long exposure is estimated from data by Chen et al. (2010), modeled by Carrington et al. (2013), and with background incidence subtracted. *From Nordberg and Fowler (2015).*

the world and millions of people are exposed. It is difficult, on a practical basis, to achieve full population protection at levels considered desirable for carcinogens in general (see earlier), but this is an ongoing and important discussion.

5.4.5 Newer Approaches to Risk Assessment and Developments for the Future

Modern biology and analytical chemistry coupled with advances in computer modeling are increasingly used as tools to address a variety of issues related to risk assessment (see Fowler, 2013). Ruiz et al. (2010) and Ruiz and Fowler (2015) used computer modeling of analytical data (from NHANES) on cadmium exposures in the US population and identified specific gender and age sections of the population with higher uptakes relative to other groups. The inclusion of molecular biomarkers of exposure and effect into future risk assessments will only strengthen mechanistic linkages between exposures at low dose levels and adverse health effects (see Fowler, 2016 for further discussion).

The NexGen program conducted in the United States (USEPA, 2014) developed several new types of high- and medium-throughput assessments. Based on the findings in that program, a number of such assessment methods are being advanced for application in the future: (1) tens of thousands of chemicals will be analyzed using quantitative structure—activity modeling/ relationships and by using rapid in vitro bioassays (e.g., ToxCast and Tox21 programs). (2) Thousands of chemicals will be evaluated using computer-driven analyses of the published literature and information stored in massive databases in order to develop new knowledge about the potential toxicity of chemicals and the causes of disease. (3) Hundreds of chemicals will be evaluated using a variety of new methods, including approaches to understand the effects of multiple chemical and nonchemical stressors. These modern approaches most probably will contribute to the enhancement of the scientific validity of future risk assessments.

In toxicology, there are increasing efforts to limit the use of laboratory animals and increase the use of human-based cell culture methods. Ethical considerations for studies in humans and animals were given in Chapter 4, Section 4.8. Considerable resources have been devoted to the development of in vitro systems during the last decades. *In vitro* assays for high-throughput screening allow the screening of entire libraries of potential toxicants for cellular changes. High-content analysis in the field of toxicogenomics permits broad genomic analyses. Such systems in combination with novel bioinformatics tools have a potential to process generated data and make them more widely applicable to safety evaluations. While the presently most widely employed animal-free risk and hazard assessment methods involve the use of chemical structures for read-across from well-characterized compounds to information-poor compounds, in vitro testing has mainly been used to support such assessments. New omics-based methods may contribute new data and be more widely applicable to hazard and risk assessment with relevance for humans in the future (Grafstrom et al., 2015).

As a result of the workshop organized by the European Commission's Joint Research Centre "AOP-informed predictive modeling approaches for regulatory toxicology", 2015 (Wittwehr et al., 2017), examples were put forward of AOP models for a number of adverse effects. A proposal was made for actively engaging the modeling community in AOP-informed computational model development. There is certainly a need to facilitate the development of computational prediction models to support the next generation of chemical safety assessment for humans, but it is of crucial importance when developing such programs, to combine mathe-matical skills with a profound knowledge of human biology, physiology, and toxicology.

A number of recent advances to improve risk assessments for metals make use of evolving approaches in toxicology and molecular biology. These approaches incorporate modern tools of molecular and computational biology that have the potential to develop more sensitive and accurate risk assessments for metals on an individual or mixture exposure basis. There is a need to integrate the new methods with established TKTD modeling to create adequate AOPs that accurately reproduce toxicity in human tissues. Validation studies, which link the modern approaches and understanding of initial molecular events to the onset of clinical outcomes are now essential to permit complete acceptance of tools for risk assessment practice. The human relevance framework described in Chapter 3 and comparisons between findings in epidemiological studies with results generated by appli-cation of AOPs may provide useful tools for such validation studies.

REFERENCES

Akerstrom, M., et al., 2013. Environ. Health Perspect. 121, 187.
Akerstrom, M., et al., 2014. J. Expo. Sci. Environ. Epidemiol. 24, 171.
Akesson, A., et al., 2014. Environ. Health Perspect. 122, 431.
Argos, M., et al., 2011. Am. J. Epidemiol. 174, 185.
Bakir, F., et al., 1973. Science 181, 230.
Berglund, F., et al., 1971. Expert group on methyl mercury in fish. Nord. Hyg. Tidskr. (Suppl. 4)

Berlin, M., Zalups, R.K., Fowler, B.A., 2015. Mercury. In: Nordberg, G.F., et al. (Eds.), Handbook on the Toxicology of Metals. Academic Press/Elsevier, Amsterdam, Boston (Chapter 46).

Budtz-Jørgensen, E., et al., 2001. Biometrics 57, 698.

Carrington, C.D., Murray, C., Tao, S., 2013. A Quantitative Assessment of Inorganic Arsenic in Apple Juice. US Food and Drug Administration. http://www.fda.gov.

Chaumont, A., et al., 2013. Environ. Health Perspect. 121, 1047.

Chen, C.L., et al., 2010. Cancer Epidemiol. Biomarkers Prev. 19, 101.

Choudhury, H., et al., 2001. J. Toxicol. Environ. Health 63, 321.

Crump, K., 1984. Fundam. Appl. Toxicol 4, 854.

Crump, K., 1995. Risk Anal. 15, 79.

Crump, K., 2002. Crit. Rev. Toxicol. 32, 133.

Diamond, G.L., et al., 2003. J. Toxicol. Environ. Health 66, 2141.

Duffus, J.H., et al., 2007. Pure Appl. Chem. 79, 1153.

Duffus, J.H., Templeton, D.M., Nordberg, M., 2009. IUPAC. Concepts in Toxicology. RSC Publishing, Cambridge, p. 179.

Duffus, J.H., Templeton, D.M., Schwenk, M., 2017. Comprehensive Glossary of Terms Used in Toxicology. RSC Publishing.

ECHA, 2012. Guidance on Information Requirements and Chemical Safety Assessment. Chapter R8: Characterization of Dose (Concentration)-response for Human Health. version 2.1. http://echa.europa.eu/documents/10162/13579/rac_carcinogenicity_dose_response_as_en.pdf.

EPA, 2017. US Environmental Protection Agency. www.epa.gov.

Fowler, B.A. (Ed.), 2013. Computational Toxicology: Applications for Risk Assessment. Elsevier Publishers, Amsterdam, p. 258.

Fowler, B.A., 2016. Molecular Biological Markers for Toxicology and Risk Assessment. Elsevier Publishers, Amsterdam, p. 153.

Fransson, M.N., et al., 2014. Toxicol. Sci. 141, 365.

Friberg, L., Kjellstrom, T., 1981. In: Bronner, F., Coburn, J.W. (Eds.), Disorders of Mineral -Metabolism. I: Trace Metals. Academic Press, New York, pp. 317–352.

Friberg, L., Elinder, C.-G., Kjellstrom, T., Nordberg, G.F., 1986. General Summary and Conclusions and Some Aspects on Diagnosis and Treatment of Chronic Cadmium Poisoning. In: Friberg, L., et al. (Eds.), Cadmium and Health: A Toxicological and Epidemiological Appraisal, vol. II. CRC Press, Boca Raton, FL, pp. 247–256.

Gaylor, D.W., et al., 1998. Regul. Toxicol. Pharmacol. 28, 150.

Grafstrom, R., et al., 2015. ATLA 43, 325–332.

Grandjean, P., Budtz-Jorgensen, E., 2015. Epidemiological approaches in metal toxicology. In: Nordberg, G.F., et al. (Eds.), Handbook on the Toxicology of Metals, fourth ed., pp. 265–280.

Hong, F., et al., 2004. Biometals 17, 573.

IARC, 2006a. Cobalt in Hard Metals and Cobalt Sulfate, Gallium Arsenide, Indium Phosphide and Vanadium Pentoxide. In: IARC Monographs on the Evaluation of Carcinogenic Risks to Humans, vol. 86. Lyon, France.

IARC, 2006b. Inorganic and Organic Lead Compounds. In: IARC Monographs, vol. 87. Lyon, France.

IARC, 2012. Monographs, vol. 100C. Lyon, France.

IARC, 2017. Dichloromethane IARC Monographs, vol. 110.

ICRP (International Commission on Radiological Protection), 1968. Recommendations of the International Commission on Radiological Protection. ICRP Publ. No. 10. Report of Committee IV on Evaluation of Radiation Doses to Body Tissues from Internal Contamination Due to Occupational Exposure. Pergamon Press, London.

ICRP, 1971. Recommendations of the International Commission on Radiological Protection. ICRP Publ. No. 10A. Report of Committee IV on the Assessment of Internal Contamination Resulting from Recurrent or Prolonged Uptakes. Pergamon Press, London.

ICRP, 1975. Report of the Task Group on Reference Man. ICRP Publ. No. 23. A Report Prepared by a Task Group of Committee II of the International Commission on Radiological Protection. Pergamon Press, Oxford.

ICRP, 1977. Recommendations of the International Commission on Radiological Protection. ICRP Publ. No. 26. Pergamon Press, Oxford.

ICRP, 1979. ICRP Publ, vol. 30 Suppl, Part 1. Limits for Intakes of Radionuclides for Workers.

ICRP, 1982. ICRP Publ, vol. 30 Suppl A, Part 3. Limits for Intakes of Radionuclides for Workers.

ICRP, 2016. Proceedings of the Third International Symposium on the System of Radiological Protection. In: Ann. ICRP, vol. 45 (1S).

Interdisciplinary Panel on Carcinogenicity, 1984. Science 225, 682.

IPCS, 2009. Principles and Methods for the Risk Assessment of Chemicals in Food. Environmental Health Criteria 240. IPCS, WHO, Geneva.

Järup, L., et al., 1998. Scand. J. Work. Environ. Health 24 (Suppl. 1), 1.

Jennings, P., 2013. Arch. Toxicol. 87, 13.

Jensen, C.S., et al., 2002. Br. J. Dermatol. 146, 636.

Jin, T., et al., 2004. Biometals 17, 525.

Kalliomaa, K., et al., 1998. Regul. Toxicol. Pharmacol. 27, 98.

Kjellstrom, T., 1985a. Renal effects. In: Friberg, L., Elinder, C.-G., Kjellstrom, T., et al. (Eds.), Cadmium and Health. A Toxicological and Epidemiological Appraisal. CRC Press, Boca Raton, FL (Chapter 9).

Kjellstrom, T., 1985b. Chapter 13: critical organs, critical concentrations and whole body dose-response relationships. In: Friberg, L., Elinder, C.-G., Kjellstrom, T., Nordberg, G.F. (Eds.), Cadmium and Health: A Toxicological and Epidemiological Appraisal, vol. II. CRC Press, Boca Raton, Fla, pp. 231—246.

Kjellstrom, T., Nordberg, G.F., 1978. Environ. Res. 16, 248—269.

Kjellstrom, T., Nordberg, G.F., 1985. Kinetic model of cadmium metabolism. In: Friberg (Ed.), Cadmium and Health: A Toxicological and Epidemiological Appraisal, vol. 1, pp. 179—197.

Kjellstrom, T., et al., 1984. Environ. Res. 33, 284—295.

Lucchini, R., et al., 2015. Neurotoxicology of metals. In: Nordberg, G.F., et al. (Eds.), Handbook on the Toxicology of Metals, fourth ed.

Menné, T., 1994. Sci. Total Environ. 148, 275.

Miettinen, J.K., 1972. Absorption and elimination of dietary mercury (Hg^{2+}) and methylmercury in man. In: Miller, M.W., Clarkson, T.W. (Eds.), Charles C Thomas, Springfield, IL, pp. 233—243.

Moffett, D., et al., 2015. In: Nordberg, G.F., et al. (Eds.), Handbook on the Toxicology of Metals, fourth ed. Academic Press, Elsevier (Chapter 10).

Nordberg, G.F., 1992. IARC Sci. Publ. 118, 3—14.

Nordberg, G.F., Fowler, B.A., 2015. Risk assessment. In: Nordberg, G.F., et al. (Eds.), Handbook on the Toxicology of Metals, fourth ed. Elsevier Academic Press, Amsterdam, Boston, pp. 461—486.

Nordberg, G.F., Strangert, P., 1976. Effects and dose—response relationships of toxic metals. In: Nordberg, G.F. (Ed.), Elsevier, Amsterdam, pp. 273—282.

Nordberg, G.F., Strangert, P., 1978. Environ. Health Perspect. 22, 97.

Nordberg, G.F., Strangert, P., 1985. In: Vouk, V., Butler, G.C., Hoel, D.G., et al. (Eds.), Methods for Estimating Risk of Chemical Injury: Human and Non-human Biota and Ecosystems. Scope and John Wiley and Sons, New York, pp. 477—491.

Nordberg, M., et al., 2004. Pure Appl. Chem. 76, 1033.

Nordberg, G.F., et al., 2005. Toxicol. Appl. Pharmacol. 206, 191.

Nordberg, G.F., et al., 2018. Pure Appl. Chem. 90, 755.

OECD, 2012. The Adverse Outcome Pathway for Skin Sensitization Initiated by Covalent Binding to Proteins. Part I: Scientific Evidence. www.oecd.org.

O'Flaherty, E.J., 1993. Toxicol. Appl. Pharmacol. 118, 16.

O'Flaherty, E.J., 1995. Toxicol. Appl. Pharmacol. 131, 297.

O'Flaherty, et al., 2001. Toxicol. Sci. 60, 196.

Rand, M.D., et al., 2016. Toxicol. Sci. 149, 385.

Renwick, A.G., 1993. Food Addit. Contam. 10, 275.

Ruiz, P., et al., 2010. Toxicol. Lett. 198, 44—48.

Ruiz, P., Fowler, B.A., 2015. 'Exposure assessment, forward and reverse dosimetry'. In: Nordberg, G.F., et al. (Eds.), Handbook on the Toxicology of Metals. Academic Press/Elsevier, Amsterdam/Boston.

Sakurai, H., et al., 1982. Scand. J. Work Environ. Health Suppl. 1, 122.

Sand, S.J., et al., 2003. Risk Anal. 23, 1059.

Scinicariello, F., et al., 2007. Environ. Health Perspect. 115, 35.

Scinicariello, F., et al., 2010. Environ Health Perspec 118, 259.

Shahristani, H., Shihab, K., 1974. Arch. Environ. Health 18, 342.

Skerfving, S., Bergdahl, I.A., 2015. Lead. In: Nordberg, G.F., Fowler, B.A., Nordberg, M. (Eds.), Handbook on the Toxicology of Metals, vol. 2. Academic Press/Elsevier, Amsterdam, Boston, pp. 911—967.

Suwazono, Y., et al., 2010. Toxicol. Lett. 197, 123.

Swedish Governmental Cancer Committee, 1984. Cancer, Causes, Prevention. SOU 1984: 64 (In Swedish with English Summary). Ministry of Health and Social Affairs, Stockholm.

Task Group on Air Pollution and Cancer, 1978. Environ. Health Perspect. 22, 1—12.

Task Group on Metal Accumulation, 1973. Environ. Physiol. Biochem. 3, 65.

Task Group on Metal Interactions, 1978. Environ. Health Perspect. 25, 3.

Task Group on Metal Toxicity, 1976. In: Nordberg, G.F. (Ed.), Effects and Dose-response Relationships of Toxic Metals. Elsevier, Amsterdam, pp. 7—111.

Thun, M., et al., 1991. Am. J. Ind. Med. 20, 629.

Travis, C.C., Haddock, A.G., 1980. Environ. Res. 22, 46.

Törnkvist, M., et al., 2008. J. Agric. Food Chem. 56.

USEPA, 2014. Next generation risk assessment: incorporation of recent advances in molecular, computational, and systems biology. In: EPA (Ed.).

USEPA, 2017a. Benchmark Dose Software. www.epa.gov/bmds.

USEPA, 2017b. www.epa.gov/iris/.

USEPA, 2018. Risk Assessment for Carcinogenic Effects. https://www.epa/fera/risk-assessment-carcinogenic-effects.

Vinken, M., 2013. Toxicology 312, 158.

WHO/IPCS (World Health Organization International Program on Chemical Safety), 1992. Environmental Health Criteria Document 134 Cadmium. WHO, Geneva.

WHO/IPCS, 1999. Principles for the Assessment of Risks to Humans Health from Exposure to Chemicals. Environmental Health Criteria No 210.

WHO/IPCS, 2009. Principles for Modelling Dose-response for the Risk Assessment of Chemicals. IPCS EHC 239.

Wittwehr, C., et al., 2017. Toxicol. Sci. 155, 326.

CHAPTER SIX

Dose—Response for Essential Metals and the Evaluation of Mixed Exposures

Abstract

There is general recognition that a number of trace metals are essential for human health. For these essential trace metals (ETMs), there is a need for recommendations aimed at protection from deficiency at low dietary intakes and protection from toxicity at high intakes. Uncertainties in the evaluations forming the basis for the recommendations have in the past led to conflicting recommendations for some population subgroups. This chapter describes principles of evaluation using a balanced approach and applying methods to achieve adequate evaluations of information on adverse effects of deficiency as well as toxicity. Application of these principles intends to make it possible to define an acceptable range of oral intakes (AROIs). When intakes are in this range a great majority of the general population will suffer no adverse effects from deficiency or toxicity. The principles include the U-formed dose—response curve and the recognition that the AROI protects only approximately 95% of the general population. Persons with genetically determined special sensitivity may have needs for higher or lower intakes than those defined by the AROI. This chapter also deals with the joint action of ETMs, other metals, and some other nonmetallic food components. It summarizes a few gene—environment interactions for metal-related health effects and points out the potential importance of this relatively new research field. The chapter finally summarizes methods for evaluation of exposure to mixtures.

6.1 ESSENTIALITY OF TRACE METALS

The foregoing chapters of this book focused on toxic effects of metallic species. These chapters included discussions on identification and assessment of risks of adverse effects from human exposures without considering possible beneficial effects from exposures to trace metals. However, a number of metals and metal compounds are essential to human health, and their essentiality must be taken into account when evaluating human exposures. This is the topic of the present chapter.

A vast number of publications and extensive knowledge exists on the roles of metallic macroelements like sodium, potassium, magnesium, and

Risk Assessment for Human Metal Exposures
ISBN: 978-0-12-804227-4
https://doi.org/10.1016/B978-0-12-804227-4.00006-6

calcium in human health and clinical medicine, as pointed out in the introductory chapter of this book. This book does not deal with this basic knowledge but focuses of the roles of trace metals/metalloids and their compounds. There is general recognition of the essentiality of the following trace metals for human health: iron, zinc, selenium, copper, manganese, molybdenum, and cobalt in the form of cobalamin (WHO, 1996; Aggett et al., 2015). In the publication by the World Health Organization (WHO, 1996), chromium was also included, but still there are diverging opinions concerning the existence of convincing evidence. Established evidence for the essentiality of manganese was not available in 1996 but has emerged later (see review by Lucchini et al., 2015; Freeland-Graves et al., 2016). Lithium and vanadium can have beneficial effects (see Bernard, 2015; Assem and Oskarsson, 2015) but are usually not included among the essential metals (EMs).

According to Mertz (1981), the dependence of the severity of signs and of the effects of resupplementation on the degree of deficiency was formulated mathematically by Bertrand (at the Eighth International Congress of Applied Chemistry, 1912). Bertrand's rule states that a function for which a nutrient is essential is very low or absent in a theoretical, absolute deficiency and increases with increasing exposure to the essential nutrient. This increase is followed by a plateau representing the maintenance of optimal function through homeostatic regulation and a decline of the function toward zero as the regulatory mechanisms are overcome by increasing concentrations that become toxic (Mertz, 1981).

Mertz (1998) set up a number of criteria for defining a metal as essential for human health. However, WHO (1996) considered that the crucial aspect is that when exposure to the element drops below a certain level, there is a reduction of a physiologically important function in the body of humans or that the element is an integral part of a molecule performing a vital function in the organism. The assessment of the toxic effects of EMs has sometimes been performed without due consideration of their essentiality, and recommendations of requirements to meet essentiality needs have not considered potential toxicity of higher intakes. Approaches in toxicological sciences were different from those used in nutritional sciences when identifying critical events and estimating uncertainties. This gave rise in the past to conflicting recommendations. A number of publications around the turn of the century (2000) pointed out the importance of a balanced approach and discussed methods to achieve adequate evaluations (IPCS, 2002; Mertz et al., 1994; Mertz, 1998; Nordberg and Skerfving, 1993; Olin, 1998;

Oskarsson, 1995; U.S. Institute of Medicine, IOM, 1998, 2000, 2001; WHO, 1996). These principles, which are now generally accepted, are the basis of the present chapter, and the following text describes and discusses them. However, despite such general acceptance, there are still a large number of recommendations and standards issued by various national and international bodies around the world (IPCS, 2002; Aggett 2010a,b; Freeland-Graves and Lee, 2012). As pointed out by King and Garza (2007), these principles need further dissemination, and it may be advantageous to get more harmonization of terminology. Abbreviations and acronyms used in this chapter are explained the first time they are used; also, Appendix lists all these abbreviations and acronyms. Table 6.1 lists current definitions of key terms.

The present chapter explains these principles for assessment of risk from essential trace elements according to the International Program on Chemical

Table 6.1 Definitions of key terms[a]

Acceptable daily intake (ADI)
Estimate by JECFA of the amount of a food additive—expressed on a body weight basis—that can be ingested daily over a lifetime without appreciable health risk.
Note 1: For the calculation of ADI, a standard body mass of 60 kg is used.
Note 2: TDI is the analogous term used for contaminants.

Provisional Maximum Tolerable Daily Intake (PMTDI)
A provisional value for TDI, see below.

Reference Dose (RfD)
Estimate of a daily exposure of the human population (including sensitive subgroups) to a defined substance that is likely to be without an appreciable risk of deleterious effect to health during a lifetime.
Note 1. The RfD can be derived from NOAEL, LOAEL, or BMDL with uncertainty factors applied to reflect limitations in the data.
Note 2. The RfD is usually reported in units of mg/kg body weight per day for oral exposures and may carry an uncertainty of perhaps an order of magnitude.
Note 3. The RfD is used in the US EPA's noncancer risk assessments

Tolerable daily intake (TDI)
Estimate of the amount of a potentially harmful substance (e.g., contaminant) in food or drinking water that can be ingested daily over a lifetime without appreciable health risk.
Note 1: For substances that are consumed rarely, but then in TDI-exceeding amounts, a provisional tolerable weekly intake may be applied as a temporary limit.
Note 2: ADI is usually used for substances not known to be harmful, such as food additives.

(*Continued*)

Table 6.1 Definitions of key terms[a]—cont'd

Tolerable weekly intake
Estimate of the amount of a potentially harmful substance (e.g., contaminant) in food or drinking water that can be ingested weekly over a lifetime without appreciable health risk. Tolerable intake is sometimes given as provisional estimates on a weekly (Provisional tolerable weekly intake, PTWI) or monthly (Provisional tolerable monthly intake, PTMI) basis.

Toxicity
1. Capacity to cause injury to a living organism is defined with reference to the quantity of substance administered or absorbed, the way in which the substance is administered and distributed in time (single or repeated doses), the type and severity of injury, the time needed to produce the injury, the nature of the organism(s) affected, and other relevant conditions.
2. Adverse effects of a substance on a living organism defined as in 1.
3. Measure of incompatibility of a substance with life: this quantity may be expressed as the reciprocal of the absolute value of median lethal dose (1/LD50) or concentration (1/LC50).

BMDL, bench mark dose, lower confidence bound; *EPA*, Environmental Protection Agency; *JECFA*, The Joint FAO/WHO Expert Committee on Food Additives; *LOAEL*, lowest observed adverse effect level; *NOAEL*, no observed adverse effect level
[a]In accordance with the International Union of Pure and Applied Chemistry (Nordberg et al., 2004, 2009; Duffus et al., 2007, 2017).

Safety document 228 (IPCS, 2002). The Food and Agriculture Organization of the United Nations (FAO)/WHO used these principles for risk assessment in their evaluations of upper levels (ULs) of intakes of essential nutrients (FAO/WHO, 2006), and they were also used for defining intakes avoiding adverse effects of deficiency (review Aggett, 2010a). However, there is still a need for full recognition of these principles by important authorities in the field and for a general understanding of the usefulness of an acceptable range of oral intakes (AROIs) designed to limit deficient and excess intakes in various age and gender groups.

6.2 DEFINING AN ACCEPTABLE RANGE OF ORAL INTAKES

6.2.1 U-Formed Dose–Response Curve

Oral intakes of an essential trace metal (ETM) which are too low lead to deficiency, and those intakes which are too high lead to toxicity. This results in the basic U-formed dose–response curve for an essential element. Because differences between individuals exist in the sensitivity to deficiency

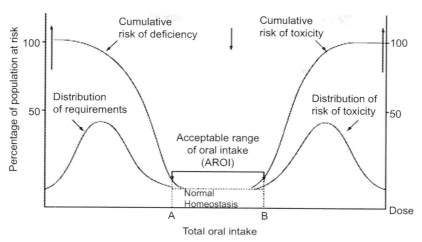

Figure 6.1 *Percentage of population at risk of deficiency and toxicity effects according to oral intake.* As essential metal (EM) intakes drop below A (lower limit of the acceptable range of oral intake [*AROI*], where 2.5% of the population under consideration will be at risk of deficiency), an increasing proportion will be at risk of deficiency. At extremely low intakes, all subjects will manifest deficiency. As EM intakes exceed B (where 2.5% of the population under consideration will be at risk of toxicity), a progressively larger proportion of the population will be at risk of toxicity. *From IPCS, 2002. Principles and Methods for the Assessment of Risk from Essential Trace Elements, Environmental Health Criteria 228, pp. 60 with permission.*

or toxicity, a curve is displayed when group or population data are described. Fig. 6.1 describes this interindividual distribution of sensitivity. The lower bell-shaped curves describe the distribution of individual sensitivity to deficiency and the distribution of requirements at low intakes. The peak represents the average requirement (AR). The right-hand part of this curve represents the level of intake that meets the needs of almost all, i.e., 95—98%, of the population at the lower limit of AROI. Another bell-shaped curve in the lower right-hand part of the figure describes the frequency distribution of toxic effect. At the intake corresponding to the upper limit of AROI, very few persons experience a toxic effect, but the frequency increases with increasing intakes to form the bell-shaped frequency distribution curve.

The upper U-formed curve is composed of a Z- and an S-formed curve (for deficiency and toxicity, respectively) describing the cumulative transformation of the distribution curves. This U-formed curve describes the risk of deficiency (low intakes) and risk of toxicity (high intakes) (see also Chapter 5, Fig. 5.1 for further explanation of the relationship between the frequency distribution and the cumulative distribution). In the middle of Fig. 6.1, at the bottom of the U, when normal homeostasis prevails, an AROI describes a zone compatible with optimal health. When the intake of an EM drops below A in Fig. 6.1, where 2.5% of the population under consideration will be at risk of (mild) deficiency, an increasing proportion will be at risk of deficiency when intakes drop further. At extremely low intakes, approaching 0, all subjects will manifest deficiency. When intakes exceed B in Fig. 6.1, where 2.5% of the population will be at risk of (mild) toxicity, a progressively larger proportion of the population will be at risk of toxicity when intakes increase further. At very high intakes, all subjects will suffer toxicity. Fig. 6.1 shows the two arms of the curve, representing deficiency and toxicity as symmetrical, but this is not always the case (see further discussion by Aggett et al., 2015.)

6.2.2 Groups With Special Sensitivity or Resistance

The low limit of the AROI represents an intake that covers the requirements of 97.5% of the population and the high limit protects 97.5% from toxicity. Special population subgroups with genetically determined sensitivity, such as those suffering from Wilson's disease, may exhibit toxicity even at intakes of copper lower than the upper limit of AROI. Other subgroups with genetically determined increased requirements, like those suffering from acrodermatitis enteropatica, require higher zinc intakes than the low limit of AROI because they lack the zinc transporter ZIP4 and therefore their intestinal uptake of zinc is impaired (reviewed by Kasana et al., 2015). When setting dietary reference values (DRVs), rare genetically determined sensitivities are not considered (see further discussion by the International Programme on Chemical Safety, IPCS, 2002 and Aggett et al., 2015). The medical profession is responsible for treatment of such patients, and DRVs set for the population as a whole cannot protect these rare cases.

Other subpopulation groups display nongenetically determined special sensitivities. Celiac disease is an example of a condition that impairs the gastrointestinal uptake of a number of nutrients including EMs such as iron and zinc. Excluding gluten from the diet of patients with celiac disease improves uptake of nutrients including ETMs. Infections and parasitic infestations cause other enteropathies with decreased uptake of ETMs. Alcoholic cirrhosis causes increased losses of zinc. Such losses occur also in diabetics. Parenteral nutrition without zinc supply causes a depletion of zinc stores and a demand for zinc (see further discussion in Aggett et al., 2015).

6.3 OTHER TERMS AND CONCEPTS USED IN RISK ASSESSMENT OF ESSENTIAL TRACE METALS

6.3.1 Terms and Concepts Used in Nutrition Science to Assess Requirements of Essential Trace Metals

6.3.1.1 Factorial Estimation of Nutrient Requirements

Estimating nutrient requirements by the factorial approach starts with an estimate of the amounts of nutrient needed for growth and tissue synthesis. It adds the amount needed to compensate for loss in various media such as urine, feces, hair, deciduous skin, menstruation, and ejaculation, as well as for pregnancy and lactation. In addition, calculations include additional amounts to maintain body depots serving as a systemic store. In order to calculate the dietary requirement, corresponding to the systemic or absolute requirement, bioavailability is considered. Calculations of required intakes to meet absolute biological needs include the use of assumed/estimated bioavailability to convert systemic requirements to dietary requirements. Data derived from biokinetic studies are crucial as a basis for factorial estimation of requirements. The quality of information on interindividual variation in absorption, distribution, metabolism, and excretion (ADME) determines uncertainty in calculated dietary requirements. It is important to describe variation in relation to factors such as age, gender, menopause, and physical activity. Dietary components like phytate, as well as other metallic compounds can influence absorption. When good data are available, including the composition of various diets and stages of deficiency and excess, and using precision measurements employing stable or radioactive isotopes, the biokinetic component of factorial estimates can be relatively good with limited measurement uncertainty; however, in other cases estimated factors are more uncertain. It is sometimes difficult to specify the uncertainties, which may be included in the judgments made during the factorial assessment and its translation into dietary requirements (King and Garza, 2007). Even in cases where there are good ADME data, it may still be difficult to relate the data on ADME to a correctly estimated systemic requirement.

6.3.1.2 Requirements for Individuals, Basic and Normative Requirements

According to the WHO (1996), the requirement for the individual is the lowest continuing level of nutrient intake that, at specified efficiency of utilization, will maintain the defined level of nutriture in the individual. The level of nutriture can be either a basal requirement or a normative requirement. The *basal requirement* is the one corresponding to the intake needed to prevent pathologically relevant and clinically detectable signs of impaired function attributable to inadequacy of the nutrient. The *normative requirement* is the one corresponding to an intake that serves to maintain a level of tissue storage or other reserves that are judged to be desirable.

6.3.1.3 Population Reference Intake, Recommended Dietary Allowance, Upper Level of Tolerable Intake and Safe Range of Population Mean Intake, Daily Reference Intake

Countries and organizations around the world use many different terms, definitions, and values when recommending dietary intakes of ETMs (Freeland-Graves and Lee, 2012). The US National Research Council developed the recommended daily allowance (RDA) as the average requirement (AR) for a defined population plus two standard deviations. The definition of the upper level (UL) of tolerable intake relates to the avoidance of any adverse effects of toxicity. The UL represents the limit of intake that does not cause any adverse effects in any person in the general population (97%−98% protection is aimed for). The RDA and UL represent the lower and upper limits of the AROI.

The population reference intake (PRI) used by EU Scientific Committee on Food (SCF, 1993) has an almost identical definition as RDA. "Adequate Intake" (AI), another term used by SCF and the European Food Safety Authority (EFSA), is a less precise estimation of AI than PRI. A term presently (2018) used in labeling of food and food supplements in Sweden (and all other EU countries) is daily reference intake (DRI). It is a legislated amount of a nutrient according to Annex XIII of regulation EU 1169/2011 (EU, 2011). The numbers listed in the Annex correspond approximately to the DRVs for nutrients set by the EFSA but do not exactly correspond to the most recent evaluations (EFSA, 2017). The DRI-values listed in the mentioned Annex are more similar to the values set by the SCF in 1993 and 2000 than to the most recently listed values (EFSA, 2017) (see also Table 7.4, Chapter 7).

Dietary recommended intakes (RDA and UL), AROI, and PRI, used in North America, Europe, and within the WHO have similarities, but there are often subtle differences in meaning, interpretation, and application. King and Garza (2007) suggested universal harmonization of terms and definitions describing nutrient-based dietary standards including the ULs based on toxicological data as well as the methods used in nutrition and toxicological risk assessment. However, there is no such harmonization agreed by the respective authorities and organizations at present.

All the concepts mentioned in the foregoing text relate to individual intakes. The WHO, in their document on trace elements in human nutrition and health (WHO, 1996), used population (group) mean intakes rather than intakes of individuals. The lower limit of the safe range of population mean intakes (SRPMI) is set so that very few (less than 3% of individuals in a defined population) have intakes below their requirement. The upper limit of the SRPMI is set to protect almost all persons from (minimal) toxicity. WHO (1996) provides a full description and discussion of the SRPMI concept; it is also described and discussed by WHO/IPCS (IPCS, 2002).

6.3.2 Toxicological Terms

Table 6.1 lists definitions: acceptable daily intake (ADI), provisional maximum tolerable daily intake (PMTDI), tolerable daily intake (TDI), tolerable weekly intake (TWI), and toxicity. The ADI is in most instances used for nutrients and TDI for contaminants, but in the past, TDI was occasionally used for additives. Because of uncertainties in the database for contaminants and some additives, provisional values are indicated by the Joint FAO/WHO Expert Committee on Food Additives (JECFA), for example, PMTDIs. The US Environmental Protection Agency (EPA) replaced ADI and TDI with the term reference dose (RfD). The term RfD was introduced in order to avoid implications that exposure to the chemical in question is completely safe or acceptable. Other toxicological terms are no-observed-adverse-effect level (NOAEL), the lowest-observed-adverse-effect level (LOAEL), and bench mark dose, lower confidence bound (BMDL). These terms are the basis for deriving ADI, TDI, and RfD. Chapter 5 describes how these terms are used and applied when estimating health-based guidance values like ADI, TDI, or RfD.

6.4 BASIC MECHANISMS OF HOMEOSTASIS

Homeostatic mechanisms exist for all the ETMs in order to maintain optimal tissue level and function. These mechanisms vary by ETM, some use mainly gastrointestinal absorption mechanisms, others biliary excretion or transport systems regulating tissue storage and urinary excretion. Metal-binding proteins such as metallothionein (MT) may also play important roles in regulating the intracellular bioavailability of EMs such as zinc and contribute to homeostasis at this level. The species of ETM is of great importance. For cobalt, only cobalamin is essential for human health, and there is no evidence that inorganic cobalt is essential. A number of publications by WHO (WHO, 1996; IPCS, 2002, 2007) and also the review by Aggett et al. (2015) give further information on homeostatic mechanisms of importance for ETMs. Section 6.3.1.1 in the foregoing text described the factorial method to estimate ETM requirements which uses data on the tissue levels considered optimal for function (systemic requirement). The concept of homeostasis is fundamental to the factorial method for estimation of requirements.

6.5 HEALTH EFFECTS OF DEFICIENCY AND EXCESS

The severity of health effects resulting from deficiency or excess varies greatly. Serious clinical effects and even death may be the result when deficiency is very pronounced or when high intakes cause severe toxicity. Fig. 6.2 shows a set of theoretical dose–response curves for effects of

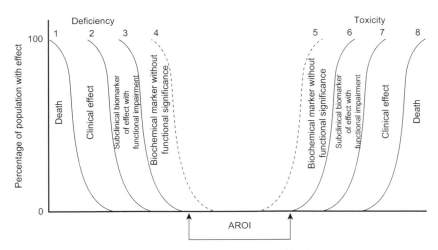

Figure 6.2 *Theoretical dose–response curves for various effects occurring in a population at various levels of intake (doses) of an essential trace metal.* The lower end of the dose–response curve for such critical effects related to deficiency (curve 3) and toxicity (curve 6) defines the range of acceptable daily oral intake (*AROI*). *Redrawn from IPCS, 2002. Principles and Methods for the Assessment of Risk from Essential Trace Elements, Environmental Health Criteria 228, pp. 60 with permission.*

deficiency and toxicity of varying severity. When defining the AROIs, it is desirable to try to find effects of similar severity at the low intake side determining deficiency and at the high intake side defining toxicity. Ideally, biomarkers of mild functional changes should be chosen as critical effects. Biomarkers known to be without functional significance should not be chosen as critical effects. The critical effect concept was introduced in Chapter 5 for toxic effects, and a similar understanding is applicable to adverse effects of deficiency. Ideally, biomarkers of similar functional importance would be available both for deficiency and toxicity and allow a balanced evaluation in relation to AROI. However, this may be difficult to achieve because of the incomplete availability and documentation of the functional significance of biomarkers. In instances where suitable biomarkers are lacking, mild clinical symptoms and signs may be the only available data.

The evaluation principles employing biomarkers of subclinical effects as the critical effect is widely used by national agencies like the US EPA and international organizations like JECFA and IPCS. It can also be applied to adverse effects of inadequate intakes as suggested by IPCS (2002), Aggett (2010b), and Aggett et al. (2015). EFSA (2004) concluded that available evidence was inadequate to set an UL for iron, but in the Nordic Nutrition Recommendations 2012 (Ministerråd, 2014), an UL for iron was established; Section 6.6 presents some of the evidence related to this question.

In risk assessment of nonessential substances and ionizing radiation, considerable efforts are devoted to stochastic effects like cancer (see Chapter 5). For such effects, it is often assumed that the dose–response curve is linear and extends down to very low doses. Thus, very low acceptable exposures are estimated for carcinogens (see Chapter 5). Carcinogenic effects of a stochastic nature are unlikely to be induced by ETMs because specialized enzymes, carriers, and chaperone systems in the human body handle all ETMs. Only when these systems are impaired, such as in certain heritable inborn errors of metabolism, will there be a risk for carcinogenicity (see further discussion below and in the review on iron by Ponka et al., 2015).

6.6 EXAMPLES OF EFFECTS OF VARYING SEVERITY

The following text gives examples of effects of varying severity in relation to the theoretical curves displayed in Fig. 6.2.

6.6.1 Lethal Deficiency

In situations when individuals are completely devoid of ETMs, severe deficiency may develop, sometimes with lethal outcome. When combined with other, usually benign conditions, severe iron deficiency may lead to severe anemia with lethal outcome in rare cases (Solomons et al., 1976). Keshan disease, with myocardial abnormalities and sometimes death, occurred in China as a result of selenium deficiency, possibly in combination with viral disease (Chen et al., 1980; Keshan Disease Research Group, 1979). Lethal outcomes of deficiency most often occur in sensitive subgroups suffering from other, usually nonlethal conditions such as infections or from combined deficiencies with other nutrients or excess of other essential or toxic metals.

6.6.2 Deficiency: Clinical Disease

Clinically observable anemia with pallor and fatigue because of iron deficiency is still common. Approximately 50% of cases of anemia among adolescents and women of childbearing age have iron deficiency according to experience in clinical practice. Although recent studies indicate that this percentage is somewhat lower (Petry et al., 2016), particularly in developing countries where infections and infestations cause many anemias, iron deficiency still is a major clinical problem worldwide. Psychomotor development is impaired in children whose mothers were iron deficient during pregnancy (Walter, 1989). Iron deficiency causes cognitive impairment by changes in the expression of growth factors and brain-derived neurotropic factors in the central nervous system (Estrada et al., 2014).

Copper deficiency sometimes gives rise to anemia. Because iron deficiency is much more common, copper deficiency anemia is often diagnosed as anemia unresponsive to iron therapy (Pettersson and Sandstrom, 1995; Sandstead, 1993). Clinical signs of zinc deficiency include growth failure, poor immunity, impaired wound healing, and impairment of special senses (Sandstead, 2015). Selenium deficiency is a cause of Keshan disease that occurs in China. Usually benign viral diseases are a probable component of this disease. Clinical symptoms, signs of cardiomyopathy, and, sometimes, deficient thyroid function characterize this disease. Kashin—Beck disease is a disease of joints and muscles occurring in the same selenium-deficient area of China where Keshan disease occurs (Alexander and Meltzer, 1995; Alexander, 2015). Patients on total parenteral nutrition with low tissue levels of selenium sometimes have muscular symptoms (WHO, 1996).

6.6.3 Subclinical Biomarkers of Deficiency and Their Clinical or Functional Significance

Biomarkers of various types are available. Enzyme levels in serum or blood cells often reflect enzyme levels in other tissues. Decreases in enzyme levels may be related to the development of adverse health effects, but there are examples of slight changes in enzyme levels that are unrelated to disease development. Other useful biomarkers are those indicating decreased body stores of ETMs that may be precursors of clinical disease.

The selenium saturation of glutathione peroxidase (GSHPx) in plasma, erythrocytes, and platelets is impaired when selenium intakes are low. Higher oral intakes are required for saturation of GSHPx in platelets than in the other mentioned media. Selenium saturation in platelet GSHPx therefore is a more sensitive biomarker than in the other media (Alexander, 2015). Selenoprotein P (SeP) requires even higher selenium intakes for full expression, and Xia et al. (2005) suggested that this protein is an even more sensitive marker of selenium status. However, knowledge is limited concerning the clinical significance of incomplete expression of SeP or incomplete saturation of platelet GSHPx.

Serum levels of ferritin decrease, serum ferritin saturation decreases, and erythrocyte protoporphyrin increases in iron deficiency. These indicators are excellent biomarkers of low iron stores. The limits of functional and clinical significance before the drop of hemoglobin levels are not well established. There is reason to believe, however, that it would be possible to establish such limits. In young women without anemia but with low serum ferritin concentrations, physical performance tests showed reductions in maximal oxygen consumption (Zhu and Haas, 1997). In another study, iron-depleted women had lower ventilator threshold when tested on a cycle ergometer compared to nondepleted females (Crouter et al., 2012).

Ceruloplasmin levels in serum and erythrocyte superoxide dismutase (ESOD) decrease when copper intake is low. Such changes are useful as indicators of copper deficiency (WHO/IPCS, 1998), but their clinical significance is not well established.

Specific and sensitive biomarkers of deficiency are lacking for some ETMs (e.g., zinc) and requirements are estimated by a factorial approach (see Section 6.3.1.1 above). The human body can maintain plasma and tissue zinc concentrations at adequate levels over long periods at low intakes by substantial reduction of endogenous losses. WHO (1996) considered this ability when estimating the physiological requirement for zinc, using data from long-term balance studies.

6.6.4 Lethal Toxic Effects

Oral intake of excessive doses of soluble salts of iron or copper give rise to severe gastrointestinal manifestations, systemic toxicity, shock, and death (Borch-Johnsen and Petersson Grawé, 1995; WHO/IPCS, 1998). Ingestion of high doses of chromate gives rise to severe, sometimes lethal, poisoning with bleeding in the gastrointestinal tract, massive loss of fluids, and cardiovascular shock. Some cases also display liver necrosis and renal tubular necrosis (Langard and Costa, 2015). Oral intake of high doses of selenium compounds like selenious acid, sodium selenite, or selenium dioxide may give rise to lethal poisoning. Symptoms and signs include gastrointestinal manifestations of various severity, hypotension, tachycardia, and cardiac failure (Alexander, 2015).

6.6.5 Clinical, Nonlethal Poisoning

High single or repeated oral doses of ETMs may cause nonlethal poisoning in some cases. Ingestion of iron salts, copper salts, chromate, and zinc salts or selenium compounds have caused such cases. Ingestion of high single or repeated doses of selenium compounds may cause nausea, vomiting, and, subsequently, hair, nail, and skin changes (Alexander, 2015). In addition, to gastrointestinal manifestations, ingestion of copper salts gives rise to hematuria and jaundice (WHO/IPCS, 1998). Intake of high oral doses of soluble iron salts that may accidentally occur in children can give rise to vomiting and diarrhea, often with bloody stools. Cirrhosis may occur later (Andersen, 1994).

6.6.6 Subclinical Toxic Effects or Biomarkers of Such Effects; Their Use as Critical Effects

Changes in enzyme levels or in levels of proteins for transport and storage may occur because of excessive exposure to ETMs and such changes may be used as biomarkers of subclinical or functional (adverse) effects. Measurements may be possible in blood or urine. If knowledge is available on the relationship between measurements of such biomarkers and the risk of adverse effects, such measurements can be used as a critical effect. Prevention of such mild changes may prevent the occurrence of more serious diseases.

A problem at present is that available information deals only with a limited number of biomarkers of potential usefulness, and there is a lack of well-established information about the clinical and functional significance of the biomarkers.

Decreased levels of ESOD (Erythrocyte superoxide dismutase) may occur in persons exposed to high dietary zinc levels. This effect is the result of influence by zinc on the intestinal uptake of copper. When considering the dose—response relationship between zinc intake and ESOD, the level of copper intake is important. Decreased ESOD may occur at relatively modest zinc intakes in persons with low copper intake (review by Sandstead, 2015), while persons with copper intake in the normal range do not display decreased ESOD until intakes are much higher. The clinical and functional importance of a decrease in ESOD is not well established. However, this biomarker is potentially useful as an indicator of acute kidney disease (Costa et al., 2016), and it seems that it would be possible to explore its use as a functional biomarker in evaluations of zinc and copper intakes. It may be a possibly useful critical effect of high zinc intake.

Excessive transferrin saturation and excessive levels of serum ferritin are biomarkers of iron overload (Ponka et al., 2015). Such excesses can be due to long-term excessive oral intakes of iron but are then usually of a moderate nature. Large excesses occur in persons with hemochromatosis, and they are of clear clinical importance. Homozygotes for hemochromatosis have marked increased risks of liver cancer and an increased risk of coronary heart disease (Bradbear et al., 1985; Niederau et al., 1985). There is no convincing documentation on the role of moderate levels of iron load in inducing disease. A relatively large proportion of the population is heterozygotic to the hemochromatosis gene, but it is unknown if they have any risk of increased iron overload. EFSA (2004) stated that there is a lack of evidence to set an UL for iron intake. The EFSA in 2015 (EFSA-NDA, 2015) considered that there is no evidence that heterozygotes for hemochromatosis are at an increased risk of iron overload. On the other hand, the Nordic Council (Ministerråd, 2014) was able to set an UL for iron intake.

There are reports of prolonged plasma prothrombin time and increased alanine aminotransferase/alanine transaminase when selenium intakes are high, and these measurements may be candidate biomarkers of such intakes (review Alexander, 2015).

6.7 SUMMARY AND CONCLUSIONS ON THE PRINCIPLES OF RISK ASSESSMENT FOR HUMAN EXPOSURES TO ESSENTIAL TRACE METALS

IPCS (2002) presented a scheme (Fig. 6.3) and table (Table 6.2) summarizing the principles for determination of the AROI. This scheme does not describe a new paradigm for assessing health risks for exposure to ETMs. It describes essentially the same principles as dealt with in the other chapters of this book for metals in general. One important difference is that for ETMs, each step includes consideration of toxicity and essentiality in a balanced approach. Ideally, a multidisciplinary team of scientists using the principles listed in Table 6.2 perform such evaluations, applying sound

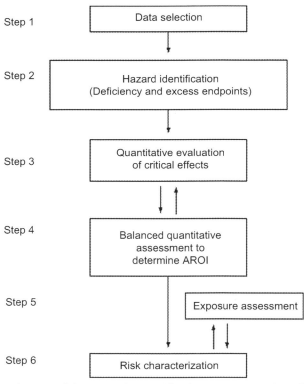

Figure 6.3 Application of the principles used for the assessment of risk from essential metals. *AROI*, acceptable range of oral intake. *From IPCS, 2002. Principles and Methods for the Assessment of Risk from Essential Trace Elements, Environmental Health Criteria 228, pp. 60 with permission.*

Table 6.2 Principles underlying the use of the homeostatic model in human health risk assessment of essential trace metals

- Homeostatic mechanisms should be identified for the selected ETM.
- Variations of the population's homeostatic adaptation must be considered.
- There is a "zone of safe and adequate exposure for each defined age and gender group" for all EMs, a zone compatible with good health. This is the AROI.
- All appropriate scientific disciplines must be involved in developing an AROI.
- Data on toxicity and deficiency should receive equal critical evaluation.
- Bioavailability should be considered in assessing the effects of deficiency and toxicity.
- Nutrient interactions should be considered when known.
- Chemical species and the route and duration of exposure should be fully described.
- Biological endpoints used to define the lower (RDA) and upper (toxic) boundaries of the AROI should ideally have similar degrees of functional significance. This is particularly relevant where there is a potentially narrow AROI as a result of one endpoint being of negligible clinical significance.
- All appropriate data should be used to determine the dose—response curve for establishing the boundaries of the AROI.

AROI, acceptable range of oral intake; *EM*, essential metal; *ETM*, essential trace metal; *RDA*, recommended daily allowance.
Slightly modified from IPCS, 2002. Principles and Methods for the Assessment of Risk from Essential Trace Elements, Environmental Health Criteria 228, pp. 60.

scientific judgment. As indicated in the table, it is very important to consider the physiological adaptation that prevents deficiency states to develop when intakes are in the lower part of the AROI.

Step 6 (Fig. 6.3), risk characterization, combines data on exposure with data on toxicity and dose—response relationships, i.e., the AROI, and evaluates if population groups are within AROI or (partly) outside the AROI. This step identifies risks of deficiency or toxicity for defined age and gender subgroups of a population and provides background information for preventive measures. For some ETMs and population groups, sufficient information is available in the scientific literature to set an AROI. However, for other ETMs and population groups, additional data have to be collected in order for an AROI to be set. Krewski et al. (2010) examined the available database for copper in order to compare the NOAEL and BMDL approaches for setting an AROI or something similar. Unfortunately, these authors found available data to be unsatisfactory for this task, partly because of the lack of several dose levels in many studies. The Nordic Council (Ministerråd, Nordisk, 2014) in the Scandinavian countries, the Institute of Medicine in the United States (IOM, 2006), EFSA in the EU (EFSA, 2017), and WHO (WHO, 1996) established intake recommendations corresponding to AROI. The Nordic Council used the terms: lower intake level (LI), average requirement (AR), recommended intake (RI), and upper intake level (UL); the IOM used recommended dietary allowance (RDA) and tolerable upper intake level (UL); the EFSA Panel on Dietetic Products, Nutrition and Allergies used population reference intake (PRI) and tolerable upper intake level (UL); and WHO used safe range of population mean intake (SRPMI).

Chapter 7 (Table 7.4) presents some of the values recommended by the organizations noted above.

6.8 THE INFLUENCE OF ESSENTIAL METALS ON EFFECTS AND DOSE–RESPONSE RELATIONSHIPS OF TOXIC METALS

The foregoing sections of this chapter dealt with the essentiality of trace metals and the relationship between daily dose and adverse effects from deficiency and excess of the same metals. The ETMs also play important roles as factors modifying the toxic effects and dose–response relationships for toxic metals. The following section (Section 6.8) will give a general discussion of the combined action of metal compounds. The present section will focus on the specific impact of EMs on dose response relationships of toxic metals, and data on these impacts will be the summarized in this section.

Lead (Pb) is the best studied toxic trace metal and a large number of publications are available concerning the influence of EMs on lead-induced changes in cells and experimental animals. The following summary gives some examples, mainly from the review by Nordberg et al. (2015a). In animals and humans, dietary deficiencies of calcium, phosphate, iron, and possibly zinc increase the uptake of Pb from the gastrointestinal tract (review Skerfving and Bergdahl, 2015). Because milk is a major source of calcium and phosphate, milk was for a long time recommended as a prophylactic against lead absorption in children, but other studies have shown that a milk diet actually increased lead uptake, this recommendation was discontinued. One of the reasons why a milk diet increases lead uptake is that it is low in iron, and a low iron intake promotes lead uptake. Several epidemiological studies reported increased risks of lead poisoning in iron-deficient children (e.g., Wright et al., 2003). Lead exposed mothers who are breast-feeding their infants transfer some lead to the infant because lead passes from the bloodstream into breast milk. However, a low calcium intake also increases lead uptake and supplementation of lactating mothers with calcium decreased the lead level in breast milk (Ettinger et al., 2006). An interaction between lead and calcium ions, inhibiting the release of neurotransmitters in the central nervous system may be an explanation for cognitive impairments related to lead. Interaction of Pb with other Ca-mediated events may be important for lead-induced oxidative stress and apoptosis. Interactions of Pb^{2+} with voltage gated Ca^{2+} channels involved in synaptic processes is an example of such an event. There is evidence of a protective effect of oral zinc supplementation on the hematological effects of lead in children (Chisolm, 1981). The interaction by zinc may be exerted on several levels: decreased lead uptake in the gut and reactivation of lead-inhibited δ-aminolevulinic acid dehydratase (ALAD).

Cadmium uptake from the gastrointestinal tract is influenced by EMs in a similar manner to that of lead. The following text summarizes information from the reviews by Nordberg et al. (2015a,b). Many animal experiments over the years have demonstrated a higher uptake of cadmium when there is a low intake of the EMs: calcium, iron, copper and zinc. For iron, there is also data on humans. There were clearly higher uptakes of iron from the gastrointestinal tract among persons with iron deficiency or low iron stores indicated by low serum levels of ferritin compared to those with normal iron status. Higher values of cadmium in blood and urine among women with iron deficiency compared to those with normal iron stores, which confirm the importance of this interaction. An explanation of this interaction is the fact that transport through the intestinal wall of both Fe^{2+} and Cd^{2+} is through the divalent metal transporter DMT1 (Tallkvist et al., 2001). When iron is lacking, there is an up regulation of DMT1 and transport of iron and cadmium is more efficient. Cadmium toxicity is changed also in other ways by zinc. Pretreatment of experimental animals by zinc can give rise to protection against toxic effects like testicular damage, ovarian damage and kidney toxicity. The induction by zinc of the low molecular mass protein MT, which binds cadmium efficiently, is a likely explanation for some of these effects, for example those on the kidney. Lin et al. (2014) reported a statistical association between low serum zinc and increased cadmium related glomerular kidney dysfunction.

Animal experiments have demonstrated selenium induced decreases of the toxicity of inorganic mercury (reviewed in Nordberg et al., 2015a).

The explanation is the binding of mercuric ions to a mercury—selenoprotein complex in plasma and tissues, thus neutralizing the toxic mercuric ion. Observations in miners in Europe (Rossi et al., 1976) and China found elevated tissue levels of mercury and selenium. The studies in China demonstrated binding of Hg to selenoprotein P (Chen et al., 2006). Selenium also influences methylmercury toxicity. Ganther et al. (1972) suggested that selenium in marine fish would protect against the toxicity of methylmercury. Although questioned initially, it has subsequently been supported to some extent (see review by Nordberg et al., 2015a), but the content of polyunsaturated fatty acids (PUFAs) is likely to be the main factor in the protection by marine fish against the neurotoxicity and cardiotoxicity of methylmercury (see Chapter 8, Section 8.9).

An interaction between two ETMs that can cause adverse health effects among domestic animals and to a lesser extent in humans is the one between molybdenum and copper. Ruminants grazing on pastures with high molybdenum content developed copper deficiency (Bremner, 1979). This is the explanation for molybdenosis, known to develop in sheep and cows grazing on molybdenum-rich land. Thiomolybdates formed in the ruminants bind copper and make copper unavailable for uptake (Mason, 1986). There is some evidence in human volunteers that molybdenum intake can decrease copper uptake in the gut. This interaction is used successfully in the treatment of Wilson's disease in humans. Tetrathiomolybdate efficiently binds copper in the gut and decreases tissue copper load in these patients (Brewer and Yuzbasiyan-Gurkan, 1992).

Potassium is a macroelement and, in principle, outside the scope of the present text. However, it is interesting that thallium and potassium have common receptor sites where they compete, and potassium is used to some extent in the treatment of thallium poisoning (review Blain and Kazantzis, 2015).

There are a number of influences by EMs on the dose—response relationships for cancer by metallic carcinogens (review by Nordberg et al., 2015a), but human evidence is limited, and this evidence will not be further described here.

6.9 THE COMBINED ACTION OF METAL COMPOUNDS, INCLUDING INTERACTIONS, PRINCIPLES, AND METHODS OF ASSESSMENT

The joint action of essential and toxic metals and other influencing factors have been studied in vivo and in vitro for several decades. Many results are of practical use in animal nutrition and some in human nutrition, but application in human health and prevention is slow and many findings with potential preventive use are still under consideration as discussed in the foregoing sections of this chapter. In the past, several international workshops reviewed the field (see below this section). In 2011, the WHO/ IPCS (Meek et al., 2011) published a framework for the risk assessment of combined exposure to multiple chemicals—further discussion of similar principles are summarized below according to the The Scientific Committee on the Toxicology of Metals (SCTM). Solomon et al. (2016) discussed risk assessment of combined exposures to chemicals and other stressors. They pointed out the need for problem formulation in their wide approach. Chapter 7 also discusses these issues briefly (see Chapter 7, Section 7.2).

The SCTM organized a series of meetings, 1972—2004, reviewing available evidence in this field and worked out consensus documents (reviewed by Nordberg et al., 2015a). The Task Group on Metal Interaction (Nordberg, 1978) considered various types of combined action of metal compounds. These basic considerations are still valid and are listed here:

Independent Action. This is an example of a noninteractive joint action. It occurs when two metals have different sites of action or different modes of action, and when they do not influence the action of each other. The dose—response relationships of the constituents of a mixture are thus independent of each other.

Similar Joint Action. This type of joint action (i.e., not a true interaction) occurs when two metals exert their action at the same site and when their modes of action are similar but do not influence the action of each other. The result of such a joint action is that the doses of the two metals should be added and the resulting effects estimated from the dose—effect and dose—response relationships of the constituents of the mixture. Such types of joint action are often observed, for example, with arsenic and lead exposure in relation to coproporphyrin excretion (Fowler and Mahaffey, 1978; Mahaffey et al., 1981) and in arsenic, lead, and cadmium exposures (Fowler et al., 2004; Whittaker et al., 2011). It is important to point out that such similar joint action (sometimes named additive action) must not at all mean a doubling of the effect. The magnitude of the effect resulting from (dose) additivity depends on the slope of the dose—effect curves.

Synergism. This occurs when the effect of the combined exposure is greater than that expected from similar joint action (additive action). A multiplicative action represents a special form of synergism. An example outside the area of metal toxicology is the greatly increased lung cancer incidence observed following cigarette smoking combined with radon daughter exposure, when compared to the carcinogenicity of either of the exposures.

Antagonism. This occurs when one factor reduces the effect of the other factor. An example is the influence of selenium on mercury toxicity (see Section 6.8).

The Task Group on Metal Interaction of SCTM pointed out that the term "interaction" thus applies only to synergism and antagonism and not to other types of joint action. Several authors and organizations published models describing the joint action of various factors in combined exposures of humans (e.g., Breslow and Day, 1980; Meek et al., 2011). The subsequent Section 6.12 of this chapter describes some models that are in practical use. Rothman et al. (2008) give further considerations and describe statistical and epidemiological methods. In the preceding Section 6.8 as well as in the following Section 6.10, the cited original publications describe the specific statistical methods used when describing the joint action of various factors influencing dose−effect and dose−response relationships.

6.10 THE ACTION OF OTHER FACTORS THAN ESSENTIAL METALS ON THE EFFECTS OF METALLIC COMPOUNDS

In addition to the impact on the effects of toxic metals by EMs, dealt with in Section 6.8, there are a number of other factors known to influence the toxic effects of metal compounds on human health.

Drugs used for treatment of metal poisoning present obvious examples of such agents. Gerhardsson and Kazantzis (2015) reviewed a number of chelating agents used for such treatment. Examples are dimercaprol—earlier widely used but now superseded by other chelating agents; sodium 2,3-dimercaptopropane-1-sulfonate (DMPS)—used in poisonings by inorganic and organic mercury, bismuth, arsenic, and lead; meso-2,3-dimercaptosuccinic acid (DMSA)—used for less severe cases of lead poisoning as well as other metal poisoning cases. These and other chelating agents increase the elimination of the toxic metallic species from the body and improve symptoms of poisoning. Other widely used drugs, like synthetic hormones used as oral contraceptives, may influence zinc and copper metabolism.

Alcohol is widely consumed in the general population. Ethyl alcohol intake increases the uptake of lead from the gastrointestinal tract and the combined exposure to lead and ethanol gives rise to higher body burdens of lead and higher risks for adverse effects than exposure to lead alone. High intake of ethanol can depress the enzyme ALAD, also a target of lead. Lead and ethanol also depress other enzymes (review Skerfving and Bergdahl, 2015). Ethanol inhibits the oxidation of mercury vapor to divalent mercuric mercury in blood, thereby decreasing the uptake and retention of mercury in the human body after exposure to mercury vapor (Chapter 8, Section 8.9; Berlin et al., 2015).

Tobacco smoking has important negative health effects in itself and the combination of smoking and exposure to metal compounds can be very deleterious. Pershagen et al. (1981) studied the joint action of smoking and exposure to airborne inorganic arsenic among smelter workers. These scientists found an age-standardized rate ratio for death from lung cancer of 3.0 for arsenic exposed nonsmokers, 4.9 for smokers without arsenic exposure, and 14.6 for arsenic-exposed smokers. According to the authors, these values indicate a multiplicative relationship. Whether this is an additive joint action or a synergistic interaction requires analysis that is more detailed. Subsequent follow-up studies in this smelter have found less pronounced effects, probably because of the decreased exposures resulting from improved working conditions.

Age and gender are other generally existing factors often influencing effects and dose—response relationships of metallic compounds.

A considerable amount of information from epidemiological studies is now available on the risks to the fetus and young child from lead exposure (see Chapter 8, Section 8.8). This is due to the passage of lead to the fetus through the placenta and the high vulnerability of the fetus because development of the function of several organs continues until after birth. Methylmercury also passes freely through the placenta. The fetal neurotoxicity of this chemical substance occurs at much lower maternal blood levels of methylmercury than those causing toxic effects in the mother (see Chapter 8, Section 8.9). Both for methylmercury and lead, fetal life and early development after birth is the most sensitive age segment of the population, and it is crucial to avoid exposures as much as possible.

Pregnant women represent a particularly sensitive section of the population, not only because of the risks to the fetus, discussed in the foregoing paragraph, but also because there is an increased risk of toxic effects on pregnant woman. Uptake of cadmium from the diet is higher in pregnant women because of an activation of the uptake mechanism for divalent metal ions (DMT1). Also in nonpregnant females of childbearing age, this mechanism for increased cadmium uptake is more often activated compared to the situation in men (see Chapter 8, Section 8.3), increasing the body burden and related health effects in women.

Other factors. The joint action of metallic compounds and various nutritional factors displays many modifications of dose—effect and dose—response relationships. This chapter does not review all these findings. Section 6.8 reviewed a few observations relating to the influence of ETMs on the toxicity of non-EMs. Other important components of the diet influencing the toxicity of metallic compounds are phytate and some dietary fibers, causing a reduction of the uptake of, for example, zinc. A low protein intake may increase the uptake of lead and cadmium (Nordberg et al., 2015a).

Human exposure to methylmercury is mainly through fish consumption (Chapter 8, Section 8.9). Accumulation of methylmercury in human tissues cause neurotoxic as well as other adverse health effects (Chapter 8, Section 8.9). Different species of fish contain different levels of PUFAs, and risks of adverse effects from methylmercury accumulation are different depending on the fish species consumed because PUFA can counteract or modify some adverse effects caused by methylmercury. Other food items also supply PUFA. In population groups with several risk factors for cardiovascular disease, methylmercury accumulation in human tissues can increase the risks for myocardial infarction. In such a population group in Finland, serum levels of PUFA modified the risk of myocardial infarction from methylmercury (Fig. 6.4). A mercury level in hair of 3 ppm was related to a statistically significantly increased risk of myocardial infarction when serum PUFA was 3% or lower. When serum PUFA was 8%, the risk was statistically significantly lower (Wennberg et al., 2012; Fig. 6.4). This is an example of a dietary factor affecting the dose—response relationship for a toxic metal compound. Textbooks on trace elements and nutrition (Mertz, 1987) describe the importance of other nutritional factors.

6.11 GENE—ENVIRONMENT INTERACTIONS

The genetically determined variation in susceptibility is fundamentally important in explaining dose—response relationships. There is genetic variation in genes regulating metal toxicokinetics and toxicodynamics. In addition, epigenetic factors that regulate gene expression may be targets

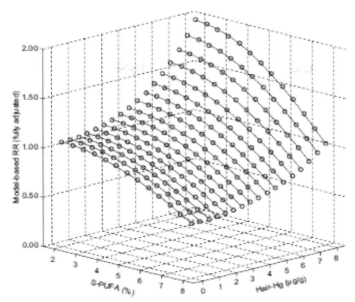

Figure 6.4 *Adjusted risk of myocardial infarction as a function of hair-Hg and long-chain n23 serum polyunsaturated fatty acids.* Model-based relative risks (*RRs*) are shown. The reference point (RR = 1.0) was set to S-PUFA = 4.0% and hair-Hg = 1.0 μg/g. Hair-Hg, amount of mercury in hair; S-PUFA, serum polyunsaturated fatty acids. *Courtesy: Wennberg, M., et al., 2012. Am. J. Clin. Nutr. 96, 706.*

for metal toxicity. Research on "Gene–environment interactions" is a part of epidemiology focusing on studies of associations between variation in one or several specific, so-called susceptibility genes and dose–effect or dose–response relationships for health effects. These studies do not require that an interaction of the kind described in Section 6.9 is detected, but any statistically significant association is of interest. Broberg et al. (2015) reviewed available evidence about such gene–environment interactions for toxic effects in humans exposed to metals. In most instances, the genetic influence is not attributable to a single gene but is polygenic, with some genes having a stronger influence than others. The first example of a gene–environment interaction was the relationship between a specific variant of the human lymphocyte antigen (HLA) system and chronic beryllium disease. Richeldi et al. (1993) found an increased prevalence of HLA-DPB1 Glu69 in patients with chronic beryllium disease. Other scientists confirmed and refined this finding of a genetically determined increased susceptibility to the disease, and this is still the best example of a well-documented gene–environment interaction. Variation in the major arsenic metabolizing gene AS3MT influences arsenic metabolism and arsenic-related toxic effects. This is another example of a gene—environment interaction (review Broberg et al., 2015). Maternal genetic variation in genes of glutathione synthesis is associated with mercury concentrations in maternal hair and possibly with relationships between methylmercury and neurodevelopmental outcomes (Wahlberg et al., 2018). An emerging field is research on epigenetic factors influencing metal toxicology. Such effects have the potential to explain associations that may occur between metal exposure early in life and toxic effects later in life.

6.12 EVALUATION OF EXPOSURE TO MIXTURES

6.12.1 Principles and Models for Assessment

Risk assessment of metallic compounds and other chemicals involves acquiring and interpreting relevant data, drawing conclusions from such data, and recommending appropriate risk management measures (Mumtaz et al., 1993). Metals are components of the earth crust, and they thus occur as natural components of human environments. They are always a component of the total exposome for humans and other organisms in the environment. While a specific metallic compound may sometimes be the dominating chemical species, present in a human working environment, exposures in the general environment more often contain a mixture of a number of metallic species and other nonmetal compounds, forming a complex mixture exposing humans by various routes. The following text summarizes methods used to assess the toxicity of such mixtures. Institutions and authorities in the United States developed and gave directions for application of these methods (ATSDR, 2001, see also Nordberg et al., 2015a):

Mixture of concern approach: there are studies of dose—response relationships of the actual mixture of concern. Such data are available only for a limited number of mixtures. ATSDR (2018) lists minimal risk levels (MRLs) for mixtures like fuel oil, jet fuels, or polychlorinated biphenyls. Occupational exposure limits are listed for asphalt fume, cotton dust, and coal dust (ACGIH, 2017; NIOSH, 2018).

Similar mixture approach: there are dose—response data for a mixture that is similar to the one that is going to be evaluated. If the evaluator judges the two mixtures similar enough, data can be used for the similar mixture to predict the dose—response relationship for the mixture to be evaluated. Obviously, this approach is dependent on the evaluator. This method can only evaluate mixtures for which there are some experimental or epidemiological data.

Hazard index approach: A hazard index (HI) is calculated by dividing the exposure level for one component of the mixture with the allowable exposure level for that chemical (for example, the MRL) and then adding the same procedure for all components in the mixture.

$$HI = Exposure\ 1/MRL\ 1 + Exposure\ 2/MRL\ 2 + Exposure\ 3/MRL\ 3 \ldots\ldots$$

HI should be below 1, otherwise the risk is likely to be higher than acceptable under assumption of an additive effect of the various components of the mixture. This principle is used also in other countries, for example, for occupational exposure levels in Sweden (see AFS, 2015, 2018).

Target organ Toxicity Dose: When data are available for target organ toxicity for various effects related to a specific target organ, e.g., hepatotoxicity, nephrotoxicity, neurotoxicity, the critical effect concept selects the most sensitive endpoint, i.e., the effect that has the lowest threshold, and this is the critical effect on which further risk assessment is based.

Weight of evidence method: De Rosa et al. (2002) partly based on Mumtaz and Durkin (1992) developed a weight-of-evidence method to take into account all available toxicological interaction data for a mixture. This method makes pairwise determinations of the joint action of components of a mixture and then weighs all these estimates together (see further description in the original publications and by Nordberg et al., 2015a).

6.12.2 Summary and Conclusions on Mixtures and Deficiencies

It should be clear from the brief overview given above that the risk assessments for essential and toxic metals on a mixture basis is a complex but extremely important area from the perspective of protecting public health. There are some general principles, borrowed from studies on toxic metals, but the issue of adverse health effects resulting from deficiencies in either dietary intakes or functional deficiencies arising from interactions between essential and/or toxic metallics requires special attention and new approaches. In particular, the issue of exposures to mixtures of toxic metals in combination with other chemical compounds released during recycling of electronic waste (e-waste) in developing countries is a case in point

(Fowler et al., 2015). These countries also often have existing human population dietary deficiencies of EMs and other nutrients. Elevated exposures of persons in poor nutritional status to mixtures of toxic trace elements released during e-waste recycling is hence a major public health concern (please see Fowler, 2017 for a review).

REFERENCES

ACGIH (American Conference of Industrial Hygienists), 2017. ACGIH Homepage. http://www.acgih.org.

AFS, 2015. Hygieniska gränsvarden 2015 (AFS 2015.7), p. 74.

AFS, 2018. Hygieniska gränsvärden 2018 (AFS 2018.1), p. 75.

Aggett, P.J., 2010a. Am. J. Clin. Nutr. 91 (Suppl.), 1433S—1437S.

Aggett, P.J., 2010b. J. Toxicol. Environ. Health Part A 73, 175—180.

Aggett, P., Nordberg, G.F., Nordberg, M., 2015. Essential metals: assessing risks from deficiency and toxicity. In: Nordberg, G.F., et al. (Eds.), Handbook on the Toxicology of Metals, fourth ed. Academic Press Elsevier, pp. 281—297.

Alexander, J., 2015. Selenium. In: Nordberg, G.F., et al. (Eds.), Handbook on the Toxicology of Metals, fourth ed. Academic Press Elsevier, pp. 1175—1208.

Alexander, J., Meltzer, H., 1995. In: Oskarsson, A. (Ed.), Risk Evaluation of Essential Trace Elements—Essential versus Toxic Levels of Intake, vol. 18. Nordic Council of Ministers, Copenhagen.

Andersen, A.C., 1994. Curr. Opin. Pediatr. 6, 289.

Assem, F.L., Oskarsson, A., 2015. Vanadium. In: Nordberg, G.F., et al. (Eds.), Handbook on the Toxicology of Metals, fourth ed. Academic Press Elsevier, pp. 1347—1367.

ATSDR (Agency for Toxic Substances and Disease Registry), 2001. Guidance Manual for the Assessment of Joint Toxic Action of Chemical Mixtures. ATSDR, US.

ATSDR, 2018. Toxic Substances Portal. https://www.atsdr.cdc.gov/substances/toxsearch.asp.

Berlin, M., Zalups, R., Fowler, B.A., 2015. Mercury. In: Nordberg, G.F., et al. (Eds.), Handbook on the Toxicology of Metals, fourth ed. Academic Press Elsevier, pp. 1013—1075.

Bernard, A., 2015. Lithium. In: Nordberg, G.F., et al. (Eds.), Handbook on the Toxicology of Metals, fourth ed. Academic Press Elsevier, pp. 969—974.

Blain, R., Kazantzis, G., 2015. Thallium. In: Nordberg, G.F., et al. (Eds.), Handbook on the Toxicology of Metals, fourth ed. Academic Press Elsevier, pp. 1229—1240.

Borch-Johnsen, B., Petersson-Grawé, K., 1995. In: Oskarsson, A. (Ed.), Risk Evaluation of Essential Trace Elements—Essential versus Toxic Levels of Intake, vol. 18. Nordic Council of Ministers, Copenhagen.

Bradbear, R.A., et al., 1985. J. Natl. Cancer Inst. 75, 81.

Brenner, I., 1979. Proc. Nutr. Soc. 38, 235.

Breslow, N., Day, N., 1980. IARC Sci. Publ. No. 32. International Agency for Research on Cancer, Lyon.

Brewer, G.J., Yuzbasiyan-Gurkan, V., 1992. Medicine 71, 139.

Broberg, K., Engstrom, K., Ameer, S., 2015. Gene-environment interactions for metals. In: Nordberg, G.F., et al. (Eds.), Handbook on the Toxicology of Metals, fourth ed. Academic Press Elsevier, pp. 239—264.

Chen, X., et al., 1980. Biol. Trace Elem. Res. 2, 91.

Chen, C., et al., 2006. Environ. Health Perspect. 114, 297.

Chisolm Jr., J.J., 1981. Ecotoxicology and Environmental Quality Series, 1—7. In: Environmental Lead: Proceedings of the 2nd International Symposium on Environmental Lead Research. Academic Press, New York.

Costa, N.A., et al., 2016. Ann. Intensiv. Care 6, 95.

Crouter, S.E., et al., 2012. Appl. Physiol. Nutr. Metab. 37, 697.

De Rosa, C.T., Hansen, H., Wilbur, S.B., et al., 2002. In: Impact of Hazardous Chemicals on Public Health, Policy, and Service. International Toxicology Books, Princeton, NJ, pp. 403—416.

Duffus, J.H., et al., 2007. Pure Appl. Chem. 79, 1153.

Duffus, J.H., Templeton, D.M., Schwenk, M., 2017. Comprehensive Glossary of Terms Used in Toxicology. RSC Publishing.

EFSA-NDA, 2015. Scientific opinion on dietary reference values for iron. EFSA J. 13 (10).

EFSA, 2004. Opinion of the Scientific Panel on Dietetic Products, Nutrition and Allergies on a request from the Commission related to the tolerable upper intake level of of iron. EFSA J. 2 (11).

EFSA, 2017. Dietary reference values for nutrients summary report. EFSA Support. Publ. 14 (12).

Estrada, J.A., et al., 2014. Nutr. Neurosci. 17, 193.

Ettinger, A.S., et al., 2006. Am. J. Epidemiol. 163, 48.

EU, 2011. Regulation (EU) No 1169/2011 of the European Parliament and of the Council of 25 October 2011 on the provision of food information to consumers. Off. J. Eur. Union.

FAO/WHO, 2006. Technical Workshop on Nutrient Risk Assessment. FAO, WHO, Geneva.

Fowler, B.A., Prusiewicz, C.A., Nordberg, M., 2015. Metal toxicology in developing countries. In: Nordberg, G.F., et al. (Eds.), Handbook on the Toxicology of Metals. Academic Press Elsevier.

Fowler, B.A., 2017. Electronic Waste: Toxicology and Public Health Issues. Elsevier Publishers, Amsterdam, p. 84.

Fowler, B.A., Mahaffey, K.R., 1978. Environ. Health Perspect. 25, 87.

Fowler, B.A., et al., 2004. Biometals 17, 567.

Freeland-Graves, J., Lee, J.J., 2012. J. Trace Elem. Med. Biol. 26, 61.

Freeland-Graves, J.H., et al., 2016. J. Trace Elem. Med. Biol. 38, 24—32.

Ganther, H.E., et al., 1972. Science 175, 1122.

Gerhardsson, L., Kazantzis, G., 2015. Diagnosis and treatment of metal poisoning: general aspects. In: Nordberg, G.F., et al. (Eds.), Handbook on the Toxicology of Metals, fourth ed. Academic Press Elsevier, pp. 487—505.

IOM (U.S. Institute of Medicine), 1998. Dietary Reference Intakes: A Risk Assessment Model for Establishing Upper Intake Levels of Nutrients. National Academy Press, Washington, DC.

IOM, 2000. Dietary Reference Intakes for Vitamin C, Vitamin E, Selenium, and Carotenoids. National Academy Press, Washington, DC.

IOM, 2001. Dietary Reference Intakes: Vitamin A, Vitamin K, Arsenic, Boron, Chromium, Copper, Iodine, Iron, Manganese, Molybdenum, Nickel, Silicon, Vanadium, and Zinc. National Academy Press, Washington, DC.

IOM, 2006. In: Otten, J.J., Hellwig, J.P., Meyers, L.D. (Eds.), Dietary Reference Intakes: The Essential Guide to Nutrient Requirements. National Academy Press, Washington, DC.

IPCS, 2002. Principles and Methods for the Assessment of Risk from Essential Trace Elements. Environmental Health Criteria 228, p. 60.

IPCS, 2007. Elemental Speciation in Human Health Risk Assessment. EHC 234.

Kasana, S., et al., 2015. J. Trace Elem. Med. Biol. 29, 47.

Keshan Disease Research Group, 1979. Chin. Med. J. 92, 471.

King, J.C., Garza, C., 2007. Food Nutr. Bull. 28 (Suppl.), S1.

Krewski, D., et al., 2010. J. Toxicol. Environ. Health Part A 73, 208.

Langard, S., Costa, M., 2015. Chromium. In: Nordberg, G.F., et al. (Eds.), Handbook on the Toxicology of Metals, fourth ed. Academic Press Elsevier.

Lin, Y.S., et al., 2014. Environ. Res. 134, 33.

Lucchini, R.C., et al., 2015. Neurotoxicology of metals. In: Nordberg, G.F., et al. (Eds.), Handbook on the Toxicology of Metals, vol. 1. Academic Press Elsevier, pp. 299—311.
Mahaffey, K.R., et al., 1981. J. Lab. Clin. Med. 98, 463.
Mason, J., 1986. Toxicology 42, 99—109.
Meek, M.E., et al., 2011. Regul. Toxicol. Pharmacol. 60, S1.
Mertz, W., 1981. Science 213 (Sept. 18.), 1332—1338.
Mertz, W., 1987. Trace Elements in Human and Animal Nutrition, fifth ed. Academic Press, New York.
Mertz, W., 1998. J. Nutr. 128, 375S.
Mertz, W., Albernathy, C., Olin, S. (Eds.), 1994. Risk Assessment of Essential Elements. ILSI Press, Washington, DC.
Ministerråd, Nordisk, 2014. Nordic Nutrition Recommendations 2012: Integrating Nutrition and Physical Activity. Nordisk Ministerråd, Nord, Copenhagen, p. 627.
Mumtaz, M., Durkin, P.R., 1992. Toxicol. Ind. Health 8, 377.
Mumtaz, M.M., et al., 1993. Fundam. Appl. Toxicol. 21, 258.
Niederau, C., et al., 1985. N. Engl. J. Med. 313, 1256.
NIOSH Pocket Guide to Chemical Hazards, 2018. http://www.cdc.gov/niosh/npg/.
Nordberg, G.F. (Ed.), 1978. Environ. Health Perspect. 25, 1.
Nordberg, G.F., Skerfving, S., 1993. Scand. J. Work Environ. Health 19 (Suppl. 1).
Nordberg, G.F., Gerhardsson, L., Mumtaz, M.M., Ruiz, P., Fowler, B.A., 2015a. Interactions and mixtures in metal toxicology. In: Nordberg, G.F., et al. (Eds.), Handbook on the Toxicology of Metals, fourth ed. Academic Press Elsevier, pp. 213—238.
Nordberg, G.F., Nogawa, K., Nordberg, M., 2015b. Cadmium. In: Nordberg, G.F., Fowler, B.A., Nordberg, M. (Eds.), Handbook on the Toxicology of Metals, fourth ed. Academic Press Elsevier, pp. 667—716.
Nordberg, M., et al., 2004. Pure Appl. Chem. 76, 1033.
Nordberg, M., et al., 2009. Pure Appl. Chem. 81, 829.
Olin, S.S., 1998. J. Nutr. 128, 364S—367S.
Oskarsson, A. (Ed.), 1995. Risk Evaluation of Essential Trace Elements: Essential versus Toxic Levels of Intake. Nordic Council of Ministers, Copenhagen, pp. 1—185. Report of a Nordic Project.
Pershagen, G., et al., 1981. Scand. J. Work Environ. Health 7, 302.
Petry, N., et al., 2016. Nutrients 8 (11).
Pettersson, R., Sandstrom, B., 1995. In: Oskarsson, A. (Ed.), Risk Evaluation of Essential Trace Elements—Essential versus Toxic Levels of Intake, vol. 18. Nordic Council of Ministers, Copenhagen.
Ponka, P., Tenenbein, M., Eaton, J.W., 2015. Iron. In: Nordberg, G.F., Fowler, B.A., Nordberg, M. (Eds.), Handbook on the Toxicology of Metals. Academic Press, Elsevier, Amsterdam, Boston, New York.
Richeldi, L., et al., 1993. Science 262, 242.
Rossi, L.C., et al., 1976. Arch. Environ. Health 31, 160.
Rothman, K.J., Greenland, S., Lash, T.L., 2008. Modern Epidemiology. Wolters Kluwer Health, Lippincott Williams & Wilkins.
Sandstead, H., 1993. Scand. J. Work Environ. Health 19 (1), 128—131.
Sandstead, H., 2015. Zinc. In: Nordberg, G.F., et al. (Eds.), Handbook on the Toxicology of Metals, fourth ed. Academic Press Elsevier, pp. 1369—1385.
SCF (Scientific Committee for Food), 1993. Nutrient and Energy Intakes for the European Community. Report of the Scientific Committee on Food, Thirty First Series. European Commission, Luxembourg, 255 pp.
Skerfving, S., Bergdahl, I.A., 2015. Lead. In: Nordberg, G.F., Fowler, B.A., Nordberg, M. (Eds.), Handbook on the Toxicology of Metals, fourth ed. Academic Press Elsevier, pp. 911—967.

Solomons, N.W., et al., 1976. Am. J. Clin. Nutr. 29, 371.
Solomon, K.R., et al., 2016. Crit. Rev. Toxicol. 46, 835.
Tallkvist, J., et al., 2001. Toxicol. Lett. 22, 171.
Walter, T., 1989. Am. J. Clin. Nutr. 50, 655—666.
Wahlberg, K., et al., 2018. Environ. Int. 115, 142.
Whittaker, M., et al., 2011. Toxicol. Appl. Pharmacol. 254, 154.
WHO (World Health Organization), 1996. Trace Elements in Human Nutrition and Health. World Health Organization, Geneva.
WHO/IPCS, 1998. Copper. Environmental Health Criteria 200. World Health Organization, International Programme on Chemical Safety, Geneva.
Wennberg, M., et al., 2012. Am. J. Clin. Nutr. 96, 706.
Wright, R.O., et al., 2003. Epidemiology 14, 713.
Xia, Y., et al., 2005. Am. J. Clin. Nutr. 81, 829.
Zhu, Y., Haas, J., 1997. Am. J. Clin. Nutr. 66, 334.

Applied Risk Assessment, Hazard Assessment, and Risk Management

Abstract

Applied risk assessment is a broad category, which covers the translation of exposure and toxicological data into risk assessments and applies this information into prevention and management or regulatory action. The term risk assessment usually implies consideration of quantitative information about dose—response relationships. When there is only qualitative or semiquantitative information about dose—response, the term hazard assessment is sometimes used. Risk and hazard assessment include a number of subcategories important for public health, discussed in this chapter. Among these are various types of risks, including critical and noncritical effects, threshold and nonthreshold effects, and severity of effects such as lethal versus nonlethal effects. In addition, the issue of sensitive subpopulations at special risk for adverse health outcomes is discussed in relation to appropriate risk assessment approaches. The central importance of high-quality exposure assessments in the development of dose—response relationship calculations is considered in the development of credible risk management regulations and practices in addressing the perceived risks. One section gives a summary of hazard assessment according to the Registration, Evaluation, Authorization and Restriction of Chemicals and the management in terms of classifying chemical substances in relation to concern from identified hazard. The value of effective risk communication to the populations impacted by any risk-based intervention is considered in relation to ethical issues and prevention of adverse effects in exposed populations.

7.1 INTRODUCTION

The term "Risk Assessment" is a general one used in risk analysis in a number of fields such as weather forecasting, engineering risk, human health risks from toxic substances, etc. This chapter and the whole of this book focuses on risks from exposure to chemicals, in particular, toxic metals, and the present chapter focuses on how to apply the information achieved in risk assessment to manage and decrease risks. As discussed in other chapters in this book, the term "risk" is usually understood as the probability of an

Risk Assessment for Human Metal Exposures
ISBN: 978-0-12-804227-4
https://doi.org/10.1016/B978-0-12-804227-4.00007-8

adverse effect (see also definition in Appendix), but it is sometimes used to include mainly qualitative evaluations of the weight of evidence for a specific adverse effect, e.g., by IARC (2012). Other organizations, e.g., the European Chemicals Agency (ECHA), use the term "hazard assessment" for qualitative or semiquantitative evaluations of the appearance of adverse effects in relation to human exposure (see further subsequent Section 7.2.5). In recent years, the chemical toxicology and risk assessment literature has increased in an exponential manner and several new regulatory approaches have emerged, intended to limit potential public health impact of chemicals. Toxic trace elements, which are found in air, food, water, and consumer goods, are an important category of public health concern since virtually all persons are exposed to these agents. Providing useful guidance on acceptable levels of exposure is complicated by a number of factors such as dose, chemical form of the element of concern and the occurence of mixtures of metallic and other substances. Diet, age, gender and genetic inheritance of the exposed persons must also be considered. Taken together, these factors are important for determining the populations at risk for toxicity as defined by one or more critical effects and hence the levels and types of regulatory actions needed to prevent these adverse health effects. The communication of health risks to the lay public is an essential component of this process since this group is frequently the element which motivates the societal decision makers/regulators to initiate protective actions. It is hence essential that risk assessments be translated into terms which are readily understood by persons with limited technical backgrounds (Section 7.4; Fowler, 2016) in order to be maximally accepted and effective.

This chapter will attempt to review how risk assessment and hazard assessment are applied in risk management using toxic trace elements as examples, since there is a robust toxicological/risk assessment literature for some of these agents. These elements are hence useful examples of where basic toxicological information has been incorporated into risk assessments for public health purposes. This background will, hopefully provide a basis for a prospective discussion of how recent advances in molecular toxicology may be used to increase the sensitivity, specificity, and precision of future risk assessment and risk management practices.

7.2 RISK CHARACTERIZATION

According to the International Union of Pure and Applied Chemistry, *risk characterization* is the outcome of hazard identification and risk estimation applied to a specific use of a substance or occurrence of an environmental health hazard (Duffus et al., 2007, 2017). Thus, both hazard assessment and risk estimation, i.e., studies of dose—response relationships are components of risk characterization.

The characterization of risk and hazard from trace metals has several important components. For many metal compounds with limited use, there is only limited information about hazards from exposure, i.e., quantitative information of the occurrence of adverse effects and qualitative estimates of risk are not possible; for metallic substances more widely used, quantitative risk estimates are possible, sometimes based on knowledge about the mode of action (MOA), toxicokinetic-toxicodynamic (TKTD) models, and adverse outcome pathways (AOPs) (see Chapters 3, 4, and 5). A risk characterization takes into account both quantitative and qualitative dimensions of risk, i.e., dose—response data, results of exposure assessment, and the severity of the critical effect. Characterization of the level of exposure (e.g., dose level), the chemical species of the element involved (e.g., oxidation state/inorganic vs. methylated, ionic vs. bound, etc.), is of basic importance. Another consideration is the sensitivity of populations exposed (e.g., fetus/children, pregnant women, senior citizens, nutritional and genetic susceptibility factors) and general factors such as severity of critical effects. In addition, the issue of deficiency vs. toxicity for essential trace metals and exposure to mixtures of metallics is an important consideration in characterizing risk since combined exposures may greatly alter risk characterization estimates due to additive, synergistic, or antagonistic interactions. Some scientists have suggested that an even wider approach is needed, i.e., to apply a systematic problem formulation to "cumulative risk assessment" for humans, i.e., the combined threats to health from exposure via all routes to multiple stressors including, in addition to chemicals, biological, physical, and psychological stressors (Solomon et al., 2016). Further discussion of this approach is not included here, because the focus of this book is on risks to human health from exposures to metals, metalloids, and their compounds.

7.2.1 The Importance of Severity of Critical Effect for Risk Management

The severity of a critical effect is a very important consideration in terms of health outcomes and the urgency of response and the resources, which must be committed to addressing underlying causes. Chapter 5 pointed out that the critical effect is often different in acute exposures than in long-term exposure. For example, acute exposures to arsine gas (AsH_3) may be rapidly lethal to exposed persons due to fulminating hemolysis and subsequent acute renal failure (Fowler and Weissberg, 1974; Fowler et al., 2015a). Control technologies must be put in place to prevent/manage such exposures in industrial settings, such as the semiconductor industry where arsine gas is used in the production of computer chips (Fowler and Sexton, 2015). The installation of such control technologies involves a substantial commitment of engineering and training resources to prevent the potentially lethal critical effect (death) from arsine gas exposure. While it is important to control acute exposures, because acute severe effects and lethality must be avoided, the lowest exposure levels that are of concern are often those occurring in long-term exposures, particularly for substances with long biological half-lives that accumulate in tissues in long-term exposures. Therefore, it is often desirable to focus the dose—response analysis on the critical effect in long-term/chronic exposures. The critical effect can be any adverse effect of importance for human health, from, on one hand, modern biomarkers detecting early cellular effects that predict functional changes and disease development to, on the other hand, a severe effect such as cancer, when no precursor biomarker is available and the cancer risk in itself is used as the critical effect. Obviously, the urgency of preventive action, as well as the extent of practical measures that it is reasonable to take, depends on the severity of the critical effect. Cancer risks, identified in epidemiological studies of population groups exposed for a long time, determine the low acceptable levels of inorganic arsenic in drinking water (see Chapter 5, Fig. 5.6 and Chapter 8, Section 8.2).

7.2.2 The Combined Consideration of the Results of Exposure Assessment and Dose—Response Assessment

Exposure assessment combined with dose—response assessment is of central importance to any risk assessment evaluation since the accuracy and fidelity of exposure assessment data will define calculation of dose to an individual, group or population. The combination of exposure assessment and dose—response assessment defines the outcome in terms of expected number of persons suffering from an adverse effect in an exposed population. As discussed below, such accurate exposure information will enable more robust overall risk assessment calculations if used in combination with similar high-quality biological response information.

The combination of exposure assessment and dose–response analysis generates quantitative estimates of how many persons exceed safe levels derived from the no-observed-adverse-effect level (NOAEL) or benchmark dose (lower confidence levels) (BMDLs) or quantitative estimates of stochastic effects (see Chapter 5) and provides estimates of the number of persons expected to display the critical effect in an exposed population. In the absence of data from humans, safety or assessment/uncertainty factors (UFs) are added in this assessment in order to arrive at an exposure level acceptable for humans (see Chapter 5, Section 5.2). Estimates of acceptable exposures, for example, by expert committees in the European Union (EU), sometimes use the margin of safety (or margin of exposure [MoE]). This is the ratio between the NOAEL in animals and the human exposure level to be evaluated (see also Chapter 5, Section 5.2.1). An MoE of 100 is usually considered acceptable for noncarcinogenic effects. The sections of the population in focus for risk management measures are those that are most vulnerable, i.e., those most susceptible and those most exposed.

Biological monitoring provides very useful information about internal exposure (internal dose) by measurements of metallic compounds in human blood or urine (Chapter 3) and such information is possible to relate to effects biomarkers forming a basis for dose–response relationships.

7.2.3 Consideration of Deficiency and Toxicity, Genetic Factors, Joint Action, and Exposure to Mixtures

A number of trace metals are essential for human health (Chapter 6), and they require recommendations aimed at protection from deficiency at low dietary intakes and protection from toxicity at high intakes. In the past, there were conflicting recommendations for some population subgroups, and present evaluations must use a balanced approach to achieve adequate evaluations of risks from deficiency as well as risks from toxicity in order to define an acceptable range of oral intakes (AROIs). When intakes are in this range, a great majority of the general population will suffer no adverse effects from deficiency or toxicity. Persons with genetically determined special sensitivity may have needs for higher or lower intakes than those defined by the AROI. The joint action of essential metals, other metals, and some other nonmetallic food components may change dose–response relationships considerably and such joint action must be taken into consideration when applying risk assessment into practice. There are also examples (Chapter 6) of genes that have been identified as increasing the susceptibility to development of disease from exposure to metals, the most well-known being the increased susceptibility to development of chronic beryllium disease by persons with a specific human leukocyte antigen variant (Chapter 6, Section 6.11). It is important when applying risk assessments in practice to consider the mentioned specific effects of joint action as well as other less well-defined effects of mixed exposures shown in experimental systems or epidemiology (Chapter 6).

7.2.4 Populations at Risk

It is well-recognized that individuals vary greatly in their sensitivity to chemical exposures. Age, gender, and nutritional status have long been used to help identify sensitive subpopulations for risk assessment purposes.

Landrigan et al. (2015) presented an overview of the unique vulnerability of infants and children to poisoning by metals. The following text summarizes a few considerations. The fetus that a pregnant woman carries has vulnerabilities that are very different from those of adult persons. Children have exceptionally heavy exposure coupled with a high vulnerability. They drink more water, eat more food, and breathe more air per kilogram of body weight compared to adults. During the first 6 months of life, they drink six times as much water per kilogram of body weight as an adult person. At an age of 1—5 years, children eat four times as much food per kilogram body weight compared to adults. Compared to exposures in adult persons, children thus have proportionately much heavier exposures to any metals that are present in water, food, or air.

In the first years of life, after birth, the metabolic pathways of children are immature, and they metabolize, detoxify, and excrete chemical substances less efficiently than adults do. Their absorption is generally greater, and they may therefore accumulate higher levels of toxic metals such as cadmium and lead in their tissues. During the 9 months of pregnancy, and the first years after birth, children undergo rapid development. Although there is some degree of plasticity, counteracting serious deviation from normal to occur, the developmental period is highly sensitive to environmental toxicants including metallic compounds. The neurotoxicity of methylmercury is perhaps the best example of the much higher sensitivity of the fetal brain. Studies performed during the methylmercury epidemic in Iraq demonstrated that the fetal brain is approximately 10 times more sensitive than the adult brain (Chapter 8, Section 8.9).

Thus, if cells are destroyed in the fetal or infant's brain by metallic compounds, the risk is high that it results in dysfunction that can be permanent and irreversible.

Recent advances in molecular biology and computational modeling have greatly increased understanding of the underlying mechanisms based on genetic differences in susceptibility, which result in differences in health outcomes for elements such as lead. Interference with the porphyrin pathway is an important mechanism of action for lead (Chapter 3). New genetic information related to this pathway has resulted in the development of systems biology approaches which will permit more refined delineations of populations at special risk and help address the question of "dose to whom" in making protective risk management decisions. One example of the use of such basic science information concerns the role of delta-aminolevulinic acid dehydratase (ALAD) alleles in mediating susceptibility to lead-induced hypertension. ALAD, which is the main carrier for lead in blood, exists as two alleles (ALAD 1 and ALAD 2) which vary in their binding affinity for lead due to a single amino acid substitution. ALAD 2 binds lead more tightly and limits susceptibility to lead-induced hypertension (Scinicariello et al., 2010). This information is very valuable in more accurately defining persons at a risk for developing hypertension in a given blood lead range and thereby allows more effective risk management strategies as discussed below.

7.2.5 Hazard Assessment and Hazard Characterization (REACH)

In several situations, the term risk assessment is also used to describe hazard identification and characterization of hazards in relation to the severity of effect and human exposures (see foregoing section).

The registration, evaluation, authorization and restriction of chemicals (REACH) regulation in the EU and the recent Lautenberg Chemical Safety for the 21st century Act (a modification of Toxic Substances Control Act) in the United States require that producers and importers of chemicals must submit toxicological information in order for the chemical to be used. REACH applies to all chemical substances, not only those used in industrial processes but also in our day-to-day lives, for example, in cleaning products, paints, as well as articles such as clothes, furniture, and electrical appliances. Therefore, the regulation has an impact on most companies across the EU. REACH places the burden of proof on companies. To comply with the regulation, companies must identify and manage the risks linked to the substances they manufacture and market in the EU. The safety measures required for safe use must be reported to ECHA, and the companies must communicate the risk management measures to the users. If the risks cannot be adequately managed, authorities can restrict the use of substances. REACH aims at stimulating the substitution of the most hazardous substances with less hazardous ones.

The REACH regulation requires registration at ECHA of all substances that are manufactured in or imported into the EU in amounts of ≥ 1 tonne/year. REACH does not apply to medicines and radioactive substances regulated by other legislation. A chemical safety assessment, including hazard assessment and hazard characterization, is required for all substances manufactured or imported in amounts of >10 tonnes/year. In the framework of REACH "Hazard assessment outcome documents" issued by EU member states are important in order to determine if available evidence forms a sufficient basis for classifying a substance as, for example, persistent, bioaccumulative, or toxic (PBT) or very persistent, very bioaccumulative (vPvB), i.e., whether the substance is of concern (see Chapter 4 concerning toxicity classification). Substances for which there is concern are placed on the "authorization list" (Annex XIV to REACH), meaning that authorization is required for their use. An example is lead chromate molybdate sulfate red, which is on that list at present (2018). Substances with hazardous properties may be placed on the candidate list of substances of very high concern (SVHCs). The REACH legislation aims to assure that risks from SVHCs are properly controlled and that these substances are replaced, when possible. SVHCs are substances classified by REACH as carcinogenic, mutagenic, or toxic to reproduction (CMR); PBT; or vPvB (see also Chapter 4). ECHA, at the request of the Commission or member states, can request a SVHC to be placed on the "restriction list" (Annex XVII to REACH). Substances on this list have various restrictions in their use; some are in practice banned from specific uses. Detailed information about the restrictions for the listed compounds is available on ECHA's web page: https://echa.europa.eu/regulations/reach/restriction.

A number of metals and their compounds are included in this list: arsenic and its compounds, including gallium arsenide and indium arsenide; cadmium and its compounds; chromium VI compounds; lead and its compounds; mercury and its compounds; nickel and its compounds; organostannic compounds. Companies are responsible for providing documentation to ECHA that appropriate safety is upheld when handling of substances. For that purpose, estimates of human exposure in various handling steps are generated by computer modeling. However, it was shown recently (Landberg, 2018) that some of these models generate lower exposure levels than those measured, thus underestimating risks. It is important to develop computer models, for example, *Stoffenmanager*, which is a widely used system, so that underestimations of risks are avoided.

ECHA is responsible for supervising also the classification, labelling and packaging (CLP) regulation (see below, Section 7.3.2), and the Biocidal Products Regulation (BPR, Regulation [EU] 528/2012). According to BPR, the approval of active substances takes place at the Union level and the subsequent authorization of the biocidal products at the member state level. Mutual recognition of evaluations allows an extension of this authorization to other member states. However, the new regulations also provide applicants with the possibility of a new type of authorization at the European Union level (Uunion authorization).

7.2.6 Threshold of Toxicological Concern

The Threshold of Toxicological Concern (TTC) is a risk assessment approach that derives a level of human intake or exposure to a chemical, perceived to be of negligible risk. This method makes judgments of the likelihood of risk despite the absence of chemical-specific toxicity data. The original Cramer decision tree was proposed in 1978 (Cramer et al., 1978) for the classification of chemical substances of concern and was the basis for the subsequent adoption of the TTC approach. Patlewicz et al. (2008) evaluated the implementation of the Cramer classification scheme. However, metal compounds and organometallic compounds are not considered suitable for assessment according to this method, and TTC is therefore not discussed further in this section.

7.3 RISK MANAGEMENT

Once an appropriate risk assessment has been conducted and decisions reached about the severity of the problem, it is important to develop an effective risk management approach to deal with the assessed risk. Section 7.2.5 (above) reviewed some management tools according to REACH and the present section will discuss other measures.

7.3.1 Source Control, Substitution, and Restriction in Use

When the risk assessment and risk characterization indicate that there are risks of concern, management of the risks is required. Reduction of exposures to toxic metals via engineering control technologies such as precipitation methods and ion exchange resins for metals in water, ventilation systems with scrubbing filters to remove airborne metal-containing particulates are common engineering approaches to reduce exposures.

In the working environment, encapsulation of production processes and the use of some of the mentioned technologies led to reduction of workroom air levels. Exposures to workers are therefore often considerably lower today than in the past (see also Landrigan et al., 2015 "Principles for Prevention of the Toxic Effects of Metals"). An exception may exist in developing countries (Fowler et al., 2015c).

For the reduction of emissions to the general environment from point sources, the *best practical means* (or *best available technology*) approach is sometimes used. It implies that an industry must use the best available technology to reduce emission of hazardous substances, provided it is economically feasible. The advantage of this approach is that resulting concentrations in various media (e.g., in ambient air, soil, rivers, lakes, and seas) around a point source will be as low as possible when the latest available cleaning techniques are used. Sometimes concentrations in the environment are achieved which are lower than those that would be permissible from a toxicological point of view. In other situations, risks to the general population may still be present, but then they are as low as achievable with the present technology. While some doubts were expressed (IPCS, 1999) concerning the effectiveness of such measures, the experience in Sweden is positive. Environmental legislation in Sweden has implemented the "best available technology approach" since the 1970s, and this has effectively reduced exposures around point sources, often achieving considerable safety margins for population groups living near such sources. This legislation is now a part of the Swedish environmental law (Miljöbalken, SFS 1998:808).

Substitution to less toxic metal compounds (e.g., essential metals in place of toxic trace metals) in industrial processes and consumer goods is another viable approach for reducing/managing risks from metal exposures. Substitution of SVHCs, particularly the many metal compounds on the restriction list (see above Section 7.2.5), is a requirement in the REACH regulation in the EU. Regulatory restrictions on usage of specific metallic compounds are a commonly used method for limiting human exposures to toxic metallic compounds. ECHA's strategy to promote substitution to safer chemicals (ECHA, 2018) intends to support informed and meaningful substitution of chemicals, including toxic metals that are of concern. ECHA's strategy is to accelerate substitution by activities complementing the stimulus provided by the chemical regulations. It includes capacity building, facilitation of funding and technical support, the use of registration, classification and risk management data for sustainable substitution, and the development of networks related to the substitution of chemicals of concern. ECHA intends to support member states and organizations in capacity building and collaborate with the Commission to ensure increased possibilities for funding. It has a central role in facilitating access to data from REACH and CLP, and it will support the formation of networks and continue to co-chair the OECD Ad Hoc Group on Substitution of Hazardous Chemicals (ECHA, 2018).

A Global Harmonized System for the classification and labeling of chemicals exists and is in concordance with the EU system. It harmonizes classification of chemicals by the types of hazard and proposes harmonized hazard communication elements, including labels and safety data sheets. Appropriate labeling is coupled with safe handling of chemicals and limitations in use of toxic substances. The CLP regulation in EU aims at fostering such responsible handling of chemicals including metallic substances The Prior Informed Consent Regulation (PIC 649/2012) implements within EU the Rotterdam Convention on prior informed consent for hazardous chemicals in international trade. ECHA administers the CLP and PIC regulations. Many regulations have been based on prior experience/risk assessment calculations and bureaucratic committee deliberations and taken a number of years for implementation. The REACH and CLP regulations in the EU places the burden of proof on companies. To comply with the regulation, companies must identify and manage the risks linked to the substances they manufacture and market in the EU. The safe use must be demonstrated to ECHA and the companies must communicate the risk management measures to the users. This legislation is now in effect in EU, its intention is to limit the occurrence of adverse effects from chemicals. Several restrictions in the use of toxic metals, decided in EU countries before the REACH regulation, have been incorporated into REACH. ECHA supervises the implementation of these rules (e.g. the "restriction list", see Section 7.2.5). An example is the ban of lead additives to petrol (see below Section 7.6). This is an example of a successful ban of a specific usage of a metallic chemical, which had a positive influence on human health; it was implemented long before the REACH regulation.

An important component of risk characterization is to provide information to the risk manager about the quality of the data forming the basis for the risk assessment, so that the manager can judge its relevance for management options such as decisions on regulatory action. The risk manager must be made aware of problems in terms of obvious data gaps in the scientific evidence in order to be able to answer possible questions relating to the risk assessment and risk control measures (for further discussion, see IPCS, 1999, 2009).

7.3.2 Permissible Exposure Limits and Guidelines

Because metals do not disintegrate in nature, a certain low-level exposure exists for human populations. Our task therefore is to define an exposure level with a small, acceptable risk. Permissible exposure levels and guidelines may be set either in terms of concentrations in exposure media (air quality standards, occupational permissible exposure limits [PELs], drinking water standards) or as amounts of substance that may be ingested (e.g., acceptable daily intake [ADI]; tolerable daily intake [TDI]).

Based on the above risk assessment/risk management considerations, PELs, guidelines and regulations have been developed for toxic trace elements over the years by various national and international public health agencies.

The risk characterization indicates how many persons in a population or a workforce (for occupational exposures) who are at risk of adverse health effects. Such information initiates risk reduction measures, which are either recommended or legislated. International organizations, and various countries or unions may issue recommended or legislated permissible exposure values. National organizations and agencies, for example, the Occupational Safety and Health Administration (OSHA) in the United States and the Work Environment Authority (Arbetsmiljöverket) in Sweden, issue limit values for levels in air of chemical substances in occupational environments (Tables 7.1 and 7.2). International organizations such as the World Health Organization (WHO) and Food and Agriculture Organization of the United Nations (FAO) issue health-based guidance values (HBGVs). They issue ADIs for food additives, TDIs or provisional tolerable weekly intakes (PTWIs), and sometimes provisional tolerable monthly intakes (PTMIs), for food contaminants. Table 7.3 gives examples of such values. The WHO also issues air pollution guidelines and drinking water guidelines. Chapter 6 discusses principles for deriving recommendations for essential metals and Table 7.4 gives some examples of population reference intake (PRI), recommended dietary allowances (RDA), and tolerable upper intake level (UL) values. These recommendations and guidelines are health based, i.e., they are based on risk assessments as described in the previous chapter of this book and do not consider other factors, that are of importance when setting standards in national legislation (see below). The risk assessments often use predetermined safety factor (or UF, see Chapter 5, Section 5.2.1). However, occupational limit values sometimes are set just below the NOAEL estimated from occupational health experience.

Under certain circumstances, the precautionary principle is the basis for exposure reduction. When exposure limitation is possible without a high cost, voluntary action may are possible, limiting exposures to levels lower than those otherwise recommended based on risk assessment. The precautionary principle (and the best practical means approach, see above Section 7.3.1) is a part of environmental legislation in Sweden and several other European countries and of the REACH regulation, implemented in EU. Ethical considerations like the paragon of virtue practiced by the ancient authorities in medicine like Hippocrates (i.e., "Do no harm") have initiated this principle.

Nongovernmental organizations sometimes issue recommendations of a precautionary nature. The "Declaration of Brescia" is an example. The Scientific Committee on the Toxicology of Metals and the Scientific Committee on Neurotoxicology, subcommittees of the International Commission of Occupational Health, issued this declaration recommending lowering of limit values of lead, manganese, and mercury (Landrigan et al., 2006, 2015).

In the United States, the OSHA and the National Institute for Occupational Safety and Health are the authorities setting the standards (national legislation) for occupational exposures. National standards consider, in addition to health-based risk assessment, practical possibilities to implement the standard. Possibilities to supervise the values by chemical analyses and economic considerations are included. Table 7.1 summarize a number of such values, limiting the concentration of metals or metallic compounds in workroom air. It is important to note that the values promulgated by these agencies do not always agree and the values may change over time, as new scientific data are accumulated and analyzed. Other countries have similar institutes and authorities. In Sweden, occupational exposure limits (OELs) are issued by the Swedish Work Environment Authority (In Swedish: Arbetsmiljöverket) in concert with EU regulations and recommendations (see later). Table 7.1 lists a selected number of values for metals and their compounds.

In the United States, the American Conference of Governmental Industrial Hygienists (ACGIH) is a nongovernmental organization issuing Threshold Limit Values (TLVs) for concentrations of chemical substances in workroom air. They also develop Biological Exposure Indices (BEIs), i.e., limits for chemical substances in biological media such as blood and urine. These recommended values are based on evaluations made by a voluntary body of independent knowledgeable individuals. They represent

Table 7.1 Selected occupational exposure limits in the United States and Sweden, 2016

Metal and compound	OSHA PEL	OSHA Calif. PEL	Sweden HGV	Comment
Aluminum metal	Total: 15 mg/m^3	Total: 10 mg/m^3 Resp: 5 mg/m^3	Total: 5 mg/m^3 Resp.: 2 mg/m^3	Total: total inhalable particles Resp.: respirable particles
Arsenic, inorganic compounds	C	0.01 mg/m^3	0.01 mg/m^3 C	C: carcinogenic
Arsine	0.05 ppm	0.05 ppm	0.02 ppm	
	0.2 mg/m^3		0.05 mg/m^3	
Barium, soluble compounds	0.5 mg/m^3	0.5 mg/m^3	0.5 mg/m^3	
Cadmium, metal and inorganic compounds	Fume: 0.1 mg/m^3 Dust: 0.2 mg/m^3	0.005 mg/m^3	Total: 0.02 mg/m^3 C,M Resp.: 0.002 mg/m^3	Total, Resp.: see aluminum C: carcinogenic M: medical biomonitoring
Cobalt and inorganic compounds, dust and fume	0.1 mg/m^3	0.02 mg/m^3	0.02 mg/m^3	
Chromium (Cr), metal and insoluble salts	1 mg/m^3	0.5 mg/m^3	0.5 mg/m^3	
Cr (II) and Cr(III) compounds		0.5 mg/m^3		
Cr (VI) compounds		0.005 mg/m^3	0.005 mg/m^3 STEL: 0.015 mg/m^3	STEL: short-term exposure limit (15 min).
Lead (Pb), inorganic compounds		0.05 mg/m^3	Total: 0.1 mg/m^3 B,M,R Resp.: 0.05 mg/m^3	B: may cause hearing loss M: medical biomonitoring R: toxic to reproduction

	HGV	OSHA	OSHA Calif.	
Nickel (Ni), metal and insoluble compounds	1 mg/m^3	Metal 0.5 mg/m^3 insoluble 0.1 mg/m^3	0.5 mg/m^3	C: carcinogenic
Soluble compounds	1 mg/m^3	0.05 mg/m^3	0.1 mg/m^3	
Nickel subsulfide (trinickeldisulfide)			0.01 mg/m^3 C	
Nickel carbonyl	0.001 ppm 0.007 mg/m^3	0.001 ppm	0.001 ppm 0.007 mg/m^3	
Platinum (Pt), metal		1 mg/m^3	1 mg/m^3	
Soluble salts		0.002 mg/m^3	0.002 mg/m^3 S	S: sensitizing
Silver (Ag)	0.01 mg/m^3	0.01 mg/m^3	Metal, insoluble: 0.1 mg/m^3 Soluble: 0.01 mg/m^3	
Zinc (Zn), ZnO	Total: 15 mg/m^3 Resp.: 5 mg/m^3	Total: 10 mg/m^3 Resp.: 5 mg/m^3	Total: 5 mg/m^3	Total, Resp.: see aluminum
Zinc chloride fume	1 mg/m^3	1 mg/m3	1 mg/m^3	
Zinc oxide fume	5 mg/m^3	5 mg/m^3	5 mg/m^3	

HGV, Sweden: hygieniskt gränsvärde (hygienic limit value); OSHA, US Occupational Safety and Health Administration; OSHA Calif., OSHA California; PEL, permissible exposure limit.
8 h time weighted average if not otherwise indicated.
Based on OSHA homepage; AFS, 2015. Hygieniska gränsvärden 2015, AFS 2015:7, pp. 74.

the opinion of these evaluation groups. Exposure at or below the level of the TLV or BEI does not create an unreasonable risk of disease or injury. TLVs and BEIs are guidelines designed for use by industrial hygienists in making decisions regarding safe levels of exposure to various chemical substances.

ACGIH has a long tradition of issuing TLVs, widely used in the United States as well as in other countries, although these values are not legally binding. The ACGIH values can be purchased on the ACGIH homepage (www.acgih.org). The scientific basis for risk assessments leading to OELs has expanded considerably in the last decades, and many of the present values are considerably lower than earlier ones. In the 1980s, most of the ACGIH TLVs were higher than the limit values in Sweden for the corresponding chemical (see below). Such a difference does not seem to exist at present; in fact, some limit values in Sweden (e.g., for beryllium) are higher than the value for the corresponding chemical in the ACGIH list (see Table 7.2).

In the EU, permissible OELs that are either indicative or binding for member states are issued by the European Commission based on criteria documents published by the Scientific Committee on Occupational Exposure Limits (SCOEL). Some EU member states like Germany and Sweden issue lists of values on a national level. Implementation of such national limit values is in harmony with the values issued by EU. Table 7.1 lists a selected number of values for some metals and their compounds according to the list valid in Sweden 2016 (AFS, 2015).

National lists of permissible OELs are issued by countries like Japan, China (Liang et al., 2006), and Russia. In the past, there were considerable differences between values in the western countries and values in the former Soviet Union (Russia) and China. However, thanks to the international

Table 7.2 Occupational exposure limits for beryllium and mercury vapor in the United States and Sweden

	OSHA	Cal. OSHA	NIOSH REL	ACGIH TLV	Sweden HGV
Beryllium and compounds	$2 \, \mu g/m^3$	$0.2 \, \mu g/m^3$	$0.5 \, \mu g/m^3$ C	$0.05 \, \mu g/m^3$	$0.002 \, mg/m^3$ $= 2 \, \mu g/m^3$
Mercury vapor	$0.1 \, mg/m^3$	$0.025 \, mg/m^3$	$0.05 \, mg/m^3$	$0.025 \, mg/m^3$	$0.02 \, mg/m^3$

ACGIH, American Conference of Governmental Industrial Hygienist; *Cal.*, California; *HGV*, hygienic limit value; *NIOSH*, National Institute for Occupational Safety and Health; *OSHA*, Occupational Safety and Health Administration; *REL*, Recommended exposure limit; *TLV*, threshold limit value.

discussions and the publication of Health Criteria Documents by the WHO International Program on Chemical Safety (e.g., IPCS, 2001, Arsenic) and its predecessors, starting in the 1970s, these differences have decreased. Advances in epidemiology, the development of new risk assessment methods such as MOA TKTD, advances in the use of biological monitoring of exposure, as well as effect biomarkers generated lot of new scientific evidence during the last several decades. This has resulted in a lowering of many OELs. In the 1980s, many values recommended in the United States by ACGIH were higher than the limit values (hygienic limit values) in Sweden (Nordberg et al., 1988). Most of the present ACGIH values are similar or sometimes lower than the PEL values issued by OSHA. No substantial difference seems to exist at present between OEL values in Sweden and the United States (see Table 7.1); as mentioned above, some Swedish values are in fact higher than the TLVs. Deveau et al. (2015) discussed the reasons in terms of methodology and access to data, explaining the differences in OELs in various countries.

In the United States, there are drinking water standards and air pollution standards, which are set by the US Environmental Protection Agency (USEPA) for a number of metals such as lead and metalloids such as arsenic (USEPA, 2018a).

Chapter 5 discussed dose—response relationships for carcinogens and briefly mentioned the unit risk concept. The USEPA (2018b) developed this concept, applicable to cancer risks. It is defined as the upper-bound lifetime cancer risk estimated to result from an agent at a concentration of 1 μg/L in water or 1 μg/m^3 in air. For example, if unit risk = 2×10^{-6}/μg/L, it would indicate two excess cancer cases (upper-bound estimate) to be expected per 1 million persons if exposed daily over a lifetime to 1 μg of the agent per liter of water or cubic meter of air. For cadmium, which the USEPA considers to be a class B1 carcinogen, the inhalation unit risk estimate is 1.8×10^{-3} (μg/m^3)$^{-1}$. The calculations of probabilities for developing cancer by USEPA use mathematical models, based on animal studies.

The WHO in collaboration with FAO has a long tradition of issuing HBGVs for additives and contaminants in food, ADI values for food additives, and TDIs or PTWIs (sometimes PTMIs) for contaminants (see Chapter 6 or Appendix for explanation of terms). IPCS (2009) reviewed methods for deriving recommendations. Table 7.3 shows examples from Fowler et al. (2015b) of such exposure limits and differences between two international agencies (the Joint FAO/WHO Expert Committee on Food Additives and European Food Safety Authority [EFSA]).

Table 7.3 Health-based guidance value or benchmark dose (lower confidence level)[a]

Metal	JECFA HBGV	JECFA Effect	JECFA Year	EFSA HBGV	EFSA Effect	EFSA Year
Arsenic	$BMDL_{0.5}$: 3 μg/ kg b.w./day	0.5% increase in lung cancer risk	2009, 2010	$BMDL_{01}$: 0.3–8 μg/kg b.w./day	1% increase in risk of lung, skin and bladder cancer. as well as skin lesions	2009[b]
Cadmium	PTMI: 25 μg/ kg b.w.	Kidney toxicity, renal proteinuria	2009, 2010	TWI: 2.5 μg/kg b.w.	Kidney toxicity, renal proteinuria	2009, 2011
Lead	Previous PTWI withdrawn	Cognitive deficit: IQ, no threshold identified	2010, 2010	Previous PTWI no longer appropriate. $BMDL_{01}$: 0.50 μg/ kg b.w./day; $BMDL_{01}$: 0.63 μg/ kg b.w./day; $BMDL_{10}$: 1.50 μg/ kg b.w./day	Cognitive deficit: IQ; Systolic blood pressure; Chronic kidney disease	2010
Mercury: inorganic	PTWI: 4 μg/ kg b.w.	Kidney toxicity	2010, 2011	TWI: 4 μg/kg b.w.	Kidney toxicity	2012[b]
Mercury: methylmercury	PTWI: 1.6 μg/ kg b.w.	Neurodevelopment	2003, 2006	TWI: 1.3 μg/kg b.w.	Neurodevelopment	2012[b]

b.w., body weight; BMDL, benchmark dose (lower confidence level); EFSA, European Food Safety Authority; HBGV, health-based guidance value; IQ, intelligence quotient; JECFA, Joint World Health Organization and Food and Agriculture Organization of the United Nations Expert Committee on Food Additives; PTMI, provisional tolerable monthly intake; PTWI, provisional tolerable weekly intake; TWI, tolerable weekly intake.

[a]BMDLs were given when a margin of exposure approach was used in the risk assessment.

[b]EFSA (2009,2012).

From Fowler, et al., 2015. Toxic metals in food. In: Nordberg, G.F., Fowler, B.A., Nordberg, M. (Eds.), Handbook on the Toxicology of Metals, fourth ed. Academic Press, Elsevier (Chapter 6) (with permission).

There is regulation in the EU limiting the levels of contaminants in food (EG466/2001). This regulation includes lead, cadmium, and mercury in foodstuffs. EU also has standards for contaminants in drinking water (98/83/EC) including some metals. Member states supervise these rules and report to the European Commission.

For essential metals, intakes, which are either too high or too low, may cause adverse health effects. Chapter 6 reviews methods used for defining an AROI and Fig. 6.3 (in Chapter 6) summarized these methods. In the United States, the National Academies through its Institute of Medicine (IOM) (now the Health and Medicine Division) and in the EU, the EU Scientific Committee on Food (SCF) and the EFSA have published recommended dietary intakes of essential metals. Although they did not use the term AROI, the range of intakes described by RDA and UL for IOM and PRI and UL for SCF/EFSA is equivalent to the AROI (for terminology, see Chapter 6 or Appendix). Derivation of a safe range of population mean intakes, defined by WHO, uses a similar approach of data handling but considers the distributions of population mean intakes instead of intakes by individuals. The range of intakes recommended is, however, similar to the AROI as indicated in Table 7.4.

Table 7.4 gives examples of recommended values for adult men, issued in the United States and EU, and by the WHO. As pointed out in Chapter 6, the legislated dietary reference intakes values in the EU (regulation 1169/2011) conform in general, but not exactly, to the values in Table 7.4. All these organizations referred to in Table 7.4 also developed recommendations for other population segments such as children, women, pregnant women, and the elderly. The intake ranges in Table 7.4 recommended by the three organizations are very similar, but some differences appear when comparing all population subgroups. Future exchange of information and international scientific discussion may further increase the agreement among recommendations.

Dermatitis due to skin exposure to metals such as chromium and nickel is a common metal-related adverse effect. This disease develops in persons who become sensitized to these metals. Chapter 3 described an AOP for chemical skin sensitization and dermatitis and Chapters 4 and 5 examined the possibilities to use this AOP for qualitative, semiquantitative, or quantitative predictions. It appears from the discussions in these chapters that qualitative and semiquantitative assessment is possible, but it is not possible to predict the concentrations of nickel that will be required for skin sensitization by the AOP model displayed in Chapter 3. As described in Section 5.4.1

Table 7.4 Comparison of intake recommendations for five essential metals in adult males from Europe,[a] North America,[b] and WHO[c]

| Essential metal | SCF/EFSA | | IOM | | WHO[c] |
	PRI	UL	RDA	UL	SRPMI
Copper (mg/day)	1.1[e]	5	0.9	10	1.3–12
Iron (mg/day)	11[f]	ND	8	45	ND[d]
Manganese (mg/day)	1–10 (a safe and acceptable range)[g]	ND	2.3 (an AI)	11	ND
Selenium (μg/day)	55[h]	300	55	400	40–400
Zinc (mg/day) (moderately available)	9.4–16.3[i]	25	11	40	9.4–45

AI, adequate intake; EFSA, European Food Safety Authority; IOM, Institute of Medicine; ND, not determined; PRI, population reference intake; RDA, recommended dietary allowances; SCF, EU Scientific Committee on Food; SRPMI, safe range of population mean intake; UL, tolerable upper intake level; WHO, World Health Organization.

[a]European Union Scientific Committee on Food (PRIs [SCF, 1993]; manganese [SCF, 2000a]; selenium [SCF, 2000b]; copper [SCF, 2003a]; zinc [SCF, 2003b]; ULs [SCF/NDA, 2006]).

[b]US Institute of Medicine Food and Nutrition Board (selenium [IOM, 2000]; copper, manganese, and zinc [IOM, 2001]; dietary reference intakes summaries [IOM, 2006]).

[c]World Health Organization (WHO, 1996).

[d]The FAO/WHO recommended a requirement of 9 mg Fe/day for an adult male (FAO/WHO, 2002) and WHO (1983) calculated a PMTDI (Provisional maximum tolerable daily intake) of 48 mg Fe/day (0.8 mg/kg b.w.). The range 9–48 can be considered as an acceptable range of oral intake for iron in adult males.

[e]EFSA (2015) considered that they were unable to set PRI because of lack of scientific evidence for copper. An AI of 1.6 mg for adult men was listed, see (EFSA, 2017). EFSA (2017).

[f]EFSA/NDA (2013) unable to set PRI for manganese, an AI of 3 mg was recommended for adults see (EFSA, 2017).

[g]EFSA/NDA (2014a) unable to set PRI. AI = 70 μg/day for adult males.

[h]EFSA/NDA (2014b) estimate derived based on range of phytate intake in European populations.

[i]Partly based on Aggett, P., Nordberg, G.F., Nordberg, M., 2015. Essential metals: assessing risks from deficiency and toxicity. In: Nordberg, G.F., Fowler, B.A., Nordberg, M. (Eds.), Handbook on the Toxicology of Metals, fourth ed. Elsevier Publishers, Amsterdam with updates.

in Chapter 5, the concentrations of nickel causing sensitization was determined by epidemiological method by patch tests in humans by Menné (1994), forming the background for the nickel directive in EU. This directive (94/27/EC) was passed in 1994 and was fully implemented in 2001. It prohibits the sale of products intended to come into direct prolonged contact with the skin that release nickel at rates $>0.5\,\mu g/cm^2$ per week. The maximum nickel release rate for piercing post assemblies is currently $0.2\,\mu g/cm^2$ per week. All forms of jewelry, watches, buttons, and zippers were initially included, and presently, the restrictions include mobile phones as well. The legislation from 1994 is now part of the REACH regulation supervised by ECHA. Nickel is placed on the REACH "restriction list" (see Section 7.2.5, above). Several studies in a number of EU countries have documented the efficient prevention of nickel sensitization that has resulted from this legislation (see Chapter 8, Section 8.10).

7.3.3 Biomonitoring Equivalents

In recent decades, the availability of large sets of biomonitoring data from human populations, for example, National Health and Nutrition Examination Survey (NHANES) in the United States has stimulated the need for an evaluation mechanism for such data. Meek (2008) and Hays et al. (2008) developed the biomonitoring equivalents (BE) approach. This method makes use of established limits in exposure media, such as air, drinking water, and food, representing acceptable risks and converts them into corresponding levels in biomonitoring media such as blood or urine. Zidek et al. (2017) described the use of BE and other methods for interpreting biomonitoring data in a biomonitoring program performed by the Government in Canada. For example, these authors showed the usefulness of a toxicokinetic model for cobalt when interpreting biomonitoring data on this metal.

7.3.4 Summarizing Comments on Risk Management

A risk management approach may thus range from doing nothing or expressing concern for potential toxicity to issuing permissible exposure levels leading to engineering solutions such as instillation of ventilation or water treatment systems, changing manufacturing practices or moving a production facility or plant away from people. The important thing is that whatever risk management solution is promulgated based on the best possible scientific data and rigorous risk assessment practices which consider the issues noted above. Risk assessments, risk characterization, and risk management are likely to be important activities for metals and metal compounds for a long time in the future because these chemical substances are natural components of the environment and many have a number of practical industrial uses. Further advances in risk assessment, integrating molecular mechanisms of action, toxicokinetic and toxicodynamic modeling, and biomonitoring, as well as improved epidemiological methods, are likely to allow more efficient and more preventive risk management for metallic compounds in the future. For other chemicals, it may be possible to decrease human exposures to negligible amounts by proper handling systems like those promoted by REACH. However, the systems, for example, computerized exposure estimations, need to be developed in a way to avoid underestimation of risks.

Since 1990s, the United Nations (UN) and WHO have been committed to strive toward sustainable development. Our Planet, our Health was the title of the report of the WHO Commission on Health and the Environment, 1992, outlining global challenges to health and the environment, the role of food and agriculture, water, energy, industry, human settlements and urbanization; transboundary, and international problems. The report recommended strategies in all these sectors for a sustainable development. The management of problems with metal contaminants is important in all the listed areas. This report was WHO's contribution to the United Nations Conference on Environment and Development in Rio the same year. Several follow-up conferences and summit meetings followed, with the latest one at the UN headquarters in November 2017.

In EU, sustainable development is recognized as an important goal. Concerning metals, the Commission ratified the Minamata Convention on the 18th of May 2017 and strengthened the restrictions on the use and emission of mercury in the EU (see Chapter 8, Section 8.9).

In Sweden, strategies and goals are in place for a sustainable development of society. One important goal is to work for a nontoxic environment. This includes a strict regulation and follow-up of metal emissions and exposures in order for these substances not to pose a threat to human health or the biological diversity. The goal is that concentrations of naturally occurring substances are close to natural occurring levels. Sustainability is a central concept for image of many companies. There is an ongoing discussion in Sweden and many other EU countries on how to introduce activities contributing to the development of a circular economy. Life cycle analyses (LCAs) of products is an important activity supporting such development.

An LCA includes studies of balances of metals in various phases of a product's life from production to waste management and recycling. Recycling of metals is preferable compared to other waste management options because it produces new raw materials without mining from geological deposits. It is important, however, to perform recycling in a good way. Recycling under favorable industrial conditions may cause minimal releases to work environments and general environments, while recycling under primitive conditions, as is sometimes the case in developing countries, may cause considerable human exposures (Fowler et al., 2015c; Fowler, 2017).

7.4 RISK COMMUNICATION

Professionals who make risk assessments and manage risks communicate with workers about the risks related to occupational environments and with the public about environmental risks. A frequently underweighted aspect of the overall risk assessment and management process concerns the development of an effective risk communication plan which is capable of informing stakeholders such as workers, the lay public, news media, legislators, and other societal decision makers of the results of the risk assessment process in "plain language." It is important to construct effective communication tools for such important groups since they may not have sufficient technical backgrounds to correctly appreciate the value of the risk assessment information being transmitted. It is hence important to make a concerted effort to communicate clearly the risk assessment findings in nontechnical terminology. According to USEPA, the following basic rules apply when communicating about environmental risks with the public (Covello et al., 2007):

1. Accept and involve stakeholders as legitimate partners.
2. Listen to people.
3. Be truthful, honest, frank, and open.
4. Coordinate, collaborate, and partner with other credible sources.
5. Meet the needs of the media.
6. Speak clearly and with compassion.
7. Plan thoroughly and carefully.

Sometimes, the public perceives the risk under consideration differently than the risk assessor. A number of factors determine the degree of outrage by the public. Some of these are: how familiar, widespread, or dreaded the risk is and if risks are controllable or not (IPCS, 1999). Methods and tools required for effective risk communication depend on the situation when and how the risk occurs. Identification of unexpected risks of severe health effects may give rise to a perception of emergency and crisis. In the United States, the Centers for Disease Control and Prevention has a website for Crisis and Emergency Risk Communication: https://emergency.cdc.gov/cerc/. This website provides detailed advice about risk communication in a crisis and downloadable wallet cards and other material for use in such situations.

7.5 ETHICAL ISSUES

There are a number of ethical issues embedded in risk analysis/risk management practices. Previous chapters of this book considered some issues of importance, including some generally accepted ethical principles (WHO, 2009). Chapter 4, Section 4.8, reviewed the application of appropriate procedures in human studies and when using animals in developing dose—response data. Considerable efforts are presently made to replace the well-established animal-based toxicity tests with in vitro assays. Ethical considerations regarding the suffering and discomfort of animals in classical animal toxicity tests is an important motivation for these efforts. Other important ethical issues relate to appropriate consideration of sensitive subpopulations and effective communication of risk assessment/risk management decisions to impact populations in a timely manner.

In general, slightly higher risks are usually accepted for occupational exposures than for exposures to the same substance in the general environment. Although the ethical principle for this practice is not altogether clear, the explanation for these differences is as follows: larger population groups including a larger age span are exposed in the general environment than in the occupational environment. Evaluation of occupational risks is often in relation to the general risk pattern for the exposed individual. An occupational risk should be small in relation to other risks for the individual. For widespread exposures in the general environment, however, the number of cases of disease caused in the population may be of concern even if the risk to the individual is negligible. In order to limit the number of cases in the population, lower risks are accepted for substances spread in the general environment.

Risk—benefit analyses often constitute part of the basis together with risk assessments and risk characterization when OELs and other limit values are legislated. It is difficult from an ethical point of view to find the balance between economic benefit and risk because different population groups may set this balance differently. This is an uncertainty when setting acceptable or permissible exposure levels. An important ethical issue at present is the level of protection afforded by the current OELs for pregnant women and their unborn children. Many OEL values are not based on sufficient information about the risk to the unborn child, because such studies are difficult to perform in humans. Animal data introduce additional uncertainty. Even for substances where data are available on risks to the unborn child, it is unclear if present rules provide sufficient safety. In Sweden, monitoring of blood lead levels is compulsory for lead workers. Lower maximum levels apply to women younger than 50 years of age than for men. Pregnant women should change to non-lead-exposed work, and if that is not possible, she will get a paid leave. These rules provide good protection, but it would of course be better and ethically more satisfying if the OELs and biomonitoring values were low enough to provide sufficient protection also for pregnant women and the unborn child.

7.6 EXAMPLES OF SUCCESSFUL PREVENTION OF ADVERSE HEALTH EFFECTS

A major goal of risk analysis/risk management for metallic compounds is the prevention of adverse health effects in the most sensitive subpopulations. This effort ideally requires an efficient integration of the knowledge gained from exposure assessment studies and risk analysis efforts with sound public health and regulatory decision making, leading to concrete preventive actions. Since the above actions are likely to include substantial costs, it is essential to communicate the value of such actions to societal decision makers in order to obtain their cooperation.

As discussed above, there has been considerable improvement in chemical analytical methods as well as in epidemiological methods and inclusion of molecular biomarker endpoints in public health in the last several decades. The advent of these innovations have made it possible to detect adverse human health effects at an earlier stage and lower exposure levels than previously and to relate such adverse effects more precisely to exposure, sometimes through biological monitoring.

A good example is the ban of the use of organic lead (tetraethyl lead) as an additive to petrol. The practice of adding tetraethyl lead to petrol was introduced in the first part of the 1900s in order to improve the octane properties of the fuel. It was then considered to cause no risks to human health and because the number of cars was small, the amount of lead released into the environment was limited. Substantial increases occurred with the expansion of the car fleet in many countries. The interference of lead in petrol with catalytic converters in cars resulted in curtailment of this practice and attendant declines in blood lead values in the general US population as documented by the NHANES survey in the 1970s. Also during this period, other epidemiological information emerged showing correlations between the levels of lead in the blood of children and the occurrence of mild effects on the brain function of the same children. Considerable scientific discussion took place concerning the causality of these findings. Ultimately, subsequent research findings confirmed this adverse effect and resulted in a ban of the use of lead additives in petrol, first in the United States and later in other countries (for review, see Landrigan et al., 2015). This change in population exposure to lead has suggested an estimated change in the IQ of children. Children in the affected countries now may have slightly higher IQ values than children born before the ban was implemented on a population basis.

REFERENCES

AFS, 2015. Hygieniska gränsvarden 2015. AFS 2015:7, p. 74.
Aggett, P., Nordberg, G.F., Nordberg, M., 2015. Essential metals: assessing risks from deficiency and toxicity. In: Nordberg, G.F., Fowler, B.A., Nordberg, M. (Eds.), Handbook on the Toxicology of Metals, fourth ed. Elsevier Publishers, Amsterdam.
Covello, V., Minamayer, S., Clayton, K., 2007. Effective Risk and Crisis Communication during Water Security Emergencies. US EPA.
Cramer, G.M., et al., 1978. J. Cosmet. Toxicol. 16, 255—276.
Deveau, M., et al., 2015. J. Occup. Environ. Hyg. 12 (Suppl. 1), S127.
Duffus, J.H., et al., 2007. Pure Appl. Chem. 79, 1153.
Duffus, J.H., Templeton, D.M., Michael, S., 2017. Comprehensive Glossary of Terms Used in Toxicology. RSC Publishing.
ECHA, 2018. Strategy to Promote Substitution to Safer Chemiscals through Innovation. ECHA, Helsinki, Finland, p. 20.
EFSA, 2009. EFSA J. 7, 1351—1356.
EFSA, 2012. EFSA J. 10, 2985.
EFSA/NDA, 2013. EFSA J. 11 (11), 3419.
EFSA, 2015. EFSA J. 13, 4253.
EFSA, 2017. Dietary reference values for nutrients summary report. EFSA Support. Publ. 14 (12).
EFSA/NDA, 2014a. Scientific opinion on dietary reference values for selenium. EFSA J. 12 (10).
EFSA/NDA, 2014b. Scientific opinion on dietary reference values for zinc. EFSA J. 12 (10).
ESA, 2012. EFSA J. 10, 2985.
FAO/WHO, 2002. Joint FAO/WHO Expert Consultation. Human Vitamin and Mineral Requirements. Rome.
Fowler, B.A., 2016. Molecular Biological Markers for Toxicology and Risk Assessment. Elsevier Publishers, Amsterdam, p. 153.
Fowler, B.A., 2017. Electronic Waste: Toxicology and Public Health Issues. Elsevier Publishers, Amsterdam, p. 84.
Fowler, B.A., Sexton, M.J., 2015. Gallium and semiconductor compounds. In: Nordberg, G.F., Fowler, B.A., Nordberg, M. (Eds.), Handbook on the Toxicology of Metals, fourth ed. Elsevier Publishers, Amsterdam, pp. 787—797.

Fowler, B.A., Chou, S.-H.S., Jones, R.L., Sullivan Jr., D.W., Chen, C.-J., 2015a. Arsenic. In: Nordberg, G.F., Fowler, B.A., Nordberg, M. (Eds.), Handbook on the Toxicology of Metals, fourth ed. Elsevier Publishers, Amsterdam, pp. 582—624.

Fowler, B.A., Oskarsson, A., Alexander, J., 2015b. Toxic metals in food. In: Nordberg, G.F., Fowler, B.A., Nordberg, M. (Eds.), Handbook on the Toxicology of Metals, fourth ed. Elsevier Publishers, Amsterdam, pp. 123—140.

Fowler, B.A., Prusiewicz, C.M., Nordberg, M., 2015c. Metal toxicology in developing countries. In: Nordberg, G.F., Fowler, B.A., Nordberg, M. (Eds.), Handbook on the Toxicology of Metals, fourth ed. Elsevier Publishers, Amsterdam, pp. 529—545.

Fowler, B.A., Weissberg, J.B., 1974. N. Engl. J. Med. 291, 1171.

Hays, S.M., et al., 2008. Regul. Toxicol. Pharmacol. 51, S4.

IARC, 2012. Arsenic, metals, fibres and dusts. In: IARC (Ed.), IARC Monographs, vol. 100C. IARC, Lyons, France.

IOM, 2000. Dietary Reference Intakes for Vitamin C, Vitamin E, Selenium, and Carotenoids. National Academy Press, Washington, DC.

IOM, 2001. Dietary Reference Intakes: Vitamin A, Vitamin K, Arsenic, Boron, Chromium, Copper, Iodine, Iron, Manganese, Molybdenum, Nickel, Silicon, Vanadium, and Zinc. National Academy Press, Washington, DC.

IOM, 2006. In: Otten, J.J., Hellwig, J.P., Meyers, L.D. (Eds.), Dietary Reference Intakes: The Essential Guide to Nutrient Requirements. National Academy Press, Washington, DC.

IPCS, 1999. Environmental Health Criteria 210. In: IPCS (Ed.), Principles for the Assessment of Risks to Human Health from Exposure to Chemicals.

IPCS, 2001. Arsenic and Arsenic Compounds. EHC 224. WHO, Geneva.

IPCS, 2009. Principles and Methods for the Risk Assessment of Chemicals in Food. Environmental health criteria 240.

Landberg, H., 2018. The Use of Exposure Models in Assessing Occupational Exposure to Chemicals. Media Tryck, Lund University, Lund Sweden.

Landrigan, P.J., et al., 2006. Med. Lav. 97, 811.

Landrigan, P.J., Lucchini, R.G., Kotelchuck, D., Grandjean, P., 2015. Principles for the prevention of the toxic effects of metals. In: Nordberg, G.F., Fowler, B.A., Nordberg, M. (Eds.), Handbook on the Toxicology of Metals, fourth ed., pp. 507—525.

Liang, Y., et al., 2006. Regul. Toxicol. Pharmacol. 46, 107.

Meek, M.E., 2008. Regul. Toxicol. Pharmacol. 52, S3.

Menné, T., 1994. Quantitative aspects of nickel dermatitis. Sensitization and eliciting threshold concentrations. Sci. Total Environ. 148, 275—281.

Nordberg, G.F., et al., 1988. Am. J. Ind. Med. 14, 217.

Patlewicz, G., et al., 2008. SAR QSAR Environ. Res. 19, 495.

SCF (Scientific Committee for Food), 1993. Nutrient and Energy Intakes for the European Community. Report of the Scientific Committee on Food, Thirty-First Series. European Commission, Luxembourg, p. 255.

SCF, 2000a. Opinion on the Tolerable Upper Level of Manganese. Report SCF/CS/NUT/UPPLEV/21 Final, Brussels, 11 pp.

SCF, 2000b. Opinion on the Tolerable Upper Intake Level of Selenium. Report SFC/CS/NUT/UPPLEV/25 Final, Brussels, 18 pp.

SCF, 2003a. Opinion on the Tolerable Upper Intake Level of Copper. Report SCF/CS/NUT/UPPLEV/57 Final, Brussels, 19 pp.

SCF, 2003b. Opinion on the Tolerable Upper Intake Level of Zinc. Report SFC/CS/NUT/UPPLEV/62 Final, Brussels, 10 pp.

SCF/NDA (SCF Scientific Panel on Dietetic Products, Nutrition and Allergies), 2006. Tolerable Upper Intake Levels for Vitamins and Minerals. European Food Safety Authority.

Scinicariello, F., et al., 2010. Environ. Health Perspect. 118, 259.

Solomon, K.R., et al., 2016. Crit. Rev. Toxicol. 46, 835.

USEPA, 2018a. Drinking Water Contaminants-Standards and Regulations. www.epa.gov.

USEPA, 2018b. Risk Assessment for Carcinogenic Effects. https://www.epa/fera/risk-assessment-carcinogenic-effects.

WHO, 1983. Iron. WHO Food Additive Series 18. WHO, Geneva.

WHO, 1996. Trace Elements in Human Nutrition and Health. World Health Organization, Geneva.

WHO, 2009. Research Ethics Committees Basic Concepts for Capacity Building.

Zidek, A., et al., 2017. A review of human biomonitoring data used in regulatory risk assessment under Canada's chemicals management program. Int. J. Hyg. Environ. Health 220 (2 Pt A), 167−178.

CHAPTER EIGHT

Examples of Risk Assessments of Human Metal Exposures and the Need for Mode of Action (MOA), Toxicokinetic-Toxicodynamic (TKTD) Modeling, and Adverse Outcome Pathways (AOPs)

Abstract

Metals are elements and intrinsic components of the earth's crust. Humans have always been exposed to naturally occurring levels in the environment and some of the metals are essential for human health. Human activities such as mining and production of metals, materials for construction of buildings, ships, automobiles, consumer items, biocides, pesticides, and medicines all involve metals. Considerable exposures of humans have occurred in the past and continue today in working environments where these activities take place. By adding to the natural geochemical cycle of metals, for example, mercury, humans have increased the quantities in these cycles. This has caused increased levels in biota, such as fish, used for human consumption. Present human exposures to metals and their compounds therefore are increased compared to the natural exposure in the ancient past. It is important to make adequate risk assessments of these exposures in order to take adequate preventive measures so that adverse human health effects are avoided. Previous chapters in this book have described methods for risk assessment; Chapter 2 deals with measurements and descriptions of exposure, internal dose, and toxicokinetics; Chapter 3 describes how to perform biomonitoring defines mode of action (MoA), target dose, and adverse outcome pathways (AOPs). Chapter 4 discusses how to identify and assess hazard, and Chapters 5 and 6 reviews methods for dose—effect and dose—response relationships;and Chapter 7 on applied risk assessment deals with the translation of exposure and toxicological data into prevention and management of risks by regulatory action. The present chapter gives examples from available data on 14 metals and their compounds, what information is available, and their use in risk assessments performed by international and national organizations preparing preventive recommendations or regulations. The 14 metals included in this chapter represent well-investigated metals/metalloids like arsenic, cadmium, lead, and mercury where risk assessments are available from established organizations. The chapter deals with cadmium in more detail than it

Risk Assessment for Human Metal Exposures
ISBN: 978-0-12-804227-4
https://doi.org/10.1016/B978-0-12-804227-4.00008-X

does with the other major metals because the cadmium section illustrates the use of toxicokinetic-toxicodynamic (TKTD) modeling in the risk assessment. The chapter also includes nickel, cobalt, and platinum, sensitizing metals in order to evaluate possible use of general knowledge on sensitization for risk assessment. A few metals are included where the database is limited such as gallium, indium, palladium, and the lanthanides (lanthanum, cerium, and gadolinium). For all the 14 metals, the chapter includes pertinent available data from the scientific literature and examples of risk assessments by recognized organizations, if available. Discussions consider the possible use of MoA, TKTD, and AOP models in the risk assessment of each metal.

8.1 ALUMINUM (AL)

8.1.1 Properties, Uses, Occurrence and Toxicokinetics

Aluminum (Al), CAS No. 7429-90-5, atomic No. 13, atomic mass 26.98, density 2.7 g/cm^3, and melting point 660.4°C, is a light, ductile metal. Exposure to air or water creates a thin film of oxide on its surface, protecting from further corrosion. It is a good conductor of heat and electricity, and it is easy to weld. It is the third most abundant element in the earth's crust, about 8% by mass. The solubility of aluminum compounds is pH dependent. Aluminum hydroxide is the least soluble compound at pH 6.2. Part of this section on aluminum is a summary of the review by Sjogren et al. (2015) where specific references are found.

Methods used for determination of aluminum in various media: inductively coupled plasma atomic emission spectroscopy (ICP-AES), inductively coupled plasma mass spectrometry (ICP-MS), and graphite furnace atomic absorption spectroscopy. Contamination is a major problem in sampling and determination of aluminum in various media because of background levels in air and precipitated dust. The world production in 2012 was 48 million metric tons.

Uses of aluminum: aluminum is used in airplanes, trains, trucks, cars, the construction industry, and in food preparation and storage. Aluminum powders are used in paints, explosives, and fireworks. Potassium alum $(KAl(SO_4)_2\ 12H_2O)$ is an adjuvant in vaccines as are aluminum hydroxide hydrated gels and aluminum phosphate. Aluminum hydroxide, aluminum phosphate, and sucralfate (sucrose sulfate aluminum complex) have been used for treatment of gastritis and ulcers. Aluminum salts have been used as phosphate binders. Alum solution is used as an intravesical irrigant for bladder hemorrhage. Aluminum salts are used topically in antiperspirants, against inflammatory skin conditions, and as an astringent. Aluminum silicates are used in cosmetics. Aluminum compounds are also used as food additives. Aluminum salts are used as flocculants in drinking water treatment.

The median **intake of aluminum in food** in adults ranges 3.6—9 mg/day in North America, Europe, China, and Japan. Aluminum-containing baking powder is high in aluminum, 2 g/100 g. Processed cheese, cake mixes, frozen dough, pancake mixes, and pickled vegetables contain high levels. Tea contains 0.67—6 mg/L. Aluminum utensils also contributes to aluminum intake. Canned soft drinks contain on average 0.7 mg/L. Drinking water contributes approximately 0.1 mg/day.

Aluminum in **ambient air** is $20-500 \text{ ng/m}^3$ in rural air and $1000-6000 \text{ ng/m}^3$ in urban air.

Workroom air levels of aluminum during aluminum powder production in the 1990s were $5-21 \text{ mg/m}^3$. During aluminum welding, it was $1-4 \text{ mg/m}^3$.

Toxicokinetics: Isotope ^{26}Al studies of intake through drinking water showed approximately 0.3% uptake. Determinations by atomic absorption in food and urine indicated 0.1—0.3% fractional absorption of aluminum in various food items. Increased absorption is seen when aluminum-containing food is taken with citrate. Absorbed aluminum is mainly bound to transferrin in plasma, and in addition, it occurs as citrate. The normal body burden of aluminum is 30—50 mg. The skeleton contains 50% and the lung 25%. Workers exposed to welding fume (sparsely soluble) have a considerably increased lung burden, and increased excretion in urine has been seen for many years after the end of exposure. Workers exposed to aluminum sulfate (water soluble) have only a small increase in lung burden, and urinary aluminum decreased quickly after cessation of exposure. The aluminum content of bone, brain, and other tissues increases with age. There is an increase in brain aluminum in dialysis dementia. There are no TKTD modeling data available for use in risk assessment. Weisser et al. (2017) discussed the data requirements for such calculations in relation to the use of aluminum adjuvants in immunizations. Excretion of aluminum is through urine (>95%), probably mainly as citrate. Biliary secretion accounts for less than 2%. Small amounts are excreted in breast milk. After intravenous injection of aluminum citrate, its half-life in blood was 1 h, in trabecular bone was 1.4 years, and in cortical bone was 29 years. Serum/plasma or urine is the most frequently used media for **biomonitoring**. Plasma aluminum in occupationally nonexposed persons was most often <5 µg/L. In Finland, 2.7 µg/L is the upper reference level for nonoccupationally exposed persons; the corresponding level in urine is 16 µg/L. Experience from uremia patients in dialysis and the risk of dialysis encephalopathy is the basis for a recommendation that serum levels of aluminum should be below 20 µg/L. Urinary aluminum levels are used in occupational biomonitoring. There is a linear relationship between aluminum levels in air and urinary levels at the end of a work shift. Neurotoxic effects have been observed in aluminum welders with urinary aluminum of 100 µg/L or higher. For soluble aluminum compounds, there is no similar evidence.

8.1.2 Health Effects

Gastrointestinal symptoms: rashes and mouth ulcers occurred in persons accidentally exposed to drinking water with pH 3 and up to 109 mg/L of aluminum.

Occupational exposure to aluminum-containing minerals, often accompanied by silica may lead to **fibrosis of the lungs, Shaver disease** (Shaver and Rydell, 1947). Occupational exposure to stamped aluminum powder, even in the absence of silica, gives rise to **fibrosis of the lungs, aluminosis**. Cases often progressed rapidly and death occurred in several cases in a few years after the onset (Ahlmark et al., 1960). Such cases are nowadays rare, but early-stage aluminum-induced pneumoconiosis still occurs (Kraus et al., 2006). Occupational aluminum exposure can also give rise to **obstructive pulmonary disease**; workers in electrolytic aluminum production exposed to a complex mixture of fluorides, aluminum compounds, and other agents may develop asthma, so called **potroom asthma**. Workroom exposure to aluminum salts such as aluminum fluoride, aluminum sulfate, and aluminum tetrafluoride has also been associated with **occupational asthma** (review: Sjogren et al., 2015).

Aluminum poisoning from other medical uses of aluminum compounds: several reports describe aluminum accumulation and poisoning symptoms in patients without chronic renal failure. Preterm infants fed intravenously had impaired neurological development related to aluminum accumulation. An aluminum-containing cement used for bone reconstruction in neurosurgery caused aluminum accumulation in brain tissue and **encephalopathy**. Intravesical alum instillations caused aluminum accumulation and **nephrotoxicity**.

Dialysis encephalopathy is a disease that occurred mainly before 1975 in dialysis patients when dialysis water contained too high (>80 µg/L) concentrations of aluminum, for example, untreated tap water. Symptoms include speech disorders, followed by dementia, myoclonus, and seizures. There were many lethal cases. The concomitant use of drugs as aluminum phosphate binders may have contributed to aluminum accumulation in tissues. Brain, muscles, and other tissues of the affected patients had elevated aluminum levels. Today dialysis fluid water is monitored, and the aluminum level is kept <10 µg/L. However, because of accidental failures of technical systems, occasional cases still occur. Some dialysis patients develop aluminum-induced **anemia** (Sjogren et al., 2015).

Several studies of aluminum welders report **neurobehavioral effects** related to aluminum exposure. The aluminum welders had inferior performance in several psychological performance tests, e.g., the digit symbol test, compared to steel welders. The aluminum level in urine of the affected aluminum welders were around 100 µg/L.

An association has been reported between the risk of dementing brain disorders including Alzheimer disease and an increased level of aluminum in drinking water. There are also reports of an increased level of aluminum in brain tissue from deceased Alzheimer disease patients. However, other studies have not found such associations, and there is no consensus on whether available studies provide sufficient evidence of an increased risk of Alzheimer disease in relation to aluminum exposure. There is no evidence for a relationship between occupational aluminum exposure and Alzheimer disease (summary by Sjogren et al., 2015).

Dialysis patients with serum aluminum >30 µg/L accumulate aluminum in **bone** tissue and have a high incidence of fracturing dialysis osteodystrophy. Persons without renal failure taking gram amounts of aluminum compounds as antacids on a long-term basis may develop osteomalacia. This is due to phosphate depletion caused by a decrease of phosphate absorption caused by aluminum binding to phosphate in the gastrointestinal (GI) tract. Premature infants given intravenous feeding with standard or aluminum-depleted feeding solutions were examined after 15 years. The children given standard solutions had decreased hip bone mineral content compared to those given aluminum-depleted feeding solutions.

Itching **skin** nodules may occur (<1%) after immunization with aluminum-containing vaccines and are related to development of sensitization against aluminum.

Inflammatory changes in the lungs of aluminum-exposed workers (see above, this section) are related to increased plasma fibrinogen levels, a known risk factor for **ischemic heart disease**. Increased risks of ischemic heart disease in aluminum workers and in population groups exposed to ambient air pollution may be related to such changes.

Aluminum phosphide is a fumigant used as insecticide. It releases phosphine in the presence of moisture and phosphine poisoning may occur.

8.1.3 Human Health Risk Assessments and Exposure Limits

Several national and international organizations have issued exposure recommendations for aluminum and its compounds. The risk assessments that form the basis for these exposure limits have all used traditional methods, for example, no-observed-adverse-effect level (NOAEL) in animals and uncertainty assessment factors. As far as we know, no TKTD- or adverse outcome pathway (AOP)-based recommendations exist.

The Joint Food and Agriculture Organization of the United Nations/ World Health Organization (WHO) Expert Committee on Food Additives (JECFA, 2011a) recommended a provisional tolerable weekly intake (PTWI) of 2 mg/kg b.w. for all aluminum compounds in food. A NOAEL of 30 mg/kg per day in rats is the basis for this value (210 mg/kg b.w. per week in rats). The WHO (2004) did not derive a health-based limit value for aluminum in drinking water, but they issued a technical value of 0.1 mg/L in large drinking water plants and 0.2 mg/L for small plants. Health Canada (2012) issued similar values. Several countries as well as independent organizations like the American Conference of Governmental Industrial Hygienists in the United States issue occupational exposure limits (OELs) and biological tolerance values in urine. The NOAEL estimation from workplace exposures in combination with available toxicological data from animal experiments sometimes considers toxicokinetic (TK) relationships. We list the following hygienic limit values (HGVs), valid at present (2018) in Sweden (AFS, 2015, 2018): aluminum metal dust (total) 5 mg/m^3, respirable 2 mg/m^3; soluble salts 1 mg/m^3; and potassium aluminum tetrafluoride 0.4 mg/m^3. Scientists in Finland (Rihimäki and Aitio, 2012) suggested a biological level of 80 µg/L in urine (preshift after 2 days without exposure) as an action limit to decrease occupational exposures.

Dialysis water should have <10 µg/L. In the United States, a maximum of 0.85 mg per dose is permitted in vaccines and the aluminum content of drugs used in total parenteral nutrition must not exceed 25 µg/L.

8.2 ARSENIC (AS)

8.2.1 Introduction/Properties

Arsenic (As), CAS No. 7440-38-2 for metallic As, atomic No. 33, atomic mass 74.9, is a metalloid. Dimethyl arsenic acid (DMA) also named cacodylic acid and monomethylarsonic acid (MMA) methylarsonic acid are organic arsenic compounds formed in the human body after exposure to inorganic arsenic. This chapter section on arsenic is in part a summary of the review by Fowler et al. (2015), and the reader is referred to that review for specific references.

There are several instrumental methods for determination of As in various media. At present, ICP-MS is the one most used. For accurate analyses, the interference of Ar—Cl in the plasma must be overcome. High-resolution ICP-MS is not sensitive to this interference. With other instruments, the interference can be overcome by use of a dynamic reaction cell or a collision cell. Speciation of arsenic compounds is possible. Fowler et al. (2015) reviewed the available methods.

8.2.2 Production and Uses

The earth's crust contains 3.4 ppm of As. It occurs in sulfide ores and is a byproduct of smelting copper and lead as arsenic trioxide (As_2O_3). Arsenic metal and other As-compounds are produced from As_2O_3. The world production in 2017 was 37,000 metric tons (USGS, 2017).

Historically, inorganic arsenic compounds were used as drugs, but their present use is limited to research on possible use in certain forms of leukemia. Organic arsenicals have been extensively used in the treatment of protozoal diseases and are sometimes still used as an antimicrobial agent in swine and poultry feed. Inorganic arsenicals are still used as pesticides and wood preservatives (copper chromium arsenate) and herbicides (monosodium arsenate and cacodylic acid (DMA)). They are used in glass manufacturing and for purification of industrial gases. Metallic As is alloyed with several other metals for improved properties. GaAs and InAs crystals are used as semiconductors in electronics, solar cells, and space research. Because of its toxicity, the use of arsenic and its compounds is restricted in the European Union (EU) (see Chapter 7, Section 7.2.5).

8.2.3 Environmental Levels and Human Exposures

Arsenic occurs in a number of chemical forms in **foodstuffs**. The highest levels of total As occurs in fish, crustaceans, and seaweed. Fish and crustaceans contain arsenobetaine and arsenocholine. Seaweeds contain arsenophospholipids and arsenosugars. The content of inorganic As in seafood is low. There is uptake of arsenic in plants from soil and irrigation water. In rice, for example, arsenic is present partly as inorganic arsenic and partly as DMA. High levels of arsenic in rice-based infant food are of concern, particularly for those with celiac disease, who need gluten-free food. The highest level of inorganic As in food is in rice. Intake of inorganic As from food in the United States is $1-20$ µg/day. Wine and mineral water may contain high levels.

Seawater and most rivers and lakes contain low levels of As. **Groundwater** is usually low in arsenic, but groundwater from arsenic-containing bedrock can be high. Some small parts of the United States and Canada have >50 µg/L, with values up to 3400 µg/L. Both DMA and inorganic forms of As occur in **drinking water**, but most is inorganic. Also in Sweden, there are some limited areas with As in groundwater used as drinking water >50 µg/L. In Mexico, Bangladesh, India, and Vietnam highly elevated levels of arsenic in drinking water occur from tube wells drilled in arsenic-containing bedrock. In Bangladesh and West Bengal, India, more than 1 million people have drinking water with elevated arsenic. In one study, 62% had levels above the WHO drinking water permissible exposure level 10 µg/L.

Arsenic in **soil** usually is $1-40$ mg/kg. In contaminated areas, it is up to 50,000 mg/kg.

In **ambient air**, arsenic occurs as particles. Volcanoes and coal combustion contributes emissions to ambient air and so does industries like metal smelters. In the United States, its levels in ambient air were $1-3$ ng/m^3 in rural areas and up to 20 ng/m^3 in urban areas (USEPA, 2012); up to 1.4 µg/m^3 occurred near a smelter in Eastern Europe. Arsenic in **tobacco** causes inhalation exposure to arsenic. In the 1950s, it was up to 40 µg/cigarette, because of the use of arsenical pesticides. In the last decades, arsenic levels in tobacco have been 3 µg/g or lower.

Workroom air in industries handling arsenic and its compounds often has elevated levels. In the past milligrams per m^3 were common. Present levels are near or lower than the present OEL of 0.01 mg/m^3.

8.2.4 Kinetics and Metabolism

Absorption after **inhalation** of As$_2$O$_3$ was 40%$-$60% of the inhaled amount (measured as urinary excretion). Insoluble compounds are absorbed slower than soluble ones. After **oral intake** of soluble trivalent or pentavalent inorganic As, more than 90% is taken up systemically. Particle size is important for the GI absorption of As_2O_3, with limited water solubility. Insoluble compounds are absorbed to a limited extent. Organic forms of As in seafood are taken up >80% after ingestion. MMA and DMA are well absorbed in the GI tract (>75%). The GI absorption of arsanilic acid is 15%—40%. **Skin absorption** is more limited. Animal experiments indicated 6.4% systemic absorption of soluble inorganic arsenic compounds after 24 h. However, accidental skin exposure causes poisoning in workers.

Transport and metabolism: The distribution of As, after exposure to inorganic forms, is different among animal species. Rats accumulate considerable levels of As in the form of DMA bound to hemoglobin in erythrocytes. Most other animal species and humans do not display such accumulation. The extent of metabolism, i.e., methylation, varies greatly among animal species; guinea pigs, marmoset, and tamarin monkeys do not methylate inorganic arsenic. Methylation requires that arsenic is in the trivalent form. In humans, methylation takes place in many tissues and to a great extent in the liver. Arsenic methyl transferase (As3MT) is of central importance for methylation. Studies are ongoing of polymorphic forms of this enzyme in relation to disease occurrence. After ingestion of low doses of inorganic arsenic in humans, urinary arsenic consists of 20% inorganic arsenic, 20% methylarsonic acid, and 60% DMA.

Arsenobetaine is distributed systemically but is quickly excreted unchanged into urine. Arsenocholine is to a great extent oxidized to arsenobetaine in vivo.

Excretion of organic arsenic compounds as well as inorganic arsenic and its metabolites is mainly through urine. Only a minor part is excreted in feces. Small amounts are also excreted in breast milk. The **biological half–life** of arsenic after systemic uptake of inorganic arsenic is 40—60 h in humans. A small proportion may have a longer half-life, 38 days. The organic forms in seafood have a half-life of less than 20 h. Ingested MMA and DMA have similarly short half-lives (summarized from Fowler et al., 2015).

8.2.5 Mechanism of Action for Arsenical Toxicity

Inhibition of mitochondrial respiration is a well-established subcellular effect of arsenic and its metabolites. It causes the formation of intracellular reactive oxygen species (ROS) causing oxidative stress with damage to DNA and other intracellular molecules. The methylation of inorganic arsenical species was originally considered a detoxification process. However, in the last 2 decades increasing evidence is accumulating concerning the formation of highly toxic trivial forms of MMA (III) and DMA(III) as intermediates in the methylation process. These intermediates probably are responsible for much of the mitochondrial toxicity and related ROS formation. Exposure to inorganic arsenic also causes derangement of porphyrin metabolism with increased excretion of uroporphyrin in humans, and these changes may contribute to cellular adverse effects. ROS formation in tissues may explain why exposure to arsenicals causes changes in antioxidant cellular defense systems, alters cell signaling pathways, and produces changes in cellular and urinary concentration of heat shock proteins, and causes apoptosis and necrosis and cancer.

8.2.6 Biomonitoring

8.2.6.1 Urine

Because all forms of arsenic are excreted in urine, the level of arsenic in urine is a good indicator of recent exposure. Inorganic arsenic exposure is of toxicological interest but not the organic forms of arsenic in fish. It is therefore useful to separate these forms when using arsenic in urine for biomonitoring. The sum of inorganic arsenic (iAs), MMA and DMA in urine is a good indicator of exposure to inorganic arsenic. Buchet et al. (2003) used hydride generation in combination with atomic absorption spectrometry (HG-AAS) and reported higher levels of the mentioned sum of values in urine samples from China compared to Belgium. Signes-Pastor et al. (2017) used ion chromatography-ICP-MS and found higher urinary excretion of iAs + MMA among children consuming rice products and higher concentration of urinary arsenobetaine (AsB) in a group consuming seafood compared to a control group.

8.2.6.2 Blood

Blood is used to a more limited extent for biomonitoring of arsenic exposures. Because of the short half-life of various species of arsenic blood, the values fluctuate in relation to ongoing exposure. Like in urine, the species of arsenic in blood reflect the exposure. All forms of arsenic (iAs, MMA, DMA, and AsB) have been detected in blood.

8.2.6.3 Hair

Arsenic in hair is used as a somewhat uncertain indicator of long-term arsenic exposure. Because arsenic may take up arsenic both directly from the environment and via the hair follicle during growth, it may be impossible to distinguish the source. IAs, MMA, and DMA, but not AsB, have been detected in hair, and it seems, thus, that arsenic from fish consumption is not reflected in hair levels.

8.2.7 Effects and Dose-–Response Relationships

8.2.7.1 Acute and Subacute Effects

It is well known that arsenic trioxide is a very poisonous substance. Inhalation of high doses can cause acute poisoning with lethal outcome. In humans, a lethal oral dose of arsenic trioxide or other inorganic arsenic compounds is 1–3 mg/kg per day. Death occurs because of multiorgan failure. In less severe acute poisoning cases, symptoms and signs are similar to those in subacute poisoning.

In subacute, oral poisoning by inorganic arsenic compounds, GI symptoms are prominent. Capillary damage leads to vasodilatation, transudation of plasma, and multiorgan failure including heart failure. In cases occurring after inhalation, respiratory symptoms are prominent with cough, tracheobronchitis, bronchial pneumonia, and nasal septum perforation. Neurotoxicity with peripheral sensory neuropathy and sometimes encephalopathy are common manifestations. Kidney toxicity includes both tubular and glomerular involvement, sometimes, cortical necrosis and anuria occur. Hepatotoxicity may occur. Hematological manifestations include anemia, thrombocytopenia, and leukopenia. Skin rash may occur (summarized from Fowler et al., 2015).

8.2.7.2 Chronic Noncardiovascular Effects

Long-term exposure to inorganic arsenic gives rise to skin changes in the form of hyperpigmentation with patches of depigmentation and palmoplantar hyperkeratosis. GI symptoms include those of gastritis and colitis. Raynaud's syndrome occurs because of peripheral vascular changes. Neurological manifestations include hearing loss, encephalopathy, and peripheral polyneuropathy. There may be hepatic and renal toxicity. Hematological changes include anemia, thrombocytopenia, and leukopenia.

8.2.7.3 Chronic Cardiovascular Effects

Exposure to inorganic arsenic may cause cardiac effects like arrhythmias, ECG changes, and pericarditis. Arsenic-exposed smelter workers and glass blowers had an increased mortality from cardiovascular diseases. Blackfoot disease is a characteristic vascular disease associated with long-term exposure to inorganic arsenic. It occurred in areas of Taiwan with elevated arsenic in drinking water. The patients suffer severe systemic arteriosclerosis with black, mummified dry foot-gangrene in severe cases. Population groups in these areas also had an increased occurrence of microvascular diseases and carotid atherosclerosis; they also had an increased mortality from cardiovascular diseases, stroke, and carotid atherosclerosis. Although Blackfoot disease was not reported in other populations exposed to inorganic arsenic, peripheral vascular disease with Raynaud's disease, microangiopathies, vasospastic tendency, and acrocyanosis were reported in smelter workers exposed to inorganic arsenic (Lagerkvist et al., 1986). There is an increased occurrence of erectile dysfunction in men exposed to inorganic arsenic in drinking water. There was in increased prevalence of hypertension in the areas with Blackfoot disease in Taiwan, as well as in areas with increased levels of arsenic in drinking water in Bangladesh and Chile.

8.2.7.4 *Carcinogenic Effects*

The International Agency for Research on Cancer (IARC, 2004) reviewed the literature and concluded that there is sufficient evidence in humans that arsenic in drinking water causes cancer of the urinary bladder, lung, and skin. Further, there are reports of increased prevalence in humans of other cancers in groups exposed to inorganic arsenic: nasal cavity, larynx, GI tract, breast, liver, kidney, prostate, and brain. In 2012, the IARC concluded that in addition to the evidence in humans, there is sufficient evidence in experimental animals for the carcinogenicity of inorganic arsenic compounds. IARC (2012) further reconfirmed that arsenic and arsenic compounds are carcinogenic to humans (IARC Group 1).

Mechanisms of carcinogenicity: ROS formation induced by inorganic arsenic may influence DNA and cause cancer (see above). Inorganic arsenic compounds show poor genotoxicity. However, As (III) reduces DNA-methylation, may perturb the transcription of genes like c-jun and c-fos, and alter histone modifications in humans (Davidson et al., 2015). Several epidemiological studies report a relationship between methylation of inorganic arsenic and the risk of cancer (see below).

8.2.7.4.1 Skin Cancer

Long-term exposure to inorganic arsenic in drinking water was shown in a dose—response relationship to be related to the risk of skin cancer in Taiwan. The occurrence of this type of cancer was also related to inhalation exposure to sodium arenite. Skin cancer risk was related to serum arsenic level and inversely related to serum beta-carotene. Methylation capacity (proportion of MMA in urinary arsenic) and genotype of certain enzymes or polymorphisms in gene promoters for IL-10 modified the risk of skin cancer induced by inorganic arsenic.

Based on the Taiwan skin cancer data, the US Environmental Protection Agency (USEPA) calculated a unit risk for inorganic arsenic in drinking water of 5×10^{-5} per µg/L (USEPA, 2012).

8.2.7.4.2 Lung Cancer

Reports, mainly in the 1980s from the United States and Sweden, show a dose—response relationship between exposure to inorganic arsenic, mainly through inhalation by smelter workers in nonferrous metal smelting operations and the occurrence of lung cancer among the workers. There was an interaction between inhaled inorganic arsenic and cigarette smoking. Also, in population groups living near the metal smelting industries, but without occupational exposure, there was an increase in lung cancer. Exposure to inorganic arsenic through drinking water increases the risk of lung cancer, particularly among smokers. Studies in Taiwan, Japan, and Argentina show a dose—response relationship between intake of arsenic through drinking water and occurrence of lung cancer. Risks were higher among those with a high proportion of MMA in urine compared to those with low MMA in urine. This indicates an importance of methylation for carcinogenesis.

Based on the US data concerning lung cancer in smelter workers exposed to inorganic arsenic through inhalation, the USEPA (2012) derived a unit risk estimate: the excess risk of lung cancer associated with a lifetime exposure to 1-µg inhaled inorganic arsenic/m^3 is 4.3×10^{-3}.

8.2.7.4.3 Cancer of the Kidneys and the Bladder (Urothelial Cancer)

Many studies have documented associations between ingestion and inhalation of inorganic arsenic and cancers of the bladder and kidney, especially urothelial cancers. These studies include population groups with elevated levels of inorganic arsenic in drinking water, patients treated with Fowler's solution, and vintners consuming arsenic-containing wine as well as copper smelter workers in the United States and Japan exposed mainly by inhalation. Cohort studies in Taiwan found significant dose—response relationships between ingested inorganic arsenic from drinking water and the risk of bladder cancer (see, for example, Chapter 5, Fig. 5.6). There is a link between the susceptibility to arsenic-induced cancer of the bladder (urothelial cancer) and specific GST (Glutathione-S-transferase) and As3MT alleles. The percentage of iAs or MMA in urine was related to the risk of developing urothelial cancer (Wang et al., 2009). Epigenetic mechanisms involving DNA methylation may be important in influencing the induction of cancer by inorganic arsenic.

8.2.7.4.4 Liver Cancer and Other Internal Cancers

Several studies reported statistically significant associations between exposures to ingested or inhaled inorganic arsenic and hepatic angiosarcoma and hepatocellular carcinoma. Such exposures were also associated with an increased risk of GI cancers, hematolymphatic malignancies, and malignant neoplasms of the brain and nervous system. One report found an increased mortality from cancer of the nasal cavity after exposure to arsenic through drinking water (Chen and Wang, 1990).

8.2.8 Risk Assessments and Recommended Preventive Measures Including Exposure Limits Set by International Organizations

WHO in their drinking water guidelines (WHO, 2011) reviewed available information on cancer risks extending down below 50 μg/L for long-term intake of inorganic arsenic through drinking water. They concluded that available data on mode of action do not provide a basis for either a linear or a nonlinear dose—response extrapolation. The report states: "In view of the practical difficulties in removing arsenic from drinking water and practical quantification in the region 1—10 μg/L, the value 10 μg/L is retained and designated as provisional."

ECHA/RAC (2017) summarized available data as follows:

The cancer mode of action of arsenic and its inorganic compounds has not been established, but it appears not to be related to direct DNA reactive genotoxicity and therefore it is possible that the arsenic carcinogenicity has a threshold exposure level. However, the available data do not allow the identification of threshold exposure levels for key events in the modes of action proposed in the scientific literature. Dose response relationships were derived by linear extrapolation. Extrapolating outside the range of observation inevitably introduces uncertainties. As the mechanistic evidence is suggestive of non-linearity, it is acknowledged that the excess risks in the low exposure range might be an overestimate.

Based on the DECOS (2012) risk estimates derived from an epidemiology study in the United States (the Anaconda copper smelter plant), the ECHA/RAC (2017) derived the following risk estimate for workers:

Based on a 40-year working life (8 h/day, 5 days/week), an excess lifetime lung cancer mortality risk $= 1.4 \times 10^{-4}$ per μg As/m^3 (derived for the inhalable particulate fraction).

An OEL was not suggested.

In Sweden, an OEL (HGV) of 0.01 mg/m^3 as a time-weighted average (TWA) is in effect since many years (AFS, 2015, 2018). According to the recent estimates by the ECHA/RAC (2017), this level would correspond to a lifetime risk of 1.4×10^{-3}, i.e., one worker out of a thousand would be expected to develop lung cancer due to the occupational exposure. This is a small fraction of the background risk of lung cancer in the general population and an even smaller fraction of the lung cancer risk among smokers. It is important, however, to make sure that arsenic workers do not smoke, because there is a synergistic effect between smoking and arsenic exposure.

It is obvious from the comments by WHO and ECHA/RAC that there is a need for better understanding of MOA and TKTD relationships for the carcinogenic effects of inorganic arsenic compounds. If robust and generally recognized models can be established, their use in interpretation of epidemiological findings and observed interactions may furnish important support for future preventive action against cancer induced by exposure to these carcinogens.

8.2.9 Arsine

(Hydrogen arsenide, AsH_3) is colorless flammable gas with garlic odor. It is formed when nascent hydrogen contacts arsenic. Because arsenic is present as an impurity in many metal ores, arsine occurs in metal industries, nonferrous metal refineries and steel industries if the ores are exposed to acid. Arsine is used in doping silicon-based chips and in the production of GaAs and InAs semiconductors.

Arsine is a powerful hemolytic poison both in acute and long-term exposure. Clinical symptoms of poisoning occur after exposure for a few hours to $0.5-10$ mg/m^3.

Symptoms include nausea, headache, poor appetite, abdominal colic, palpitation on exertion, and blood-colored urine and jaundice. With longer exposures, anemia is a prominent feature. Arsenic in urine is elevated. Blockage of renal tubule by hemoglobin can cause renal failure.

Animal experiments have shown anemia, porphyrinuria, and changes in the immune system.

An OEL (TWA) of 0.05 mg/m^3 is used in Sweden (AFS, 2015, 2018).

8.3 CADMIUM (CD)

8.3.1 Introduction/Properties

Cadmium (Cd), CAS No. 7440-43-9, atomic No. 48, atomic mass 112.4, density 8.6 g/cm^3, melting point 321°C, is a silvery or bluish white metal, with oxidation state +2; cadmium oxide and cadmium sulfide are insoluble in water while cadmium chloride and cadmium nitrate are soluble in water. Cd^{2+} has some chemical similarities to zinc but is considerably more thiophilic than zinc. In metallothionein (MT), the tetrathiolate binding of Cd is three orders of magnitude stronger than it is for Zn. The most used analytical method for determination of Cd in various media is ICP-MS. It is important to ascertain adequate quality control of chemical analyses in order to avoid erroneous values. Parts of this chapter section represent a summary of the information in Nordberg et al. (2015, 2018), where specific references can be found if not given in the text here.

8.3.2 Production and Uses

Cadmium occurs in ores and soil together with zinc in ratios 1:100 to 1:1000. It is a by-product to zinc, copper, and lead production from sulfide ores containing these elements. The world production, presently taking place largely in Asia, has increased from less than 200 metric tons in the 1930s to around 20,000 metric tons around the year 1990 and since then has remained almost constant. The recycling of cadmium is approximately 25% after year 2000. In 2016, the world production was 23,000 metric tons (USGS, 2017). In recognition of its toxicity, the Swedish Government has since the 1970s restricted the most dispersive uses of cadmium such as for plating, most of the uses as a stabilizer in plastics and as pigments. These rules are now a part of the EU legislation. Cadmium is on the restriction list according to REACH. An extension of the EU battery directive (2006/66/EC) prohibits the use (with few exceptions) of NiCd batteries in cordless tools in the EU. Outside of EU, cadmium is still used for plating of steel, in plastics and paints, in NiCd batteries, and in alloys with copper. Cadmium telluride is increasingly used worldwide in thin-film solar panels. CeS can replace some Cd pigments and Ba—Zn or Ca—Zn stabilizers replace Cd stabilizers in plastics.

8.3.3 Environmental Occurrence and Human Exposures

Environmental pollution with cadmium, although in a limited scale, has taken place for several thousand years, ever since humans started to produce metals from ores. Metal mining and smelting in the 20th century has contributed to environmental contamination, particularly in areas adjacent to such industries. The use of fossil fuels has further contributed to environmental contamination. The cadmium content in coal varies; the use of cadmium-containing coal in the past for heating and energy production contributed to environmental contamination because flue gas cleaning was inefficient. Dispersive uses also contribute to environmental cadmium levels. Cadmium production increased substantially during the 20th century (see above Section 8.3.2). An increase in cadmium in wheat occurred in Sweden from 1920 to 1970, but there has been no further increase in Sweden in later decades. Ambient air levels are higher in cities than in rural areas. The values in European cities show a decreasing trend during the last decades with less than 1 ng/m^3 in the last decade in Stockholm, Sweden.

Cadmium levels in natural water are low, in the ng/L range. In uncontaminated soil, cadmium levels are usually below 1 mg/kg. In drinking water, levels are below 5 µg/L.

Human **cadmium exposures in the general population** are mainly from food. They vary greatly in different parts of the world. Population groups in several Asian countries, living in cadmium-contaminated areas and consuming locally grown cadmium-contaminated rice have suffered adverse health effects (see Section 8.3.6.3). Concentrations in rice ranged up to 4 mg/kg in such areas. In Japan, general dietary cadmium intake in the Japanese population has decreased from 59 to 113 µg/day in the 1960s to approximately 25 µg/day in 2005. In European countries and the United States, intakes are usually 20 µg/day or lower.

For smokers, inhalation of **cadmium in cigarette smoke** contributes significantly to the body burden of cadmium. Smoking 20 cigarettes per day corresponds to an uptake of 2 µg of Cd, i.e., more than the amount of cadmium taken up from food in uncontaminated areas.

Cadmium levels in **workroom air** were high in the past. Often 200 µg/m^3 was measured in the 1960s and 5−10 µg/m^3 in the 1980s. Section 8.3.7 gives information on the present OEL.

8.3.4 Toxicokinetics

8.3.4.1 Absorption and Uptake

Cadmium **absorption in the GI tract** is dependent on a number of factors. Animal studies showed that deficient intake of protein, iron, calcium, and zinc increases the uptake. A low fiber content also increased uptake. Choudhury (Choudhury et al., 2001) used a TK model described in Chapter 2 and found that an average fractional uptake from the diet of 5% in men and 10% in females was the best fit to measure biomonitoring data (see Chapter 2, Section 2.6.2.1; Fig. 2.10). Fransson et al. (2014), however, found somewhat lower values based on similar calculations in Sweden. An explanation for the higher uptake in women of childbearing age compared to men is the fact that women often have lower iron stores than men because of menstrual iron losses. Flanagan et al. (1978) found that volunteers (mainly women) with low body iron stores (serum ferritin less than 20 µg/L) had four times higher fractional absorption of cadmium than those with normal iron stores. The molecular explanation probably is an upregulation of the divalent metal transporter 1 (DMT-1) in the mucosal cells by low iron (Tallkvist et al., 2001). An influence of zinc transporters on intestinal cadmium absorption is also likely (Rentschler et al., 2014).

Cadmium in air occurs as a particulate aerosol. Chapter 2, Section 2.3.3.2, describes general principles for **deposition and uptake of inhaled particles**. Depending on the particle size and solubility, a variable proportion of inhaled cadmium will be absorbed systemically. Transport to the pharynx and transfer into the GI tract is the route for poorly soluble particles deposited on the mucociliary escalator in the bronchial tree.

Oberdorster (1992) studied the in vivo solubility on clearance following deposition in the lung of cadmium chloride, cadmium sulfide, and cadmium oxide instilled endotracheally into rat lungs, and then he collected lung tissue, bronchoalveolar lavage fluid, and bronchoalveolar lavage cells over a 30-day period. Despite the difference in water solubility—with chloride being readily soluble and both sulfide and oxide being poorly soluble—all three compounds had similar lung retention half-times. The compartmentalization of dose in the lungs and systemic distribution (kidney, liver) were different, though, and indicated the importance of in vivo dissolution. Cadmium chloride readily distributed to lung tissue and systemic organs, where it was presumably bound to MT. Cadmium sulfide, however, remained largely in lavage cells, where it was slowly dissolved and redistributed to lung tissue; in the timeframe of the study, clearance to the systemic circulation did not occur. Cadmium oxide, which is also poorly water soluble, proved to be soluble in lavage cells (mostly macrophages), so cadmium uptake and MT binding occurred in lung tissue, as did clearance to liver and kidney. These observations demonstrate the importance of in vivo solubility for tissue and systemic uptake of particulate cadmium.

A range of systemic uptake 7—40% has been estimated for inhaled cadmium-containing particles (summary by Nordberg et al., 2015). The lower range of uptake applies to larger cadmium-containing particles with low solubility, and the upper part of the range applies to small and soluble particles.

8.3.4.2 Transport and Distribution

Transport of cadmium, absorbed in the lung or the GI tract, takes place via blood to other organs. In the blood, cadmium is mainly in the blood cells. However, cadmium in blood plasma plays a more important role in the transport process. In plasma, cadmium is partly bound to MT, and because of the small size of this protein, it is filtered through the glomeruli. This is an efficient carrier mechanism for cadmium into the kidney where Cd-MT is taken up in the renal tubular cells (see TK model in Chapter 2, Fig. 2.9). This explains why the kidney has the highest concentrations of Cd among bodily organs. Cadmium bound in plasma to larger proteins is transported to the liver and most other organs including bone tissue. The blood—brain and placenta barriers protect the brain and the fetus from high cadmium concentrations. There is a dose dependence of cadmium binding in plasma with a larger proportion bound to larger proteins at higher doses. Thus, the ratio between kidney and liver cadmium is dose dependent. There is proportionally more cadmium in the liver at higher doses, but ultimately, the kidney always has the highest cadmium concentration among body organs. Approximately 50% of the body burden of cadmium in humans is found in the kidneys at the exposure level (intake 12 μg/day) occurring in Sweden (summarized from Nordberg et al., 2015, 2018).

8.3.4.3 Excretion, Biological Half-Life

Cadmium accumulates in the human body with age. Daily excretion in feces and urine is only 0.01—0.02% of the body burden. Urinary cadmium is proportional to the body burden and the accumulation of cadmium in the kidney. When cadmium-induced tubular dysfunction occurs, cadmium is released from the renal tubular cells, and there is a dramatic increase in urinary excretion. Fecal cadmium is, to a large extent, unabsorbed cadmium in the diet, passing out with feces. True fecal excretion therefore is difficult to measure in humans. Animal studies showed a relationship to body burden for true fecal excretion, particularly at lower doses. The biological half-life of cadmium in the human body is long. It is comparatively short in blood with 100 days for a fast component and 7—16 years for a slow component. It is longer for bodily organs. Animal studies showed that the half-life is dependent on the level of exposure with longer half-life at higher exposures (until cadmium-induced kidney dysfunction occurs). An explanation is that the induction of MT in tissues binds cadmium and prolongs the half-life. For population groups in Sweden with background exposures, the half-life in tissues such as muscles, bone, kidney, and liver was estimated to be 10–40 years (Kjellstrom, 1979). Akerstrom et al. (2013), based on studies of human kidney biopsies, calculated a biological half-life for cadmium in the kidney cortex of 21 years when the cadmium level in the cortex was 8 mg/kg and 43 years when the kidney cortex level was 23 mg/kg.

8.3.4.4 Toxicokinetics Model for Cadmium

Chapter 2, Fig. 2.9, describes a physiological TK model of cadmium absorption, tissue accumulation in the kidney and other organs, and excretion. It was further developed by Choudhury et al. (2001) and applied by Diamond et al. (2003) for calculations of relationships between intake, kidney cortex levels, and urinary cadmium levels in women (women are more vulnerable than men who require higher intakes to reach the same kidney accumulation of cadmium). Based on the Berkeley Madonna modeling of data from the National Health and Nutrition Examination Survey (NHANES) (Ruiz et al., 2010), these differences in cadmium uptake between males and females begin in early childhood and continue into later life suggesting that the risk of adverse health effects should be considered over the course of a lifetime. A cadmium concentration in the kidney cortex of 84 µg/g wet weight is reached after 55 years of dietary intake of 1 µg/kg b.w. per day, and the corresponding urinary cadmium concentration is 1.4 nmol/mmol creatinine (Diamond et al., 2003). Assuming a background oral intake from food of 0.3 µg/kg b.w. per day, exposure to industrial air with 2.7 µg/m^3 from the age of 20–60 years will give rise to 84 µg/g wet weight in kidney cortex.

Amzal et al. (2009) described a one-compartment TK model for oral intake and urinary excretion of cadmium. Based on their data, an intake on 0.6–1 µg/kg b.w. per day corresponds to a low probability of reaching urinary cadmium 2 nmol/mmol creatinine after life-long exposure at this intake level.

Risk assessment evaluations in Section 8.3.7 of this chapter make use of these values.

8.3.5 Biomonitoring

Chapter 3 described the general principles and terminology in biomonitoring (biological monitoring). Blood and urine are the most frequently used media for biomonitoring of cadmium, and the following text gives a detailed description of these biomarkers. Blood and urine are also used for effects biomonitoring, using, for example, determinations of proteins and enzymes in urine as indicators of kidney dysfunction. Cadmium in hair, placenta, cord blood, or feces is used to a limited extent for biomonitoring. Cadmium can also be measured in vivo in the liver and kidney, but the instruments are not widely available and detection limits do not allow quantitation of tissue levels occurring in the general population in Europe (see Nordberg et al., 2015). The bone mineral density is used in studies of osteoporosis and clinical biomarkers of osteomalacia in severely affected population groups. Section 8.3.6 will describe the various effect biomarkers used in the epidemiological studies.

8.3.5.1 Cadmium in Blood

In the blood, cadmium occurs mainly in the blood cells. Binding forms for cadmium in blood plasma were studied in animal experiments using radio-isotopes, allowing studies at much lower levels than those possible to detect by chemical determinations. Some recent studies report cadmium levels in blood plasma or serum determined by ICP-MS, but the values are near to the detection limit and such measurements require careful consideration of possible contamination. All values for blood cadmium (BCd) discussed here are whole blood values.

"Normal" or reference values for cadmium in the blood among non-smokers with background exposures in the general environment are below 1 µg/L in most countries. In Japan, such values were approximately 2 µg/L in the 1990s. In smokers, values are higher due to uptake of cadmium from cigarettes (see Section 8.3.3).

Section 8.3.4.3 described a fast and a slow component of cadmium elimination from the blood. The fast component explains why blood values fluctuate in relation to recent exposure during the last months. The slow component of BCd reflects the uptake of cadmium in body organs. In life-long exposures, this component of BCd represent a substantial proportion of the BCd value. BCd thus reflects both exposure during recent months and long-term accumulation of cadmium body burden. An even better indicator of body burden would be calculations of cumulative BCd values calculated from blood values from repeated sampling or time integrated values. Unfortunately, no such values are available.

The BCd values are used for occupational biomonitoring in some countries. The blood values are better than urine cadmium values for biomonitoring of current exposure.

8.3.5.2 Cadmium in Urine

"Normal" or reference values for cadmium in urine are available from several populations around the world. Values vary depending on age and sex and smoking status but are usually below 1 nmol/mmol creatinine (<1 μg/g creatinine or <1 μg/L adjusted to specific gravity 1.024) in nonsmokers. However, 1−4 nmol/mmol creatinine was reported in some Japanese uncontaminated areas (Ezaki et al., 2003; Suwazono et al., 2000). Creatinine-adjusted values are used here despite the bias discussed below, because most reports include no other values.

Cadmium in urine is a widely recognized biomarker of cadmium accumulation in the kidney and cadmium body burden. Since the 1970s, several studies in industrial workers and persons exposed in the general environment have shown a curvilinear relationship between urinary cadmium and cadmium in the kidney cortex (summarized by Nordberg et al., 2015). This relationship holds up to the level in kidney cortex when cadmium induces tubular dysfunction. When the cadmium level in the kidney cortex reaches the critical concentration that induces renal tubular dysfunction, the tubular cells in the kidney lose their ability to take up CdMT from the tubular fluid. With more severe damage, the cells release their content of cadmium into urine. The relationship between kidney cadmium and urine cadmium changes dramatically. Urinary cadmium is a reliable biomarker of accumulation in the kidney cortex up to the level causing tubular dysfunction. However, at low-level urine cadmium, several factors unrelated to cadmium accumulation in the kidney cortex may influence the relationship. These include diuresis and sampling conditions.

Creatinine adjustment compensates for the variable hydration of individuals in a group, but it is not perfect and introduces an error in the opposite direction. Akerstrom et al. (2013) used repeated urine sampling to demonstrate the erroneous associations found in urine samples from the same individual. Such erroneous statistical associations in epidemiological studies can be avoided. Barr et al. (2005) recommended that urinary cadmium be expressed per liter and adjusted with creatinine, based on the regression coefficient between the two analytes. Despite the existence of this clear recommendation, recent papers still use traditional creatinine adjustment, for example Eom et al. (2017).

Timing of sampling is a factor influencing urinary cadmium values. Akerstrom et al. (2014) found a diurnal variation in urinary cadmium with 50% higher values in the morning than in the afternoon.

8.3.6 Effects and Dose—Response Relationships With Special Reference to Toxicodynamics and Toxicokinetic-Toxicodynamic Relationships

Cadmium exposure may cause both acute and chronic toxic effects. Acute effects were more common in the past; chronic effects are in focus for the present scientific discussion. Inhalation of 5 mg/m^3 of cadmium oxide fume for 8 h may cause acute lethal poisoning. Ingestion of 15 mg/L in drinking water gives rise to acute poisoning with vomiting and other GI symptoms, but fatalities do not usually occur (see summary by Nordberg et al., 2015). The following text will focus on the adverse effects on human health caused by long-term exposure to cadmium. Because of its cumulative properties, tissue levels of cadmium increase for a long time (decades) in continuous exposure.

8.3.6.1 Respiratory Effects

Airborne cadmium is in the form of a particulate aerosol (Section 8.3.4.1, above). Respiratory effects are due to deposition of cadmium-containing particles on the mucosa or alveolar membranes of the respiratory tract, and their dissolution and uptake in tissues. The size and solubility of the particles determine the deposition pattern and tissue dose in the respiratory tract (see Chapter 2). Section 8.3.4.1 (above) emphasized the importance of in vivo solubility (which may be different from solubility in water) for the uptake into lung tissues (and further for systemic absorption) of cadmium from particles. While there are OELs specifying levels for respirable particles (see Section 8.3.7), TKTD models of respiratory effects resulting from inhalation of cadmium compounds occurring in occupational environments, cigarette smoke, and aerosols in the general environment are not available.

Observations, mostly in the past, of the occurrence of respiratory effects in industrial workers in relation to measured air levels show that long-term (years) cadmium exposure by inhalation may give rise to disorders of the respiratory system: chronic inflammation of the nose, pharynx, and larynx; olfactory disturbances; chronic obstructive lung disease; and emphysema. Elinder (1986) reviewed the literature and estimated that several years of inhalation of workroom air, i.e., 8 h per day, 5 days per week, of 20 μg/m^3 respirable particulate cadmium was the lowest exposure giving rise to lung effects. Based on the data published by Cortona et al. (1992), the Scientific Committee on Occupational Exposure Limits (SCOEL, 2010) in the EU estimated a lowest-observed-adverse-effect level (LOAEL) for respiratory effects corresponding to a cumulative exposure of workroom air (respirable particles) of 500 $\mu g/m^3$ years corresponding, for example, to 25 years exposure to 20 $\mu g/m^3$. The SCOEL considered this exposure to correspond to a urinary cadmium level of 3 nmol/mmol creatinine. Nordberg et al. (2018) reviewed some more recent studies on respiratory effects but considered that it was difficult to untangle the effects of cadmium from those of smoking.

8.3.6.2 Kidney Effects

The kidney is the organ that accumulates the highest concentration of cadmium in the body (Section 8.3.4), and the kidney cortex has the highest levels in the kidney. It is usually considered to be the critical organ in long-term cadmium exposures. There is considerable evidence from both humans and experimental animals (Nordberg et al., 2015, 2018; EFSA, 2009) showing that long-term exposure to cadmium gives rise to tubular changes in the kidney and related low molecular mass proteinuria. Because there is a large variation in the human population, the level of cadmium in the kidney cortex that causes tubular proteinuria varies from 80 to >200 mg/kg (0.71 to >1.78 mmol/kg). Diamond et al. (2003) estimated that in the US population, 84 $\mu g/g$ wet weight in the kidney cortex corresponds to the lower confidence limit for the lower 10% of the population, representing the most sensitive individuals. This value is higher than the 95% upper value of cadmium in the kidney cortex from background dietary exposures (Choudhury et al., 2001). Diamond et al. (2003) concluded that cadmium-related risks from dietary cadmium in the United States would be negligible in the absence of other exposures. Urinary cadmium of 1.4 nmol/mmol creatinine corresponds to 84 $\mu g/g$ wet weight in the kidney cortex and the dietary intake, giving rise to these levels is 1 $\mu g/kg$ b.w. per day (Section 8.3.4.4, above).

Epidemiological studies measuring increased urinary excretion of marker proteins such as beta-2-microglobulin (B2M), α-1-microglobulin (A1M), and retinol-binding protein (RBP) as well as the enzyme N-acetyl-β-D-glucosaminidase (NAG) in relation to urinary excretion of cadmium showed clear and statistically significant relationships (Nordberg et al., 2015, 2018; EFSA, 2009). The relevance of increased excretion of these biomarkers is documented by follow-up studies of population groups in Japan (Nishijo et al., 2006; Elinder and Nordberg, 2017). Both EFSA (2009) and JECFA (2011a,b) used dose—effect relationships derived from the meta-analysis performed by EFSA (2009) in their risk evaluations. Both organizations derived a starting point at 4—5 nmol/mmol creatinine of urinary cadmium for their estimates of safe exposure levels (see later Section 8.3.7). A weakness of the meta-analysis is the exclusion of several studies of high quality (because they did not use B2M but other biomarkers, or they did not report creatinine adjusted values). Nordberg et al. (2018) included these studies in their assessment. The CadmiBel study (Buchet et al., 1990) shows statistically significant associations between urinary cadmium and RBP, NAG, B2M, amino acids, and calcium in urine at 2−4 µg/day of urinary cadmium, corresponding to slightly lower numbers in terms of µg/g creatinine (nmol/mmol creatinine). A study in China (Jin et al., 2004) found statistically significantly increased urinary levels of NAG, B2M, albumin, and RBP in the same range of urinary cadmium. A study in Sweden (Akesson et al., 2005) found statistically significant associations between low molecular mass (LMM) proteins in urine and urinary cadmium <1 nmol/mmol creatinine. In Japan, Suwazono et al. (2010) reported benchmark dose, lower confidence level-five percent (BMDL-5) values for LMM effects of 1.5−3.2 nmol/mmol creatinine. It is unclear at present whether the associations between cadmium in urine at <1−2 nmol/mmol creatinine and increased LMM protein excretion are causal, partly because of uncertainties in the relationship between urinary cadmium and kidney cortex cadmium at low levels of urine cadmium (Bernard, 2016; Section 8.3.5.2). Another uncertainly is the possible confounding by smoking, because tobacco smoke contains cadmium and other components in the smoke may influence kidney tubule cells (Haddam et al., 2011; Chaumont et al., 2011). Another phenomenon that may influence the relationship is co-excretion of proteins and cadmium (Chaumont et al., 2012). Nordberg et al. (2018) discussed these uncertainties and concluded that for statistical associations reported at urine cadmium below 2 nmol/mmol creatinine causality is uncertain.

High occupational cadmium exposures give rise to glomerular kidney effects with decreased glomerular filtration rate (GFR) and increased serum creatinine (Jarup et al., 1998; Nordberg et al., 2015). The relevance is uncertain for associations between urine cadmium and slightly decreased eGFR reported at lower exposures (Nordberg et al., 2018). Increased urinary albumin excretion related to urinary cadmium, shown in China, was reversed after cadmium exposures decreased (Liang et al., 2012).

8.3.6.3 Bone Effects

Excessive exposure to cadmium through consumption of cadmium-contaminated rice gave rise to the itai-itai disease, a combination of kidney dysfunction, osteomalacia, and osteoporosis with bone fractures. Most of the patients were multiparous females who fell ill after menopause. They all lived in an area of Toyama prefecture in Japan where rice paddies were contaminated by cadmium from river water receiving effluents containing cadmium from a lead mine. Most cases were diagnosed during 1967–70. Totally, 190 cases are officially recognized (review Nordberg et al., 2015). There are reports of clinical cases of osteomalacia also in workers with high occupational cadmium exposures (Kazantzis, 1979).

Mechanisms explaining the bone effects in itai-itai disease include a deficient renal synthesis of active vitamin D metabolites as in classical renal osteomalacia. Losses of calcium and phosphate into urine because of deficient reabsorption in renal tubules and losses during pregnancies and lactation contribute to skeletal decalcification. The average level of urinary cadmium was >30 nmol/mmol creatinine in itai-itai patients. Low dietary intakes of vitamin D, calcium, iron, and zinc may also have contributed.

During the last 2 decades, a number of studies have investigated a possible link between lower cadmium exposures and osteoporosis. Nordberg et al. (2018) reviewed 20 studies on this subject published after 1999. Studies with relatively high exposures (Nordberg et al., 2002; Jin et al., 2004; Wang et al., 2003; Nawrot et al., 2010; Chen et al., 2009) showed decreased bone mineral density in relation to urinary and sometimes also BCd. These observations are likely to represent causal relationships. Chen et al. (2009) included subjects with urine cadmium >20 nmol/mmol creatinine and found a statistically significant decrease in bone mineral density in all subgroups with urine cadmium >5 nmol/mmol creatinine (women) but not in groups with lower urine cadmium. Studies with lower exposures display a complex pattern. Some studies (e.g., Akesson et al., 2006; Thomas et al., 2011; Engstrom et al., 2011) report statistically significant associations between urine cadmium and bone effects at lower urinary cadmium levels, while other studies (e.g., Trzcinka-Ochocka et al., 2009; Wallin et al., 2005) do not find such effects (review Nordberg et al., 2018).

8.3.6.4 Cancer

The IARC updated their assessment of cadmium and cancer in 2012 (IARC, 2012) and confirmed their previous classification of cadmium as a human carcinogen (IARC Group 1). It is based on clear findings in animal experiments by Takenaka et al. (1993) showing lung cancer in rats exposed to cadmium chloride via inhalation and epidemiological studies in industrial workers with increased occurrence of lung cancer and other cancer forms in the respiratory tract (Thun et al., 1985; Stayner et al., 1992; Sorahan and

Esmen, 2004). A number of other epidemiological studies reported statistically significant positive associations between occupational or environmental cadmium exposure and risk of cancer in the prostate, kidney, bladder, breast, and endometrium (review by IARC 2012). The IARC considers that there is sufficient evidence in humans and in animals for the carcinogenicity of cadmium and its compounds (review IARC, 2012; Nordberg et al., 2018). Dose—response relationships for cadmium exposure and cancer occurrence in humans are uncertain.

In addtion to IARC, other organizations also classified cadmium as a carcinogen. In the EU, the Classification, Labelling, and Packaging (CLP) regulation classified cadmium and some cadmium compounds in Group 1B. In the United States, the EPA classified cadmium as a possible human carcinogen by inhalation (Group 1B) based on limited evidence of lung cancer in humans and sufficient evidence in animals (see Chapter 4 concerning classification of carcinogenicity).

8.3.6.5 Other Effects

Anemia occurring in itai-itai disease patients is sometimes severe and persistent with markedly decreased serum erythropoietin levels.

Experimental studies in animals indicated links between cadmium and *diabetes*, but epidemiological studies show variable findings.

Several epidemiological studies report a statistically significant association between biomarkers of cadmium exposure (cadmium in blood or urine) and *cardiovascular disease* (e.g., Barregard et al., 2016), but studies in workers exposed to higher doses of cadmium by inhalation found no statistically significant associations. Nordberg et al. (2018) considered that more evidence is needed in order to establish causality and dose—response relationships.

Experiments in animals showed *reproductive effects and endocrine disruption* after cadmium exposure, but findings in epidemiological studies were not separated from effects of smoking and it cannot be stated with any certainty whether an effect of cadmium exists at low background exposures.

8.3.7 Risk Assessments and Recommended Preventive Measures Including Exposure Limits Set by International and National Organizations

JECFA recommended a provisional tolerable monthly intake (PTMI) of 25 µg/kg b.w. (JECFA, 2011b). This is a lowering of the recommended average daily intake from the previous 1 to 0.8 µg/kg b.w. The long biological half-life of cadmium motivates the change from a PTWI (weekly) to a

PTMI (monthly) recommendation. This recommendation used a BMDL of 5.24 μg/g creatinine of urinary cadmium, derived from a meta-analysis (see Section 8.3.6.2) as a point of departure (POD) and estimated the corresponding dietary intake by the one-compartment TK model by Amzal et al. (2009), using the fifth percentile dietary intake corresponding to the POD.

The EFSA (2009) recommended a TWI of 2.5 μg/kg b.w. (corresponding to an average daily intake of 0.36 μg/kg b.w.) based on a POD of 4 nmol/mmol creatinine (μg/g creatinine) of urinary cadmium derived from a meta-analysis (Section 8.3.6.2). The EFSA used an adjustment factor of 3.9 to compensate for the use of group means instead of individual values in the meta-analysis and arrived at a urinary cadmium 1 nmol/mmol creatinine. By the model by Amzal et al. (2009), the EFSA derived a weekly intake of 2.5 μg/kg b.w.

In the United States, ATSDR (2012) issued a minimal risk level (MRL) for chronic oral exposure of 0.1 μg/kg b.w. per day. It was derived from a POD of urinary cadmium of 0.5 μg/g creatinine.

In the EU, the SCOEL (2010) published a recommendation of an OEL of 4 μg/m^3 (respirable fraction) for cadmium oxide in air, based on the lowest inhalation exposure giving rise to respiratory effects (Section 8.3.6.1), i.e., 12.5 μg/m^3 during 40 years and a default extrapolation factor of 3.

The International Union of Pure and Applied Chemistry (IUPAC) Task Group on Risk Assessment of Effects of Cadmium on Human Health (Nordberg et al., 2018) selected the kidney effects (LMM proteinuria) as the critical effect and noted that bone effects occur at exposure levels similar to those giving rise to kidney effects. LMM proteinuria is caused, in a susceptible subsection of the population, by long-term cadmium exposure giving rise to urinary cadmium of 2 nmol/mmol creatinine. Population exposure should be kept sufficiently low to prevent higher urinary cadmium. The daily oral intakes corresponding to a low probability of reaching such a urine value in women (susceptible subsection of population) is 0.6—1 μg/kg b.w. (estimate based on TK calculations referred to in Section 8.3.4.4, above). Because of uncertainties concerning dose—response relationships, a numerical value for a no-effect level could not be determined and the Group recommended that cadmium exposures be kept as low as possible.

For cadmium, both early assessments by IPCS (1992) and the recent risk assessment by an IUPAC Task Group (Nordberg et al., 2018) used TKTD calculations of exposures related to kidney effects. Because risk assessments for cadmium are good examples of the use of TKTD calculations, they are described and referred to in this section on cadmium.

8.4 COBALT (CO)

8.4.1 Introduction/Properties

Cobalt (Co), CAS No. 7440-48-4, atomic No. 27, atomic mass 58.9, density 8.9 g/cm^3, melting point 1495°C, is a silver grey metal with magnetic properties. Its most common oxidation state is +2 but can also be +3, 0, −1 (RSC, 2018). Metallic cobalt in various alloys, the oxides, and divalent salts are of toxicological interest. *Vitamin B12* (cyanocobalamin and hydroxocobalamin) is a biologically important cobalt compound, essential for human health. In this compound, cobalt is complexed with four pyrole nuclei joined in a corrin ring, similar to porphyrins. Determination of cobalt in various matrices is possible with HG-AAS, ICP-AES, or ICP-MS. At present, the latter is most common. This chapter section is partly based on the review by Lison (2015), and the reader is referred to that review for specific references.

8.4.2 Production and Uses

The world production of cobalt metal was 82,000 metric tons in 2011, and it is increasing. **Uses:** Historically, the use of cobalt compounds for blue glass and pottery is documented in ancient Chinese culture (B.C.), and this use is still ongoing. Presently, the leading use of cobalt metal and cobalt oxides is in NiCd and Li-ion rechargeable batteries. Another important use of cobalt is in steel and alloys. So-called superalloys consist of cobalt, chromium, and other metals. Hard metals (or cemented carbides) are composite materials containing tungsten carbide and cobalt metal. Hip and knee replacement prostheses are made from Vitallium (CoCrMo). Cobalt-based nanoparticles are used in electronics, magnetic fluids, catalysis, and nanomedicine. Cobalt salts were previously used as an additive to beer and in the treatment of anemias (see below).

8.4.2.1 Vitamin B$_{12}$—An Essential Cobalt-Containing Compound

Cobalt in the form of vitamin B$_{12}$ is essential for human health but other forms of cobalt are not. In humans without additional exposure, the major part (about 85%) of the human body burden of cobalt (total approximately 1.1 mg) is in the form of vitamin B$_{12}$. Plasma levels of cobalt are <200 pg/mL and of vitamin B$_{12}$ 200−900 pg/mL. The daily requirement of vitamin B$_{12}$ is about 1 μg. Under normal circumstances, humans efficiently take up vitamin B$_{12}$ through the GI tract. However, when this uptake mechanism is impaired, deficiency occurs. Treatment is by large doses

(1000 µg/day) of the vitamin, thus overcoming the lack of specific uptake mechanism. Cobalt constitutes 4.3% of the vitamin and the cited dose corresponds to 43 µg of cobalt. Slightly impaired uptake is common in older people and some vitamin supplements contain up to 200 µg/day (9 µg of Co). Most of the treatment dose passes unabsorbed into feces and the plasma and body content of the vitamin remain in the normal range.

8.4.3 Environmental Occurrence and Human Exposures

Dietary intake of cobalt by humans is 5—50 µg/day. Most of the intake is usually in inorganic form. Vitamin B12 is only a minor part except in persons treated with the vitamin because of deficient uptake (see above). Pennington and Jones (1984) reported 3.4—11.6 µg/day as the range of intake in the United States. Some dietary supplements used by athletes supply up to 1000 µg/day of soluble cobalt compounds (Unice et al., 2012).

Addition of cobalt sulfate to beer, as done in the past, produced beer with values up to 1.1 mg/L.

Levels of cobalt in ambient air are low <40 ng/m^3. In sea water, there is 0.3 µg/L, and in lakes and ground water, there may be a few micrograms per liter. In drinking water, it is below 5 µg/L.

Air levels in **occupational environments** range 0.01—1.7 mg/m^3. Exposures in the hard metal industry and among diamond polishers may cause exposures of health concern. For OELs, see below. There is also exposure to the skin of cobalt workers.

Hip and knee arthroplasties made from Vitallium (CrCoMo) may release cobalt locally and systemically. Metal-on-metal (MoM) hip arthroplasties, particularly in patients with failing prostheses may give rise to considerably elevated cobalt levels in periprosthetic fluid and blood serum. **Consumer exposure** to the skin may occur from products containing cobalt, e.g., inexpensive jewelry.

8.4.4 Toxicokinetics

This section deals with inorganic cobalt, while a previous paragraph summarizes information on vitamin B$_{12}$.

Lung retention and systemic uptake of cobalt-containing airborne particles depend on size and solubility. Pottery plate painters using a soluble pigment have increased blood and urine values, but not those using an insoluble pigment. **Dermal absorption** through dissolution in sweat occurs in workers in the hard metal industry and for soluble cobalt compounds on the skin. The GI **absorption** of inorganic cobalt varies from 5% to 45%. Children and adolescents have higher uptakes than older people. Women have higher uptake than men, probably related to iron status. Iron deficiency increases cobalt uptake by increasing the expression of transporters in the mucosa of the GI tract. **Systemically absorbed cobalt** reaches all tissues in the body with the highest concentration in the liver, kidneys, and thyroid. There is no accumulation with age. **Excretion** is mainly through urine with a smaller proportion in feces. The biological half-life is approximately 1 week. Unice et al. (2012) presented a biokinetic model describing blood and urine values after oral intake of soluble inorganic cobalt supplements.

8.4.5 Biomonitoring

Reference (or normal) values of cobalt in blood are <0.5 μg/L. For urine, they are <2 μg/L (or <2 μg/g creatinine). In **occupational exposures** in the hard metal industry, the cumulative airborne exposure during the work week (in one study, 5–150 μg/m^3) is correlated to the urinary cobalt in Friday afternoon samples. The relationship between air and urine values varies among industries and depends on the particle size and solubility of cobaltous air pollution.

Follow-up programs for patients with MoM hip **prostheses** recommend measurements of cobalt in blood, serum, plasma, or urine. A blood cobalt level of >7 μg/L appears to predict local failure of the prosthesis (Hart et al., 2014).

8.4.6 Effects and Dose–Response Relationships

Irritation and sensitization sometimes results from cobalt exposure. Cobalt carbonyl is a strong irritant causing respiratory manifestations after inhalation and mucous membrane reactions in the GI tract if ingested. Sensitization to cobalt may occur in part of the workforce in industries with cobalt exposures, not only in the classical cobalt industries but also in polyester resin manufacture, in cement workers, and in workers exposed to cutting fluids where cobalt has been dissolved. Sensitized workers may develop asthma (see later) or dermatitis upon skin contact with cobalt. Chapter 3, Fig. 3.5, describes a general AOP for allergic dermatitis caused by skin sensitizers. As far as we know, an analysis of the applicability of this AOP for cobalt-induced allergic dermatitis has not been published. Cobalt skin allergies usually are combined allergies with nickel and chromium. Sensitization to cobalt may also occur as a result of contact with consumer products such as hair dyes, antiperspirants, crayons, and jewelry. Allergic dermatitis due to cobalt occurs more frequently in Europe than in the United States.

Hard metal asthma is the disease identified in workers in the hard metals industry with symptoms like wheezing, cough, and shortness of breath that were relieved after removal of the workers from the working environment. Similar symptoms have occurred in a relatively small proportion (less than 5%) of workers in other industries with exposure to cobalt metal or cobalt compounds. Sauni et al. (2010) found that the occurrence of such **cobalt asthma** correlated with air cobalt levels in working environments. Some of the patients with these cobalt-induced diseases have increased IgE against a complex of Co with albumin, indicative of a type I allergic reaction. However, other researchers (Kusaka et al., 1986) have found positive results in a lymphocyte transformation test, indicating a role for cellular immunity. Compared to noncobalt-exposed persons, there is an accelerated decline in FEV-1 (forced expiratory volume in 1 second) with age in workers suffering from these diseases.

Hard metal lung disease occurs in a small percentage of workers in the hard metal industry. It is a giant cell interstitial pneumonia with clinical presentation as acute alveolitis or chronic interstitial fibrosis. Although most cases occurred in the hard metal industries, some cases occurred among diamond polishers exposed to cobalt metal powder with iron and diamond dust. Examination of hard metal lung disease (HMLD) cases by high-resolution computed tomography shows reticulation, traction bronchiecstasis and peripheral cystic spaces with a mid and upper lung distribution. There is no clear relationship between the occurrence of disease and the duration and intensity of exposure. The possible involvement of sensitization and immunological changes for the induction of the disease remains to be established. Occasionally, patients have both cobalt dermatitis and HMLD. The existence of genetic susceptibility is suggested by the finding of an association between HMLD and Glu-69 polymorphism of the HLA-DP beta chain (Potolicchio et al., 1997), but confirmation is required.

Hematopoiesis: cobalt salts in doses of 1 mg/kg b.w. given to animals increases erythropoiesis. Mechanisms involve stabilization of hypoxia inducible factor, HIF1α, which is usually degraded under normal oxygenated conditions. Cobalt salt administration is suspected to be misused by some athletes as an alternative to blood doping for enhancing aerobic performance (Lippi et al., 2005). Oral treatment with cobalt chloride (6–12 mg Co per day and sometimes higher doses) was used in the past for treatment of anemias. Polycythemias occurred among heavy drinkers of cobalt-fortified beer.

Myocardial effects: animal experiments have shown myocardial degeneration and ECG changes after injection or oral treatment with cobalt compounds or inhalation of cobalt.

In humans, an outbreak of cardiomyopathy occurred in the 1960s among heavy beer drinkers consuming beer with cobalt additives. Clinical observations included heart failure, polycythemia, and thyroid lesions with up to 50%. Outbreaks occurred in Quebec, Canada, in Minneapolis, the United States, and in Belgium. Up to 1.1 mg/L of cobalt occurred in beer, and a heavy beer drinker thus consumed several milligrams per day. This dose is high, but not higher than the dose used in the past in the treatment of anemia. The combined effect of cobalt, ethanol in beer and nutritional factors has therefore been considered of importance, as an explanation for the pronounced cardiac effects. A few cases of cardiomyopathy and an increased occurrence of decreased left ventricular heart function have been reported in cobalt-exposed industrial workers.

Thyroid: in the past, patients given 20–30 mg of cobalt in the treatment of anemia often developed goiter as a side effect. Thyroid changes were seen in the drinkers of cobalt containing beer in Quebec. Animal studies have confirmed the toxic effect of cobalt chloride on the thyroid.

Neurotoxic effects: in patients with orthopedic prostheses, mainly MoM hip replacements, there are several case reports of elevated blood or serum levels of cobalt and neurotoxic effects such as headache, anxiety, peripheral neuropathy, optical nerve atrophy, tinnitus, deafness, hand tremor, diminished coordination, slow cognition, poor memory, and convulsions. Blood, serum or plasma levels up to 600 µg/L were reported. Signs and symptoms resided after surgical revision of defective prosthesis. Some of these cases also had hypothyroidism and cardiomyopathy (see above).

Patients treated in the past with high doses of cobalt compounds for anemia reported neurotoxic effects. There is also limited evidence for neurotoxic effects in industrial cobalt workers. Intravenous injection in rabbits (Apostoli et al., 2013) of high doses of cobalt salt (but not of chromium salts) could reproduce neurotoxic effects (auditory and optic manifestations).

Systemic toxicity observed in patients with high blood levels of cobalt because of metal release from orthopedic hip replacements is named *arthroprosthetic cobaltism* because there is reason to believe that the increased systemic cobalt levels and not the chromium levels cause the symptoms (Tower, 2010)—see also information above.

Gessner et al. (2015) reviewed reported cases of this disease involving symptoms of the cardiovascular system (60%), audiovestibular system

(52%), peripheral motor–sensory system (48%), thyroid (48%), psychological functioning (32%), visual system (32%), and the hematological, oncological, or immune system (20%). Brown et al. (2015) reviewed the literature including a few small studies of groups of persons with MoM hip replacements. These authors concluded that a consensus has not been reached on the levels of cobalt or chromium that serve as triggers for either removal of the device or closer monitoring of the patient.

Medicines and Healthcare products Regulatory Agency in the United Kingdom recommends that MoM implantees are followed up annually for 5 years postsurgery with Co and Cr in blood, and imaging for patients who experience painful replacements. A follow-up after 3 months after the first test is recommended for patients with Co or Cr in blood >7 μg/L.

Reproductive and developmental effects: rats with dietary cobalt 265 mg/kg and mice with 100–400 mg/L of Co in drinking water displayed degenerative changes in testicles. Mice, but not rats, inhaling 3 mg/m^3 cobalt sulfate showed reduced sperm motility. There were increases in preimplantation losses in the dominant lethal assay when male mice were exposed to 400 mg/kg of cobalt chloride in the diet. Oral cobalt chloride (12–48 mg/kg per day) affected postnatal survival and development of pups. Several developmental alterations were seen in fetuses of mice and rats treated with cobalt sulfate (0–100 mg/kg per day).

Genotoxicity and carcinogenicity: there are a large number of studies in vitro and in animals of the **genotoxicity and mutagenicity** of hard metals and other cobalt compounds. The IARC (2006) in their review of genotoxic and mutagenic effects concluded that there is strong evidence that the WC-Co mixture is mutagenic in vitro and in vivo in rat cells. De Boeck et al. (2001) examined the genotoxic effects of occupational exposure to cobalt-containing dust at the current OEL 20 μg/m^3. Workers who smoked and were exposed to hard metal dust had elevated 8-OHdG (8-hydroxydeoxyguanosine) and micronucleus values, but workers exposed solely to cobalt did not show increased genotoxic effects.

Animal experiments with cobalt oxide, cobalt alloys, particularly tungsten carbide, showed local tumors after injection or tracheal instillation, but some inhalation studies were negative. Cobalt sulfate inhalation in rats and mice produced alveolar and bronchial neoplasms. According to the evaluation of cobalt sulfate by the National Toxicology Program in the United States, there was some evidence of **carcinogenic** activity in male rats, and clear evidence in female rats and in male and female mice.

Studies in **humans** included cohorts of workers exposed to cobalt from Sweden, France, and Denmark, some with combined exposure to tungsten carbide. According to the IARC (2006), these studies showed that there is inadequate evidence for carcinogenicity in humans of cobalt metal in the absence of tungsten carbide and that there is limited evidence for **carcinogenicity in humans** in the presence of tungsten carbide. Together with animal evidence, such exposures were classified by the IARC in their Group 2A, i.e., probably carcinogenic to humans.

8.4.7 Risk Assessment and Recommended Preventive Measures

Cobalt and its compounds are skin-sensitizing agents, but available information is not sufficient to recommend precautions for limiting skin exposures to the general public. It appears that it would be possible to perform studies similar to the ones performed with nickel (see Section 8.10) in order to develop efficient prevention.

The use of cobalt-containing alloys in arthroplastic surgery causes increased internal exposure to cobalt, particularly for certain types of prostheses and when there is failure of the prosthesis. An increasing number of reports of arthroplastic cobaltism appear in the international scientific literature. It is important to further investigate the occurrence of this condition in epidemiological studies and to establish a relationship between cobalt in blood and symptoms as a basis to establish criteria for revision. In some countries, there are recommendations for follow up of patients with devices that are likely to release cobalt, including biomonitoring of cobalt in blood. Similar programs may be considered by other countries.

Respiratory diseases such as cobalt asthma and HMLD occur after occupational exposure to airborne cobalt-containing dust, sometimes in combination with tungsten (in the hard metal industries). The dose–response relationship for induction of these diseases is unclear, partly because of the lack of established TKTD models or AOPs. The extent of protection offered by current OELs is uncertain. The values recommended or legislated for cobalt metal and its inorganic compounds vary.

In the United States, the Occupational Safety and Health Administration (OSHA) permissible exposure limit is 0.1 mg/m^3; OSHA California lists 0.02 mg/m^3, and this is the value currently in use in Sweden. The Swedish HGV list (AFS, 2015, 2018) further classifies these compounds as carcinogenic, sensitizing, and with dermal uptake. Cobalt sulfate and cobalt chloride are also classified as reprotoxic.

8.5 GALLIUM (GA)

Gallium (Ga), CAS No. 7440-55-3, atomic No. 31, atomic mass 69.735, is a member of Group 13 of the Periodic Table of Elements. It has valence states of +2 and +3. It can be measured by atomic emission spectroscopy, X-ray fluorescence, and ICP-MS. The world production of Ga in 2017 has been estimated to be 315 tons (USGS, 2018).

8.5.1 Uses

Gallium has a number of uses in the semiconductor industry in relation to high-speed circuits, light-emitting diodes (LEDs), photovoltaic cells, anticancer and antimicrobial agents (Fowler and Sexton, 2015), and more recently, flexible Ga-In circuits (Liu et al., 2014).

8.5.2 Dispersion in the Environment

Gallium has been reported in open ocean seawater, smelter-damaged soils, river sediments, and well groundwater near a semiconductor manufacturing plant in Taiwan (Fowler and Sexton, 2015).

8.5.3 Work Environment

Gallium is encountered in the work environment of semiconductor-manufacturing facilities (Fowler and Sexton, 2015) as a result of polishing of computer chips and cleaning of ovens used in the production of GaAs chips.

8.5.4 Human Exposures

In addition to occupational exposures, humans may be exposed to gallium in air, food, and water (Fowler and Sexton, 2015).

8.5.5 Toxicokinetics

Gallium is bound to transferrin in the blood and distributed to a number of organ systems with major concentrations in the liver, kidneys, skeleton, bone marrow, and spleen (Fowler and Sexton, 2015). Urine is the main route of excretion from the body with lesser amounts in the feces. Lactating mothers have been shown to efficiently transfer gallium into breast milk (Wappelhorst et al., 2002).

8.5.6 Biomonitoring

Biomonitoring studies on optoelectronic workers in Taiwan (Liao et al., 2004) have reported elevated Ga levels in blood and urine.

8.5.7 Acute Toxicity

The acute toxicity of gallium compounds varies with both the gallium moiety and the anionic component such as nitrate or arsenide (IARC, 2006).

8.5.8 Target Organ System Effects

8.5.8.1 Kidney

The kidney is a major target for gallium toxicity on an acute in vitro and in vivo or longer term exposures (Aoki et al., 1990; Conner et al., 1993; Fowler et al., 2005; Fowler and Sexton, 2015; NTP, 2000).

8.5.8.2 Immune System

The immune system is also a major target for gallium toxicity, and exposures result in suppression of both humoral and cellular-based immune function (Burns and Munson, 1993).

8.5.8.3 Lung

Gallium compounds such as GaAs and Ga_2O_3 have been shown to produce extensive lung inflammatory responses following acute intratracheal or inhalation exposure protocols (Goering et al., 1988; NTP, 2000).

8.5.8.4 Irritation

Gallium compounds are also skin and eye irritants and must be handled with appropriate protective measures (Science Lab, 2013).

8.5.9 Carcinogenicity

The IARC (2006, 2012) classified gallium arsenide (GaAs) as carcinogenic to humans based on limited evidence of carcinogenicity of GaAs in animals in combination with the fact that GaAs releases inorganic arsenic in the body after uptake. Inorganic arsenic is a well-established carcinogen for humans (IARC, 2012).

8.5.10 Human Risk Assessment

A number of essential components of standard risk assessment practice are currently available. These include information to support hazard assessment, exposure assessment, and experimental and human toxicity data which provide consistent biomarker information data and thus a scientific basis in support of mechanism/mode of action-based risk assessments for this metal. To date, no such risk assessments have been published.

8.5.11 Human Health Risks

It is clear from the above information that gallium is clearly a toxic element and that there are attendant health risks to a number of major organ systems. The use of gallium is increasing in a number of products and processes thus increasing the likelihood of more extensive human exposures and associated risks to health unless appropriate protective measures are put in place.

8.6 INDIUM (IN)

Indium (In), CAS No. 7440-74-6, atomic No. 49, atomic mass 114.8, is member of Group 13 of the Periodic Table of Elements. It has valence states of +1, +2, and +3. It can be measured by atomic emission and atomic absorption spectroscopy, neutron activation analysis, polarography, and ICP-MS (see Fowler and Maples-Reynolds, 2015). The world production of indium has steadily increased over the last 30 years to 759 metric tons in 2015 (USGS, 2015).

8.6.1 Uses

Indium has a number of uses in the semiconductor industry in relation to high-speed circuits, LEDs, photovoltaic cells, optoelectronics, flat-panel plasma television screens, solders, alloys, and more recently, nanomaterials (Fowler and Maples-Reynolds, 2015) and flexible Ga-In circuits (Liu et al., 2014). The use of indium arsenide is restricted in the EU (see Chapter 7, Section 7.2.5).

8.6.2 Dispersion in the Environment

Indium has been reported in open ocean seawater, air, soils near smelters, and rain water (Fowler and Maples-Reynolds, 2015).

8.6.3 Work Environment

Indium has been reported in the work environments of a manufacturing plant in Japan (Miyaki et al., 2003) and optoelectronic manufacturing facilities (Liao et al., 2004) in Taiwan. The workroom air limit in Sweden at present is 0.1 mg/m^3 (AFS, 2018).

8.6.4 Human Exposures

In addition to occupational exposures, humans may be exposed to indium in air, food, and water (Fowler and Maples-Reynolds, 2015).

8.6.5 Toxicokinetics

Indium is bound to transferrin in the blood and distributed to a number of organ systems with major concentrations in the liver, kidneys, skeleton, bone marrow, and spleen. Urine is the main route of excretion from the body with lesser amounts in the feces (Fowler and Maples-Reynolds, 2015).

8.6.6 Biomonitoring

Blood and urine values of indium are useful biomarkers of indium exposures (Fowler 2012). Biomonitoring studies on optoelectronic workers in Taiwan (Liao et al., 2004) have reported elevated levels of indium in blood and urine. Indium has also been reported in samples of blood, serum, and spot urine in workers exposed to respirable particles containing indium compounds in Japan (Miyaki et al., 2003). Nakano et al. (2009) reported serum indium levels of 0.9 to >20 ng/mL in Japanese workers in an electronic factory.

8.6.7 Acute Toxicity

The acute toxicity of indium compounds varies with both the indium moiety and the anionic component such as chloride (Fowler et al., 1983; Bustamente et al., 1997) or phosphide (IARC, 2006).

8.6.8 Target Organ System Effects

8.6.8.1 Kidney

The kidney is a major target for indium toxicity on an acute or longer term basis (Aoki et al., 1990; Conner et al., 1993, 1995; Fowler et al., 2005; Fowler and Maples-Reynolds, 2015; NTP, 2001).

8.6.8.2 Developmental Toxicity

The developing fetus is a major target for indium toxicity, and acute exposures have been reported to result in both teratogenic and embryo-lethal effects (see Fowler and Maples-Reynolds, 2015).

8.6.8.3 Lung

Indium compounds have been shown to produce extensive lung inflammatory responses and fibrosis following acute intratracheal or inhalation exposure protocols (Morgan et al., 1995; NTP, 2001).

8.6.8.4 Irritation

Indium compounds are also skin and eye irritants and must be handled with appropriate protective measures (ScienceLab, MSDS, 2013).

8.6.9 Carcinogenicity

Based on findings in a long-term carcinogenicity study in rats (NTP, 2001), the IARC (2006) determined that indium phosphide is a probable human carcinogen (IARC Group 2A).

8.6.10 Human Risk Assessment

A number of essential components of standard risk assessment practice are currently available. These include information to support hazard assessment, exposure assessment, and experimental and human toxicity data which provide consistent biomarker information data, which is a scientific basis in support of mechanism/mode of action-based risk assessments for this metal. To date, these modern tools of risk assessment have not been applied to risk assessments for indium compounds.

8.6.11 Human Health Risks

It is clear from the above information that indium and its compounds are toxic and that there are attendant health risks to a number of major organ systems. The probable carcinogenicity of indium phosphide forms a basis for special protection against this compound. The use of indium is increasing in a number of products and processes, thus increasing the likelihood of more extensive human exposures and associated risks to health unless appropriate protective measures are put in place.

8.7 THE LANTHANIDES (INCLUDING LANTHANUM, LA; CERIUM, CE; AND GADOLINIUM, GD)

The lanthanides (or lanthanoides) include lanthanum (La) with atomic number 57 and the 14 subsequent elements in the periodic table with numbers 58–71 (cerium, Ce; praseodymium, Pr; neodymium, Nd; promethium, Pm; samarium, Sm; europium, Eu; gadolinium, Gd; terbium, Tb; dysprosium, Dy; holmium, Ho; erbium, Er: thulium, Tm; ytterbium, Yb; lutetium, Lu). All these elements together with scandium (Sc) and yttrium (Y) are included in the group of elements named rare-earth elements (REEs). The discoverers of these elements named them rare-earth elements because they thought that these elements existed only in very low concentrations in the earth's crust.

Later research has shown that many of these elements are not rare. In fact, cerium is the 25th most abundant element in the earth's crust, adjacent to copper; most of the REEs are more abundant in the earth's crust than gold. The total world production of REEs, taking place mainly in China, exceeds 120,000 metric tons (USGS, 2017). Their uses include permanent magnets in wind turbines (NdFeB alloys or SmCo) and smaller REE magnets in CD and DVD units. Nd, Sm, and Pm are REEs often included in such magnets. They also have many other uses (see below). Although our toxicological knowledge of these elements is very limited, their increasing use in various technologies makes it important to discuss the need for risk assessment related to present and possible future uses. This chapter section will deal mainly with the three elements: lanthanum (La), cerium (Ce), and gadolinium (Gd).

8.7.1 Lanthanum (La)

Lanthanum (La), CAS No 7439-91-0, rel. atomic mass 138.9055, density 6.17 g/cm^3, melting point 920°C, a silvery white metal that tarnishes rapidly in air. The review by Wedeen et al. (2015) is a partial basis for the following text, and specific references can be found there. Lanthanum forms compounds mainly in the +3 oxidation state, e.g., lanthanum oxide, La_2O_3; lanthanum hydroxide, $La(OH)_3$; lanthanum sulfate, $La_2(SO_4)_3$; lanthanum nitrate, $La(NO_3)_3$; and lanthanum carbonate, $La_2(CO_3)_3$. Lanthanum sulfate and nitrate are soluble in water to a variable extent, but lanthanum hydroxide and carbonate are insoluble in water. La in various media can be determined by ICP-MS.

8.7.1.1 Production and Uses

Lanthanum occurs in the earth's crust together with other REEs. Although the element is not rare, it is a challenge to find deposits that are economically feasible to mine and process. Lanthanum is produced from the minerals bastnäsite and monazite. Bastnäsite occurs at Bastnäs, Sweden, and in China and the United States. Lanthanum production occurs mainly in China from bastnäsite. The total world production of lanthanum exceeds 30,000 metric tons (USGS, 2017). China is also a major user of La with applications in electronics manufacturing. Japan and the United States are other major users. La is used as an additive to glass and as a glass-polishing agent. It is a major component of mischmetal and a minor one in certain steel alloys. Lanthanides are phosphors in cathode ray tube displays and fluorescent lamps. La is an electrode component in some nickel–metal hydride batteries. La-compounds are used for defluoridation and removal of arsenate from water. Lanthanum carbonate is approved for use as a drug to reduce phosphate in patients with renal failure (Wedeen et al., 2015).

8.7.1.2 Environmental Levels and Human Exposures

Ambient air concentrations of La are in the range $0.05-30 \text{ ng/m}^3$. La concentrations up to 600 ng/L were reported in coastal, estuarian, and sea water. Concentrations in soil range $1-50$ mg/kg, similar to the average in the continental crust (32 mg/kg). Fertilizers derived from apatite often contain REEs and may contaminate soils.

Concentrations of La were up to 9 μg/L in drinking water in the Netherlands. Studies of the daily dietary intake of La are available only from China, where La compounds and other REEs are used as fertilizers. In China, the mean dietary intake of total rare earth oxides (REOs) was 0.13 mg, which is only 3% of the Chinese acceptable daily intake (ADI) for REOs. La-carbonate is taken orally in gram amounts as a drug by kidney patients (see Section 8.7.1.4). Levels of La in workroom air are not reported, but increased tissue levels in deceased metalworkers indicates that exposure occurs. No OELs are legislated or recommended.

8.7.1.3 Toxicokinetics

La compounds including lanthanum carbonate are poorly absorbed via the GI tract. Lanthanum carbonate binds phosphate in the GI tract forming lanthanum phosphate eliminated in feces. The small proportion of systemically absorbed La is partly accumulated in bone. After 2 years of treatment of patients with kidney failure with lanthanum carbonate in daily oral doses of gram amounts, La concentration in bone was only 1.9 mg/kg and plasma lanthanum was 0.09 ng/mL. **Biomonitoring** in lanthanum-treated patients is by determinations of lanthanum in blood plasma to check that they do not absorb too much lanthanum. Most patients have plasma levels below 2 ng/mL (Spasovski et al., 2006).

8.7.1.4 Toxicity and Human Health Effects

Lanthanum compounds have a low **acute toxicity** by the oral route. Lanthanum sulfate, lanthanum trinitrate, and lanthanum triiodide are irritating to the skin and eyes; labeling is required according to the CLP regulation in the EU; lanthanum nitrate is also very toxic to aquatic life, and inhalation of lanthanum triiodide may cause respiratory irritation. Some patients taking lanthanum carbonate orally develop GI disturbances. Experience of **systemic toxic effects** in patients treated with lanthanum carbonate indicates that effects on bone morphology may occur in some patients treated for a long time. There are also reports of effects on cerebral function in some patients after long-term treatment (Wedeen et al., 2015;

Altman et al., 2007). When side effects are identified, a change of phosphate binder is necessary. There is no recognized efficient chelator to remove excess lanthanum from the body.

Dufresne et al. (1994) reported a case with findings of X-ray-dense deposits in the lungs after long-term inhalation of lanthanum. A risk of pneumoconiosis may exist in workers exposed for a long time to lanthanum occupationally, although such cases are rare.

8.7.2 Cerium (Ce)

Cerium (Ce), CAS No 7440-45-1, rel. atomic mass 140.116, density at room temperature 6.77 g/cm^3, melting point 799°C, is a silvery white metal that tarnishes in air and burns at 150°C to cerium(IV)oxide, ceria (CAS 1306-38-3). Its oxidation states are +3 and +4 (RSC, 2018). It is the most abundant of the lanthanides, and the earth's crust contains 66 ppm of Ce. It can be determined in various media by ICP-MS.

8.7.2.1 Production and Uses

Production of cerium is from the same minerals as for lanthanum (see above). The world production of Ce is approximately 20,000 tons (2016). Cerium metal is a component of mischmetal, used in flints for lighters. It has also been used as a component in arc carbon for carbon-arc lamps. Cerium oxalate is a yellow pigment used in glass. Ceria (cerium dioxide, CeO_2, cerium (IV) oxide) is used as a colorless glass constituent and glass polish, and in catalytic converters. CeO_2 nanoparticles are used as an additive to diesel fuel in order to improve fuel combustion and decrease exhaust emissions of NOx, but there is a simultaneous dramatic increase in emissions of ultrafine particulates, CO, hydrocarbons, and volatile organic compounds (Cassee et al., 2011). Nanoscale cerium compounds are also used as surface protection agents and in medical applications (Cassee et al., 2011). Cerium(III)oxide is used in self-cleaning ovens and in catalytic converters (RSC, 2018).

8.7.2.2 Human Exposures

Human exposures to cerium compounds occur in occupational settings, for example, glass polishers, but no measured concentration or legislated OELs are available. In the general environment, ambient air (PM10) concentrations of cerium increased from approximately 10 to 40 ng/m^3 when nanocerium was introduced as an additive in diesel fuel, used in city busses in Newcastle, UK (Cassee et al., 2011). No recommended or legislated air levels are available.

8.7.2.3 Toxicokinetics

Adult rats absorb Ce compounds poorly after oral exposure, while suckling animals absorb a considerable proportion of ingested Ce into the tissues of the GI tract. Inhaled particulate Ce is poorly soluble and behaves in relation to particle size as described in Chapter 2, i.e., with deposition of fine particulates deep in the lung. Clearance of lung Ce is by a first rapid phase corresponding to mucociliary transport and a slower phase with a half-life of 100—190 days in rodents. Greatly elevated levels of Ce were found in lung tissue of deceased workers occupationally exposed to Ce at unknown concentrations in workroom air (review by EPA, 2009; Cassee et al., 2011). Elimination of absorbed cerium is mainly via feces with less than 10% via urine. No TK model for Ce compounds is available (EPA, 2009).

8.7.2.4 Acute Toxicity

Acute toxicity of orally administered Ce compounds is low, requiring doses of 500—1000 mg/kg b.w. in rats to produce toxicity. Single-dose/short-term inhalation of CeO_2 at concentrations above 50 mg/m^3 produces toxicity. Intravenous injection of 1.3 mg/kg b.w. of cerium chloride gave rise to increased protein synthesis and increased lipid peroxidation in cardiac muscle in female rats (data summarized by EPA, 2009).

8.7.2.5 Risk Assessment

Epidemiological studies in India suggest an association between cerium in the soil and the incidence of endomyocardial fibrosis (summarized by EPA, 2009). A case—control study in 10 European heart centers found an association between toenail cerium and first myocardial infarction (Gomez-Aracena et al., 2006). As mentioned, cardiac muscle changes were found in animals exposed to Ce compounds, but the EPA (2009) concluded that available human and animal evidence was insufficient to derive a reference dose for oral cerium exposure (see above Section 8.7.1.2 concerning Chinese ADI for REOs).

Derivation of **reference concentration for human exposure**: a number of case reports found accumulation of cerium containing particles in the lungs after long-term occupational exposure to cerium fumes or dust. A 13 weeks inhalation study of CeO_2, 2 μm MMAD particles, in rats, summarized in EPA (2009), reported an increase of alveolar epithelial hyperplasia. A BMCL10 of 8.7 mg/m^3 in female rats was taken as POD and converted to 0.86 mg/m^3 for 24 h 7 days per week chronic exposures. EPA (2009) derived a reference concentration (RfC) of 0.9 μg/m^3 from this information. A low confidence in this RfC was expressed because of the lack of a chronic study. However, it is obvious that the RfC derived for 2-μm particles is not relevant for nanoscale cerium particles. Dale et al. (2017) showed that the cerium containing nanoparticles in exhaust from diesel engines have different characteristics compared to CeO_2 nanoparticles in diesel fuel. This observation further underlines the conclusion by Cassee et al. (2011) that the health effects related to the use of CeO_2 nanoparticles, including new composition of diesel emissions, are not known at present.

8.7.3 Gadolinium (Gd)

Gadolinium (Gd), atomic number 64, rel. atomic mass 157.25, CAS No 7440-54-2, density 7.9 g/cm^3, melting point 1313°C, oxidation state +3, is a soft silvery white metal that reacts with oxygen and water. It can be determined in various media by ICP-MS.

8.7.3.1 Production and Uses

Production of Gd is from the same minerals as La. Gd metal is a (usually minor) component of alloys with iron or chromium. Certain magnets and electronic components contain Gd. Gd chelates are useful contrast agents (GdCAs) in magnetic resonance imaging (MRI). There are two categories of GdCAs, linear and macrocyclic. Macrocyclic GdCAs form cage-like structures with Gd(III) enclosed in the cavity of the complex. The macrocyclic GdCAs have lower dissociation constants and are therefore more stable than the linear GdCAs (Rogosnitzky and Branch, 2016).

8.7.3.2 Environmental Levels and Human Exposures

When producing various Gd-containing products, some occupational exposures occur, but the levels are unknown. There are no legislated OELs. In preparation for MRI, GdCAs are injected intravenously into the patient in doses, usually 0.05—0.3 mmol/kg b.w. Patients with normal kidney function excrete GdCAs (see below) and waste water from hospitals contain elevated concentrations of Gd, also traceable in rivers used as recipients of such water (see, e.g., Song et al., 2017).

8.7.3.3 Toxicokinetics

Like the situation for other REEs, oral absorption of Gd compounds is limited. Frenzel et al. (2008) found that the linear GdCAs released even more Gd^{3+} in human blood plasma in vitro than predicted from their stability constants, while the macrocyclic GdCAs were stable for 15 days.

Solubility of inorganic Gd compounds in water and in blood plasma is dependent on pH. For example, $GdCl_3$ is soluble at pH = 5, but insoluble at pH = 7.4 (i.e., the pH of blood). This means that dechelation of GdCAs may cause release of ionic Gd, which may precipitate in the blood stream. GdCAs are efficiently excreted in the urine of patients with normal renal function, but tissue retention occurs in patients with impaired renal function. Therefore, restrictions apply in the use of GdCAs in persons with decreased renal function. In recent years, increasing evidence indicates that there is retention of a variable proportion of GdCAs in various tissues including the brain even in patients with normal renal function. Such retention is more pronounced for linear GdCAs than for macrocyclic ones. Frenzel et al. (2017) demonstrated increased retention of Gd after repeated injection of linear GdCAs compared to macrocyclic compounds in rats with normal kidney function.

8.7.3.4 Toxicity

The acute oral toxicity of Gd compounds is low, similar to other REEs with LD50 in rats and mice of >1000 mg/kg (Bruce et al., 1963). Intravenously injected inorganic Gd compounds are toxic at lower doses. Spencer et al. (1997) reported toxic effects in terms of hepatocellular and splenic necrosis in rats after intravenous injection of $GdCl_3$ 0.14 or 0.35 mmol/kg b.w. and minimal deposits of $GdCaPO_4$ in kidney and lung vasculature at 0.07 mmol/kg. In patients with renal impairment, given GdCAs during MRI examinations, a condition developed named nephrogenic systemic fibrosis (NSF). This condition is characterized by fibrotic infiltration of the skin and other organs. The recognition of this condition led to changed practices for use of the GdCAs and the occurrence of NSF has decreased. However, there is recognition of an increased accumulation of Gd in tissues such as bone, the kidney, and the brain, after repeated use of the linear GdCAs, even in patients with normal kidney function. Patients suffering joint complaints expressed concern and the term gadolinium deposition disease was coined (Ramalho et al., 2016). Animal experiments (see above Section 8.7.3.3) demonstrated brain accumulation of Gd after repeated dosing of the linear agents.

8.7.3.5 Risk Assessment

There is incomplete characterization of occupational and environmental exposures to Gd and its compounds, and there are no known health risks. GdCAs used in MRI caused a number of cases of NSF, but restrictions in the use of these agents have decreased the number of such cases. In the last few years, brain accumulation of Gd was identified as a potential problem. Although clinical disease related to such accumulation has not been documented; the EMA (2017) decided to restrict the use of some linear GdCAs and suspended the authorizations of others. These rules are now applicable in all EU member states. The macrocyclic compounds can continue to be used in their current indications but in the lowest doses that enhance images sufficiently and only when unenhanced body scans are not suitable.

8.8 LEAD (PB)

8.8.1 Introduction/Properties

Lead (Pb), CAS No. 7439-92-1, atomic No. 82, atomic mass 207.19, density 11.3 g/cm^3, melting point 327.5°C, is a member of the Group 14 of the Periodic Table of Elements. It has valence states of +2 and +4. It can be measured by atomic emission spectroscopy, X-ray fluorescence, and ICP-MS.

8.8.2 Production and Uses

The world production of Pb in 2017 has been estimated to be 11.58 million tons (USGS, 2018).

Lead has been used in a number of industries for centuries including batteries, water piping, gasoline additives, paint, lead shot and ammunition, solders, and radiation shielding. In more recent years, it has been used in shielding in cathode-ray tube monitors and solders in a number of electronic products ultimately contributing to e-waste (Fowler, 2017). The use as an additive to gasoline is now prohibited in most countries around the world, including all EU countries and the United States. The use of lead is restricted in the EU (see Chapter 7, Section 7.2.5).

8.8.3 Dispersion in the Environment and Human Exposures

Due to its extensive historical uses, lead has been reported in open ocean seawater, smelter-damaged soils, river sediments, and well groundwater (NAS/NRC, 1993; Skerfving and Bergdahl, 2015). It is found in a number of both private and public water systems (NAS/NRC, 1993; Skerfving and Bergdahl, 2015). Global lead emissions into the environment peaked in 1960—80, when approximately 400,000 metric tons per year were emitted, partly because of its use in petrol. However, considerable lead pollution causing human exposure has occurred through history; during the Roman

Empire, lead was used for water piping and lead acetate as a sweetener of wine. Although lead exposures of general population groups in industrialized countries have decreased in the last 2 decades, the remaining exposures are probably considerably higher than the natural background in prehistoric times. Patterson et al. (1991) estimated that the human body burden of lead around 1990 was approximately 1000 times higher than that of prehistoric humans and exposures from the general environment are approximately proportionate. Considering the decrease in exposures in the last 2 decades, the present exposure is perhaps 100 times higher than that in prehistoric times, and because of the delay in body burden decrease, the present body burden is perhaps 200—500 times that in prehistoric times.

8.8.3.1 Work Environment

Lead is encountered in a number of work environments including smelters, radiator repair shops, and semiconductor manufacturing facilities (NAS/ NRC, 1993; Skerfving and Bergdahl, 2015) as a result of use of lead solders in the electronics industry and production of lead batteries.

8.8.3.2 Human Exposures

In addition to occupational exposures, humans may be exposed to lead in air, food, and water (Skerfving and Bergdahl, 2015). Considerable exposure of the general population including children in towns and cities occurred because of the widespread use of lead additives in petrol. Because most countries in the world have now discontinued this use, lead exposures have decreased.

8.8.4 Toxicokinetics

Lead is primarily bound to delta-aminolevulinate dehydratase (ALAD) in the blood and distributed to a number of organ systems, with major concentrations in the liver, kidneys, skeleton, bone marrow, and spleen (NAS/NRC, 1993; Skerfving and Bergdahl, 2015). The skeleton is the major site of lead deposition in the body (NAS/NRC, 1993), where retention is pronounced; the biological half-life in the cortical bone is as long as 10—20 years. In target tissues such as kidney and brain, lead is bound to a number of other lower molecular mass proteins (Fowler et al., 1993; Quintanilla-Vega et al., 1995; Smith et al., 1998). Urine is the main route of excretion from the body with lesser amounts in the feces. Lactating mothers have been shown to efficiently transfer lead into breast milk. Toxicokinetic models for lead are available (Skerfving and Bergdahl, 2015).

8.8.5 Biomonitoring

Lead biomonitoring studies on workers (Skerfving and Bergdahl, 2015) and the general US population (CDC, NHANES, 2012) have reported elevated lead levels in blood and urine, respectively. Fewtrell et al. (2004) reported, from various parts of the world, PbB in children (μg/L): 98—111 in Africa; 22—90 in the Americas; 68—154 in Eastern Mediterranean; 35—67 in Europe; 74 in SE Asia; and 27—66 in Western Pacific. Studies that are more recent show somewhat lower values: a geometric mean value of 32 μg/L in Ecuador and 14—20 μg/L in Europe (Hruba et al., 2012).

8.8.6 Acute Toxicity

The acute toxicity of lead displays similar symptoms as subacute toxicity. The absorbed dose determines the severity of symptoms.

8.8.7 Target Organ System Effects

8.8.7.1 Skeletal System

As noted above, the skeletal system is the major site of lead deposition in the body (Nordberg et al., 1991; NAS/NRC, 1993) and associated with a number of adverse health effects in bones and teeth (Skerfving and Bergdahl, 2015).

8.8.7.2 Kidney

The kidney is a major target for lead toxicity in both experimental animal models (Fowler et al., 1980) and humans (Fowler, 2010; Fowler et al., 1980; NAS/NRC, 1993; Skerfving and Bergdahl, 2015).

8.8.7.3 Immune System

The immune system is also a major target for lead toxicity, and exposures result in variable suppression of both humoral and cellular based immune function (Skerfving and Bergdahl, 2015).

8.8.7.4 Hematopoietic System

The hematopoietic system is a major target for lead toxicity at both low-dose and higher dose levels (Silbergeld and Fowler, 1987; Fowler, 2010). In particular, the enzyme ALAD which catalyzes the second step in the heme biosynthetic pathway is remarkably sensitive to inhibition (Fowler, 2010; Skerfving and Bergdahl, 2015), but other enzymes such as ferroche-latase which catalyzes the insertion of Fe^{2+} into the porphyrin ring to form heme are also sensitive to lead inhibition (Fowler, 2010). Chronic high-dose lead exposure may result in anemia (Silbergeld and Fowler, 1987; Skerfving and Bergdahl, 2015) because of these combined inhibitory effects of lead on the heme biosynthetic pathway (NAS/NRC, 1993; Skerfving and Bergdahl, 2015). Fig. 3.3 in Chapter 3 describes the enzymes in the heme-synthesis pathway that are inhibited by lead.

8.8.7.5 Cardiovascular System

The cardiovascular system is also highly sensitive to lead-induced hypertension (Scinicariello et al., 2007, 2010) which is mediated in part by the binding of lead to ALAD, which is the major carrier protein for lead in blood (Skerfving and Bergdahl, 2015). The affinity of this protein for lead is mediated in part on a genetic basis which in turn mediates lead-induced hypertension on an ALAD allelic basis (Scinicariello et al., 2010).

8.8.7.6 Nervous System

Both the central and peripheral nervous systems are sensitive to lead toxicity (NAS/NRC, 1993; Skerfving and Bergdahl, 2015). At lower lead dose levels, decrements in IQ are the known endpoints of concern, while at elevated dose levels, lead-induced "wrist drop" due to peripheral neuropathy with muscle weakness, lead-induced encephalopathy may be major clinical manifestations. The critical effect in population exposures is cognitive deficits with decreased IQ. In the past, PbB levels of 100 μg/L were not associated with adverse effects. However, recent studies published after 2004 concluded that an increase of PbB from 24 to 100 μg/L was associated with a reduction in IQ by 3.9 points (Lanphear, 2005). The National Toxicology Program (NTP, 2012), based on an extensive review, reached similar conclusions. These findings indicate that PbB levels even below 100 μg/L impacts negatively on brain development in children. Despite the decrease in PbB that has occurred because lead is no longer used as an additive to petrol, lead levels in the range of 20—100 μg/L still occurs in many countries around the world, and such levels impact negatively on IQ, thus contributing to global disability-adjusted life year (DALY) estimates (see below Section 8.8.9).

8.8.8 Human Risk Assessment

A number of essential components of standard risk assessment practice are currently available. Existing OELs and limit values for humans in the general environment use epidemiological data as the basis. Available information supports hazard assessment, exposure assessment, and experimental and human toxicity data which provide consistent biomarker information data which provide a scientific basis in support of mechanism/mode of action-based risk assessments for this metal. To date, there are no published such risk assessments for human exposures. For lead, this is already possible via integrating data from the extensive literature on molecular mechanisms of lead toxicity with the lead analytical data, human demographics, clinical data, nutritional status, and genetic polymorphisms information from the NHANES database to identify subpopulations at special risk for adverse outcomes (AOs) such as lead-associated hypertension (see Scinicariello et al., 2010).

8.8.9 Human Health Risks

It is clear from the above information that lead is a very toxic element and that there are attendant health risks to a number of major organ systems. As mentioned in Chapter 1, the WHO (2009) estimated that globally 143,000 deaths and nearly 9 million DALYs were caused by lead exposure in 2004. Epidemiological studies and evaluations after 2004 (see Section 8.8.7 above) support the notion that additional low-exposure effects of lead occur in addition to those identified in 2004. It is therefore quite possible that an estimate of the number of DALYs caused by present lead exposure globally would arrive at a similar or even higher number despite the decreases of lead exposures of the general population that has taken place because of the discontinued use of lead additives in petrol. The use of lead is increasing in a number of products and processes such as recycling of batteries and e-waste in developing countries thus increasing the likelihood of more extensive human exposures and associated risks to health unless appropriate protective measures are put in place.

8.9 MERCURY (HG)

8.9.1 Introduction/Properties

Mercury (Hg), CAS No. 7493-97-6, atomic No. 80, atomic mass 200.6, density $13.6 \, g/cm^3$, melting point $-38.9°C$, boiling point $356.6°C$, is a silver white metallic liquid, with oxidation state $+1$ or $+2$. Calomel, mercurous chloride is a monovalent mercury compound. Mercuric chloride is divalent. This section of the chapter is in part a summary of the review by Berlin et al. (2015) where specific references are cited.

8.9.2 Production, Uses, Restrictions, and Substitutes

The world **production** of mercury was 2500 metric tons in 2017 (USGS, 2018), and it has decreased from 7000 to 8000 metric tons per year in the 1980s. The main producer is China, **using** mercury as a catalyst in coal-based manufacture of vinyl chloride monomer and in other manufacturing industries. In some parts of the world, mercury is used in the recovery of gold in small-scale mining. At present, conversion is ongoing of chlor-alkali production from mercury to nonmercury technologies. The closure of the world's mercury-cell chlor-alkali plants, which used to cause considerable emissions to the atmosphere, now makes a large quantity of mercury available to the global market for recycling, sales, or storage. Due to export bans in Europe and the United States, considerable quantities of mercury are stored in safe deposits in these countries. The present use in the United States is limited to 40 tons in two remaining chlor-alkali plants, dental use and in manufacturing of electronic and fluorescent lighting (USGS, 2018).

In the EU, production of mercury stopped in 2003 and the exports from the EU in 2011. The use of mercury in the EU is decreasing. EU rules **restrict** use in products, such as batteries, lamps, nonelectronic measuring devices and in chlor-alkali production (see Chapter 7, Section 7.2.5). EU countries are acting to further decrease anthropogenic emissions of Hg and its compounds according to the Minamata convention, ratified by the EU in 2017.

Apart from the intentional uses, there are unintentional emissions of mercury into the air from coal burning (for heating, cooking, power and steam generation, and industrial process plants), cement clinker production, nonferrous metals production, and waste incineration.

Substitutes: Ceramic composites substitute for dental amalgam. "Galistan," an alloy of gallium, indium, and tin, replaces the mercury used in traditional mercury thermometers, and digital thermometers have replaced traditional thermometers. Newer membrane cell technology replaces mercury-cell technology at chlor-alkali plants. LEDs that contain indium substitute for mercury-containing fluorescent lamps. Lithium, nickel—cadmium, and zinc—air batteries replace mercury-zinc batteries in the United States; indium compounds substitute for mercury in alkaline batteries; and organic compounds substitute for mercury fungicides in latex paint (USGS, 2018).

8.9.3 Environmental Occurrence and Human Exposures

8.9.3.1 Geochemical Mercury Cycle, Mercury in Ambient Air, Water, Sediments; Uptake in Biota

The United Nations Environment Programme (UNEP, 2013) estimated that the global release of mercury to the atmosphere had increased by a factor of three in the last century. A rapid increase of mercury concentrations in marine species after the mid-19th century is likely to be caused by anthropogenic emissions. In the last 3 decades, the release of mercury to the atmosphere from its specific uses has decreased considerably, particularly from the United States and Europe, but the unintentional uses and releases from sources such as coal burning are still increasing in Asia. According to the UNEP (2013), the major contributors to the global emission of mercury to the atmosphere are artisanal gold mining, burning of coal, production of nonferrous metals, and cement production.

Elemental mercury in the atmosphere is oxidized to divalent mercury by ultraviolet (UV) light, ozone, and bromine. This oxidation process is more efficient in the arctic than at other locations, and this means a larger deposition of mercury in this region. Deposition of divalent mercury is both by dry and wet deposition (rain). In water, bacteria in the upper part of the bottom sediments methylates mercury, forming monomethyl and dimethylmercury. Divalent water-soluble mercury is also reduced in water environments to mercury vapor. Dimethylmercury and mercury vapor are volatile and enter the atmosphere. An equilibrium exists between these different forms of mercury in the environment. Methylmercury is very efficiently bioaccumulated in the marine food web. Predatory species like tuna and shark contain high concentrations of methylmercury (Bjerregaard et al., 2015).

Because fish, particularly predatory species of fish, contain high levels of mercury in the form of methylmercury, fish intake determines the human intake of methylmercury. Natural water contains low concentrations of mercury usually $1-10$ ng/L. However, much higher levels are present in bottom sediments. Atmospheric mercury levels range from a few nanograms per cubic meter in remote areas and up to 20 ng/m^3 in urban areas. Even if these levels appear low, mercury can travel through air around the globe with the jet stream. Emissions from coal-fired power plants are an important contribution to the global mercury cycle (see above). Considerable human exposure takes place by use of mercury in artisanal and small-scale mercury mining. Such activities expose, not only the mining and refining workers but also their families. It also contributes a considerable part of global mercury circulation. Mercury contamination of lakes and rivers cause methylmercury accumulation in fish that may be used for human consumption.

8.9.3.2 Human Exposure from Food, Dental Amalgam, and Skin Creams

As mentioned, a major proportion of mercury in fish is in the form of methylmercury. High concentrations occur in tuna and swordfish sometimes exceeding 1 mg/kg. Terrestrial animals and other food items have much lower levels of mercury. Methylmercury intake thus is related to fish intake. The daily intake of inorganic mercury is low, less than 10 μg/day. For persons with amalgam tooth fillings, intake is higher. Chewing releases mercury vapor from the amalgam and the mercury vapor is inhaled and absorbed into the blood. The amount of mercury released from amalgam varies (see below, Section 8.9.5). In some exceptional cases, for example, in people using chewing gum, it can be considerable (urine values up to 50 μg/g creatinine).

The use of **skin creams** to lighten the skin is widespread in Asia where a large proportion of the population use such creams. Some brands contain mercury iodide, but the extent of this use is not presently known (Wallander et al., 2015).

8.9.3.3 Working Environment

Exposure to a combination of mercury vapor and divalent mercury is common in chlor-alkali plants. Mercury exposures also occur in the fluorescent lamp manufacturing industry. The numbers of workers in the EU and United States in such mercury-exposed occupations are decreasing. Mercury is still to a limited extent used in dentistry, but this use is also decreasing. Dentists and nurses are exposed to mercury vapor. A large number of artisanal mercury miners in the developing countries are exposed to high, uncontrolled levels of mercury vapor (see Section 8.9.7 for OEL value).

8.9.4 Toxicokinetics and Metabolism

8.9.4.1 Mercury Vapor and Inorganic Divalent Mercury

Metallic mercury vapor is to a limited extent taken up through the skin. In whole-body exposures 1% of the total uptake was through the skin (and 99% through uptake from inhaled mercury vapor). Inhaled **mercury vapor** is not soluble in water and reaches the alveolar space in the lungs. Uptake in the lung is 80% of the inhaled amount by diffusion through the alveolar membrane. For a short time after uptake, mercury vapor exists in blood dissolved mainly in erythrocytes from where it diffuses into the brain and other tissues. The brain of humans and other primates accumulates the highest level in the body soon after exposure to mercury vapor. In erythrocytes, catalase mediates the oxidation of mercury vapor to divalent mercury. Ethanol influences the extent of absorption because it inhibits catalase, the mercury-oxidizing enzyme in red blood cells (Nielsen-Kudsk, 1965). The blood transports divalent mercury to the kidneys, where it accumulates. A dominating proportion of mercury in the human body after exposure to mercury vapor is present as divalent mercury. The uptake of orally ingested liquid metallic mercury is extremely limited ($<$0.01%) and it passes out with feces.

Divalent mercury salts in contact with skin are taken up in the skin and may cause sensitization; only a minor proportion is taken up systemically. Dusts containing **divalent salts of mercury** deposit in the respiratory tract according to size (see Chapter 2); uptake is more limited than for mercury vapor, but specific information is lacking. After oral ingestion in humans, uptake of divalent mercury is approximately 2% of the dose. After uptake, the blood transports divalent mercury to many organs in the body including the kidneys where it accumulates in the kidney tubules. In blood, mercury distributes about equally between blood cells and plasma. Among organs, the kidneys invariable accumulate the highest level of divalent mercury. Divalent mercury does not transfer across the blood—brain and placental barriers easily, and the level in the brain and fetus is lower than in other tissues. The biological half-life of mercury varies among organs. The longest half-life is in the parts of the brain. The high uptake of mercury in the brain after exposure to mercury vapor compared to exposure to divalent salts of mercury explains why the brain is the critical organ after vapor exposure and the kidney after exposure to divalent salts of mercury.

Excretion of mercury, both after exposure to mercury vapor and exposure to divalent mercury salts is mainly through urine and feces. Small amounts are excreted with sweat and with milk during lactation. A larger proportion is excreted in urine at relatively high doses compared to low doses.

Mercury in blood and urine are good **indicators of recent exposure**, after inhalation of mercury vapor and most probably also after inhalation exposure to divalent mercury containing dust.

Roels et al. (1987) described relationships between levels of mercury vapor in air and blood or urine levels in workers. Blood sampling was at the end of a work shift, and urine values taken the following morning. The relationship between air level ($\mu g/m^3$) and whole-blood value ($\mu g/100$ mL) was: blood value $= -0.14 + 0.048 \times$ air level; for urine values ($\mu g/g$ creatinine), the corresponding relationship was: urine value $= 10.2 + 1.01 \times$ air level.

8.9.4.2 Methylmercury

Uptake into blood of inhaled methylmercury compounds is approximately 80%. Orally ingested methylmercury is also well absorbed. The uptake through skin is considerable. After uptake, methylmercury binds to erythrocytes. >90% of methylmercury in blood is in erythrocytes. Methylmercury is distributed to many tissues in the human body. It traverses the placenta and accumulates in the fetal brain. The brain accumulates the highest levels, about 10% of the body burden in humans and other primates. Other animal species accumulate much less in the brain, for example, 1% of the body burden in rats. An explanation for the efficient transfer of methylmercury into the brain is probably due to its binding to cysteine and that this complex uses the methionine pathway into the brain (see Chapter 2, Section 2.4, and review by Berlin et al., 2015). Methylmercury is slowly biotransformed to divalent mercury in the body. Methylmercury levels in various human tissues follow similar kinetics, and one-compartment model for the kinetics of methylmercury is applicable (see Chapter 2). Hair takes up high levels of methylmercury and is a useful indicator of body burden. The biological half-life of methylmercury in the human body as derived from studies of levels in hair from exposed persons is 33–189 days (Chapter 2, Section 2.5.3). Excretion is mainly through bile. Excreted methylmercury is partly demethylated in the gut by intestinal microflora to divalent mercury. This form of mercury is poorly absorbed in the intestine and thus excreted in feces. Methylmercury entering the intestine through bile is efficiently reabsorbed, thus contributing to enterohepatic recirculation of methylmercury. Rand et al. (2016) demonstrated the importance of intestinal microflora for the biological half-life of methylmercury in humans. As mentioned, a small proportion of methylmercury is demethylated in human tissues and the divalent mercury formed is excreted mainly in urine. In total, the dominating excretion route for methylmercury is into feces. Mercury in blood cells or whole blood and mercury in hair are good **indicators of body burden** and accumulation in the critical organ (the brain). The levels of mercury in maternal hair are a good indicator of methylmercury levels in fetal brain (the critical organ).

8.9.5 Biomonitoring

Mercury in urine is useful for biomonitoring of recent exposure to **mercury vapor and divalent mercury salts**. According to the SCOEL (2007), the mean level of mercury in urine of persons without occupational exposure in Germany is 0.4 µg/g creatinine, and the 95th percentile of mercury in urine is 2.2 µg/g creatinine. For persons with 10 amalgam fillings, the mean level in urine is 1.45 µg/g creatinine. The SCOEL (2007) recommended a biological limit value of 30 µg/g creatinine for occupational mercury exposure. Air exposure in the occupational environment that gives rise to 30 µg/g creatinine in urine will be to some extent dependent on how many amalgam fillings the worker has.

Mercury in blood is another useful biomarker of ongoing exposure to mercury vapor. In Norway, Simic et al. (2017) reported a mean level of mercury in whole blood: 3.19 µg/L, upper 90th percentile 8.42 µg/L. Persons living in an inland community, eating fish three times per month or less, had an upper level less than 5 µg/L. The SCOEL (2007) recommended a biological limit value of 10 µg/L for occupational exposures to mercury vapor and divalent mercury salts. In Norway, the occupational exposure to mercury vapor that gives rise to such a blood level will, to a considerable extent, depend on the fish consumption habits of the worker.

Mercury in whole blood, in erythrocytes, or in hair is a good indicator of the body burden of **methylmercury** and of the accumulation in the brain (the critical organ). In pregnant women, mercury in blood or in hair is a useful indicator of the level in the fetal brain and the risk of adverse effects in the child after delivery. The JECFA (2007) (see below, Section 8.9.7) estimated a BMDL = 14 µg/g of mercury in maternal hair for adverse neurodevelopmental effects of methylmercury on children at the age of 6 years.

8.9.6 Effects and Dose–Response Relationships

8.9.6.1 Mercury Vapor and Divalent Mercuric Mercury

Inhalation of high concentrations of **mercury vapor** may occur if liquid mercury is spilled in confined spaces. A few hours of inhalation gives rise to **acute poisoning** with severe lung symptoms and, in exceptional cases, lethal outcomes. There are no acute poisoning cases from ingestion of metallic mercury. Long-term exposure to lower levels of mercury vapor in occupational environments gives rise to **chronic poisoning.** Symptoms from the central nervous system (CNS) dominate in such poisoning with tremor and erethism, i.e., severe behavioral and personality changes, increased excitability, loss of memory, and insomnia. There are changes in brain signaling with changes in visual evoked potentials and in conduction velocities of peripheral nerves. In severe cases, there are also inflammatory changes in the gums and salivation. Reduced color vision and contrast sensitivity is likely to be related to the accumulation of mercury in the retina. Effects on the kidney and other organ (see below) occur because of the divalent mercury formed in blood from mercury vapor. Mercury vapor traverses the placenta, thus, there is reason to believe that exposure to the fetus may give rise to adverse effects if pregnant women are exposed to mercury vapor. Data from nonhuman primates indicates that levels of mercury in the fetal brain, much lower than those giving rise to similar effects in the adult brain, can cause changes in brain tissue and behavioral changes in the offspring.

Studies of mercury levels in air of working environments and the occurrence of symptoms like history of nervousness, loss of appetite, weight loss, and shyness, indicate a relationship down to approximately 50 $\mu g/m^3$ of mercury in air and at higher exposure classical symptoms like tremors and insomnia.

Several epidemiological studies have studied relationships between mercury levels in urine and results of test in neuropsychological performance. Meyer-Baron et al. (2002) performed a meta-analysis considering 44 such epidemiological studies. 12 studies were eligible for inclusion in the analysis. The authors found significant effect sizes at mean urinary mercury of 18–34 $\mu g/g$ creatinine. Considering all available evidence, Berlin et al. (2015) considered that an exposure level giving rise to detectable health effects in a group of exposed workers may fall somewhere between 10 and 30 $\mu g/g$ creatinine.

The ingestion of large doses of **divalent mercury salts** accidentally or with suicidal intent gives rise to **acute poisoning** with corrosive effects on the mucous membranes of the GI tract with vomiting, bloody diarrhea, circulatory collapse, and death. If the patient survives the first phase, there is necrosis of the tubular epithelium in the kidney, anuria, and uremia. Similar high doses of monovalent mercury salts, for example, calomel (mercurous chloride) are considerably less toxic. **Chronic poisoning** caused by exposure only to mercuric mercury is rare. The most common exposure, particularly in working environments, is exposure to a combination of dusts of mercuric mercury salts in combination with mercury vapor. This is the typical environment in chlor-alkali manufacturing factories. The kidney is usually regarded as the critical organ in chronic exposure to divalent mercury salts and kidney effects are critical effects. However, in some situations, effects on the thyroid and immunological effects are observed at lower exposures than the kidney effects. Skin exposure to mercury and **mercury compounds** can give rise to sensitization and dermatitis. Kidney effects are both caused by a toxic effect on the kidney tubules—increased urinary excretion of NAG and alpha-1 globulin occurs in mercury-exposed workers. Cases of nephrotic syndrome occur because of a toxic effect of mercury on the cells of the basal membrane of the glomerulus and the induction of antibodies again the basal membrane. Hultman and Pollard (2015) summarized available evidence on immunological effects of inorganic mercury, including skin sensitization, glomerulonephritis, and the earlier reported cases of acrodynia (pink disease), i.e., puffy, painful pink hands and feet in mercury-exposed children and the "Baboon syndrome"—mercury-induced skin eruptions or generalized skin rash after previous sensitization. Cases are reported of immunologically mediated effects after exposure via mercury-containing skin creams, dental amalgam, and thimerosal skin injection. However, dose—response relationships are not known. Changes in thyroid hormones in chlor-alkali workers indicate an adverse effect on the thyroid, possibly by an inhibitory effect on deiodinase enzyme. Such changes were reported in groups of workers with mean urinary mercury 10—27 µg/g creatinine.

8.9.6.2 Methylmercury

There is no specific acute poisoning syndrome after exposure to methylmercury, but there is a long latency (one to several weeks) between exposure and the appearance of symptoms after the uptake of a toxic dose. Regardless of whether the toxic dose is taken up on a single occasion or as repeated exposure, the symptoms and signs of **poisoning** are similar. In adults, mild poisoning cases have sensory disturbances with paresthesia in the extremities, in the tongue and lips. More severe poisoning cases display ataxia, concentric constriction of visual fields, and seizures. Pregnant women exposed to methylmercury give birth to children with infantile cerebral palsy in severe cases and psychomotor retardation in less severe cases. Despite severe poisoning in the children, exposed pregnant women may be symptom free. An outbreak of this disease occurred in population groups living near Minamata Bay, Japan; the first cases identified in the late 1950s. This disease was named **Minamata Disease** (Harada, 1968). Fishermen and their families ate fish caught in the bay where a chemical plant discharged mercury in various chemical forms into the bay. Methylmercury, either produced from other forms of mercury by a natural biomethylation process or possibly released as such from the factory, was bioaccumulated in the aquatic food chain to such an extent that consumption of fish from the bay resulted in cases of severe poisoning. More than 2000 cases are recognized. A large number of epidemiological studies describe dose—response relationships between the body burden of methylmercury and symptoms of poisoning (review by Berlin et al., 2015). The body burden (reflecting the level in the nervous system and brain) can be calculated from measurements of methylmercury in blood or hair. Chapter 5, Figs. 5.4 and 5.5, described such relationships for short-term exposures and calculations of dose—response relationships for long-term exposure. From the point of view of risk assessment for the population as a whole, the critical effect (i.e., the effect occurring at the lowest dose) in the most sensitive section of the population is of interest. For methylmercury, the fetal brain is considered most sensitive. Extensive studies in methylmercury-exposed population groups in the Faroe Islands have found clear relationships between mercury levels in maternal blood, cord blood, or maternal hair and decreased performance in neuropsychological tests by the children. Budtz-Jorgensen et al. (2001) used various benchmark response (BMR) levels and mathematical models when calculating BMDL (5% lowest limit). When using BMR 10%, these authors obtained BMDL values for maternal hair from 9.3 to 16.7 µg/g. A review of the literature is also available from U.S. National Research Council (2000).

In population groups with low dietary intakes of polyunsaturated fatty acids, there are some data indicating a relationship between such intake, mercury in hair, and risks of myocardial infarction. In Chapter 6, Fig. 6.4, risks for myocardial infarction are shown in relation to mercury levels in hair 1—8 µg/g. More information from other population groups on such relationships would be of interest for confirmation.

There has been a considerable expansion in the last decades of the knowledge base concerning molecular toxicological mechanisms of mercury-induced effects in animals and in vitro and for toxicokinetics of mercury and its compounds in humans. It is, however, notable that no TKTD or AOP model is sufficiently established for use in risk assessment by national or international organizations performing risk assessment and preparing recommendations for preventive measures.

8.9.7 Risk Assessments and Recommended Preventive Measures Including Exposure Limits Set by International Organizations

The SCOEL (2007) listed classifications of mercury vapor: toxic by inhalation; danger of cumulative effects; very toxic to aquatic organisms; and may cause long-term adverse effects in the aquatic environment. Mercuric oxide and mercuric chloride were classified in the same category for ecotoxicity: very toxic if swallowed; toxic: danger of serious damage to health by prolonged exposure in contact with skin and if swallowed; causes burns.

The SCOEL (2007) summarized available data and found that a NOAEL in animals, after repeated inhalation of mercury vapor, is in the range $0.1-0.2$ mg/m^3. In humans exposed in the working environment, consistent CNS effects and kidney effects of an adverse nature start to appear with urinary mercury levels above 20 mmol/mol creatinine ($=35$ µg/g creatinine). Based on a meta-analysis (Meyer-Baron et al., 2002), The SCOEL considers that the difference in performance between exposed and controls corresponds to 5%–7% performance decrease. Assuming that higher working exposure in the past might be the reason for the effects in some studies, a critical level of 30 µg/g creatinine can be recommended to avoid possible behavioral effects. They recommend a biological limit value of 30 µg/g creatinine and an OEL of 0.02 mg/m^3 of mercury in workroom air. The biological monitoring of mercury exposures is superior to air monitoring as it is more closely related to health effects.

The JECFA (2007) reviewed epidemiology studies in children exposed to methylmercury in food in the Faroe Islands and the Seychelles (Budtz-Jorgensen et al., 2001) (see above, Section 8.9.6.2); The U.S. National Research Council (2000) made similar assessments. Children aged 5.5–7 years were assessed for neurodevelopmental endpoints in relation to measured maternal hair Hg. The JECFA derived a BMDL/no-observed-effect-level of 14 mg/kg (14 µg/g) for concentrations of mercury in maternal hair in the studies of neurodevelopmental effects, which was calculated from a daily Hg intake of 1.5 µg/kg b.w. A total uncertainty factor (UF) of 6.4 resulted in the (weekly) PTWI value of 1.6 µg/kg b.w.

8.10 NICKEL (NI)

8.10.1 Introduction/Properties

Nickel (Ni), CAS No. 7440-02-01, atomic No. 28, atomic mass 58.71, density 8.9 g/cm^3, melting point 1453°C, is a silver white transition metal. It exists in five oxidation states -1, $+1$, $+2$, $+3$, and $+4$, with $+2$ being the most common form. Among the compounds, nickel carbonyl, Ni $(CO)_4$, CAS No 13463-39-3, is a volatile liquid. Several chemical analytical methods are available for Ni determination in various matrices, e.g., ICP-MS. Parts of this section on nickel is a summary from the review by

Klein and Costa (2015), and the reader is referred to their text for references when other sources are not specified.

8.10.2 Production and Uses

Mining of nickel-containing sulfide or oxide ores occur in several countries. The world production of nickel metal is increasing and reached 2 million tons per year in the mid 2010s (http://www.insg.org/prodnickel.aspx). In addition to this primary production, more than 300,000 tons of nickel is recycled. The uses of nickel include steel and alloy production, electroplating, production of nickel—cadmium and nickel—hydride batteries, other electronic components, engine parts, various tools and household items, coins, jewelry, and medical devices.

8.10.3 Environmental Occurrence and Human Exposures

Direct **exposure of the skin** is common by contact with nickel-containing items such as buttons, jewelry, eating utensils, and coins. Such contact may give rise to allergic contact dermatitis, occurring in a variable but relatively high percentage of persons in western countries (see below). Depending on the technical characteristics of the metallic objects, they release Ni into body fluids like sweat and enter the epidermis. Some high-quality Ni-containing surgical steel qualities release so small quantities of Ni that they can be used without risk for sensitization, while other objects release too much Ni to be safe. The limits for release are regulated in the EU (see Section 8.10.7 below).

Because oil and coal contains nickel, fossil fuel combustion contributes substantially to the environmental dispersion of nickel. Nickel smelters and industries using nickel are other important sources of emissions into the environment. Natural emission sources are volcanos and rock shear processes. Reported nickel concentrations in **ambient air** varies up to 10 ng/m^3 in the United States (Chen and Lippman, 2009). Nickel in cigarettes range up to 0.5 μg per cigarette and smoking contributes to exposure via the respiratory tract. However, only 1.1% of the nickel in cigarettes is in the smoke while the major part stays in the ash. Nickel in soil varies widely and high levels may occur in areas contaminated by local sources reaching mass fractions up to 50 g/kg in extreme cases.

Nickel values in **drinking water** vary with averages of 2—7 μg/L and occasional values up to 35 μg/L. In nickel mining areas, values may extend up to 200 μg/L in drinking water. The WHO guidance value for nickel in drinking water is 70 μg/L. The limit in the EU according to the Council Directive on water quality (EC, 1998) is 20 μg/L. In the United States, the EPA has set a maximum contaminant level of 0.1 mg/L. Nickel in food generally ranges 0.1−0.5 mg/kg fresh food. Nuts and cocoa have higher values in the 5−10 mg/kg range. Average estimates of total **daily dietary Ni intakes** are 200−300 μg, but in certain circumstances, intakes up to 1000 μg may occur because of leaching from cooking ware, kitchen utensils, and water piping. A reported value of 0.8 μg/L in breast milk is approximately 10 times lower than values for nickel in infant formula (Klein and Costa, 2015). The EFSA (2015) estimated a BMDL-10 for systemic contact dermatitis (SCD) and expressed a concern that current levels of acute dietary exposure to Ni may cause eczematous flare-up skin reactions in Ni-sensitized individuals (see further details Section 8.10.6 below).

Occupational exposures results from elevated levels of Ni in air in mines, refineries, smelters, factories, and chemical plants. Welding in stainless steel releases nickel causing exposure of workers. The SCOEL (2011) proposed OELs intended to be implemented in European countries (Section 8.10.7): nickel metal 0.005 mg/m^3 (respirable fraction); soluble nickel compounds 0.005 mg/m^3 (respirable fraction); soluble and poorly soluble nickel compounds (inhalable fraction) 0.01 mg/m^3. In Sweden, the most recent occupational exposure values (AFS, 2015, 2018) are: nickel metal 0.5 mg/m^3; nickel compounds (except nickel carbonyl and trinickelsulfide) 0.1 mg/m^3; trinickelsulfide (nickel subsulfide) 0.01 mg/m^3; nickel carbonyl 0.007 mg/m^3.

8.10.4 Toxicokinetics

8.10.4.1 Dermal Uptake

Skin contact with Ni-containing objects gives rise to Ni uptake in the skin. Nickel chloride solution applied to the skin accumulates in the *stratum corneum* and the hair shafts (review by IPCS, 1991a). Despite the considerable local uptake of nickel, systemic uptake through the skin is very limited. There are several studies of the release of Ni from objects and studies using patch tests on human skin to find out the concentrations of nickel giving rise to sensitization and elicitation of local dermal reaction (see below).

Inhalation of aerosols containing nickel leads to **uptake through the respiratory route**. The deposition of an inhaled Ni-containing aerosol uptake in tissues of the respiratory tract and subsequent systemic uptake varies depending on the particle size and solubility of the Ni compound (see Chapter 2, Section 2.3.3).

8.10.4.2 Uptake From Food and Drinking Water

Uptake of nickel **from food or drinking water** occurs to a varying extent in the GI tract and is dependent on the water solubility of the nickel compound (EFSA, 2015). Uptake is approximately 1% or less of nickel in food while uptake of ionic nickel (Ni^{2+}) in drinking water on an empty stomach may be 40 times higher. It is likely that binding of Ni^{2+} ions to various ligands in food explains the difference.

8.10.4.3 Transport and Distribution

Nickel is bound to albumin and nickeloplasmin in blood plasma. Transferrin also binds nickel. Nickel is carried through membranes by DMT-1. Transport by DMT-1 involves also several other divalent metals, and interactions with these metal ions (e.g., Fe^{2+}) occur. Cellular uptake processes for nickel includes macropinocytosis and clathrin-mediated endocytosis. After absorption from drinking water in humans, concentrations in serum were the highest 1 h after intake. Studies in humans indicated **biological half-lives** in serum and urine in the range 20–40 h. Nickel is widely **distributed** in tissues. It traverses the placenta barrier. In human autopsy studies, the ribs, lungs, thyroid, adrenals, and kidneys had the highest concentrations (review by IPCS, 1991a,b; EFSA, 2015).

8.10.4.4 Excretion

Excretion of nickel is mainly via urine. Excretion through sweat can also be important. Fecal nickel mainly represents unabsorbed nickel.

8.10.4.5 Toxicokinetic Models

A physiologically based toxicokinetic model is available for exposure to soluble nickel compounds through the GI tract. It calculates urinary and serum values, but not other tissue values. Calculations of the relative deposition of nickel compounds in the respiratory tract of experimental animals in comparison with humans are available (Oller and Oberdorster, 2010; SCOEL, 2011).

8.10.5 Biomonitoring

Blood, serum, plasma, or urine nickel values can be useful in biomonitoring of exposures and related health effects. Because of the possible contamination from nickel-containing steel needles, often used for blood collection, precautions may be advisable such as using plastic cannulas or allowing some blood to flow for other sampling purposes, before collection into tubes for metal analysis. Values of nickel in Norwegian men and women only exposed via the general environment were 0.49 μg/L (median), upper 90 percentile 1.47 μg/L in whole blood (Hansen et al., 2017). The IARC (2012) summarized available biomonitoring data: in Italy: blood mean value 2.3 μg/L (range 0.6—3.8); serum mean value 1.2 (range 0.2—3.7); urine mean value 0.9 μg/L (range 0.1—3.9). In Japan, the urine mean value was 2.1 μg/L (range 0.2—57). In Nikel, Russia (where a nickel smelter is located), urine mean value was 4.9 μg/L (range 0.3—62); in Apatity, Russia, the urine mean was 2.6 μg/L; in Tromso, Norway, the urine mean was 1.4 μg/L (range 0.3—6.0). Elevated values occur in persons with nickel-containing medical devices such as orthopedic implants and cardiovascular stents. In occupational exposures, there are also increased nickel values in biomonitoring media. For occupational exposures, SCOEL (2011) recommended a biological guidance value for nickel in urine: 3 μg/L.

8.10.6 Effects and Dose—Response Relationships

Very low (deficient) dietary intakes of nickel may reduce growth and change lipid metabolism in rats, but proof of an essential role of nickel in humans is lacking.

8.10.6.1 Skin Effects

Dermal contact with nickel-containing items causes uptake of nickel in the skin and may cause sensitization. *Ni-induced allergic contact dermatitis* is a *delayed type (type IV) hypersensitivity reaction.* After uptake into the skin, Ni serves as a hapten and is bound to endogenous peptides. Antigen-presenting cells mediate a proliferative response of T-lymphocytes. Skin-specific dendritic (Langerhans) cells are the critical cell type of antigen-presenting cells (Res et al., 1987). Ni interacts with endogenous components in the antigen-presenting grove of the human lymphocyte antigen molecule, thereby changing the antigenicity of these peptides. As a result of this induction process, Ni-specific T-cell clones occur in patients with Ni sensitivity. Exposure of these cells to haptenized nickel causes activation/elicitation (Emtestam and Olerup, 1996). Activation/elicitation leads to inflammation and skin symptoms like dermatitis with itchy, popular erythema.

Thus, we know these mechanisms for some time. Nickel may be seen as a prototype of an agent eliciting a type IV sensitivity reaction. Such nickel-induced effects confirm the AOP for skin sensitization introduced in Chapter 3, Section 3.4.3, Fig. 3.5. However, in order to elicit this reaction, Schmidt et al. (2010) showed that an additional molecular event is required, i.e., a specific interaction of Ni with an innate immune receptor: toll-like receptor 4 (TLR4). This interaction is required in order to induce nuclear factor-kappa-B activation and proinflammatory cytokine production. In humans, Ni is capable of inducing both the haptenization and the interaction with TLR4, but the same molecular interactions do not occur in some animals, for example, common mice strains (Schmidt et al., 2010).

Nickel serves as an example illustrating the *AOP for chemical-induced skin sensitization and contact dermatitis* displayed in Chapter 3, Section 3.4.3. The molecular initiating event for nickel has two components: (1) haptenization and (2) interaction with TLR4. The AO is skin symptoms occurring as a result of inflammation caused by proliferation of activated T-cells in combination with induction of inflammatory cytokines like nuclear factor-kappa-B.

Patch tests detect *sensitization to nickel*. Reported dose—response relationships in terms of exposure levels in patch tests and related detection of skin reactions in humans formed the basis for proposals of legislation limiting skin exposure to nickel in the EU (see below and Section 8.10.7). Menné (1994) concluded that trace amounts of nickel present in the general environment do not induce nickel sensitization. He further stated that elicitation of nickel dermatitis is unlikely for concentrations $<0.1-1$ $\mu g/cm^2$ in contact with the skin during occluded exposure and 15 $\mu g/cm^2$ when nonoccluded. A nonsensitizing nickel concentration of 0.5 $\mu g/cm^2$ per week was suggested for consumer items made of nickel alloys. Highly sensitized individuals might react to 0.5 ppm nickel (0.0075 $\mu g/cm^2$) when exposed on inflamed skin under occlusion.

Sensitization to nickel is very common. Mortz et al. (2002) performed patch tests on 1146 school-children (aged 12—16 years) in Odense, Denmark, 1995—97. 19.4% of the girls and 10.3% of the boys showed a positive reaction to one or more allergens, the most common being nickel sulfate (13.7% of girls and 2.5% of boys). These authors found a highly significant association between contact allergy and hand eczema, but not with atopic dermatitis or inhalant allergy. Other studies also report that sensitization to nickel is common in both children and adults and that it often leads to hand eczema, ill health and time off from work (e.g., Garg et al., 2013). Denmark implemented legislation to limit the dermal exposure to nickel already in 1992, i.e., earlier than in the EU as a whole. Jensen et al. (2002) found that the odds ratio for nickel sensitization was 3.34 ($P = .004$) for girls who had their ears pierced before 1992 when compared to girls without ear piercing. The corresponding odds ratio for girls who had their ears pierced after 1992 was 1.20 ($P = .52$). Garg et al. (2013) found decreasing trends for nickel sensitization in several EU countries after implementation of the legislation limiting dermal exposure to nickel.

Systemic contact dermatitis (SCD) may occur in persons sensitized to nickel, who ingest food or drink containing concentrations of nickel that activates a flare-up of skin symptoms. The EFSA's Panel on Contaminants in the Food Chain (the EFSA CONTAM Panel; EFSA, 2015) identified the data of Jensen et al. (2003) in human volunteers as the most sensitive and adequate study basis for a reference point (RP) for acute oral intake of nickel (soluble compounds) in risk assessment. From the data in Jensen et al. (2003), the panel derived a BMDL-10 of 0.08 mg Ni per person, corresponding to 1.1 μg Ni/kg b.w. as an RP for SCD elicited in Ni-sensitive humans after acute oral exposure to Ni. The Panel noted that this value of 1.1 μg Ni/kg b.w. is in the same range as the lower confidence bounds of the ED-10 values calculated in the meta-analysis by Jensen et al. (2006).

8.10.6.2 Pulmonary and Systemic Toxicity

Upon inhalation of volatile *nickel carbonyl* ($Ni(CO)_4$), the compound rapidly decomposes, giving rise to toxicity to the lungs and brain both in experimental animals and humans. In humans, initial respiratory effects may be mild or transient in the first 2—3 days following nickel carbonyl exposure, but subsequently, clinical symptoms including cough, shortness of breath (dyspnea), and worsening symptoms of pneumonia and acute respiratory distress may appear. Alveolar damage in the lungs is maximal 4—6 days after $Ni(CO)_4$ exposure. Other symptoms of such severe poisoning include myalgias, fatigue, weakness, delirium, and convulsions. Urinary nickel values 18 h postexposure is a useful basis for judging the severity of nickel carbonyl poisoning: mild, 60—100 μg/L; moderately severe, 100—500 μg/L; and severe >500 μg/L. Because of the high toxicity of nickel carbonyl, a low occupational exposure value is in effect for this substance (Sections 8.10.3 and 8.10.7).

Rhinitis, sinusitis, and formation of nasal polyps, as well as perforation of the nasal septum, occur among workers inhaling *Ni-containing aerosols*, occurring, for example, in nickel smelting and roasting. High-level exposures may cause lung fibrosis and pneumoconiosis. Cases of airway hypersensitivity and asthma also occur, although they are rare.

A long-term study with inhaled nickel sulfate in rats (NTP, 1996c) showed inflammatory reaction in lungs at nickel mass concentrations of 0.06 mg/m^3 and higher, whereas no effects were observed at 0.03 mg/m^3.

Similar experiments with metallic nickel (Oller et al., 2008), Ni_3S_2 (NTP, 1996b), or NiO (NTP, 1996a) found inflammatory changes or fibrosis in the lungs at the lowest tested dose 0.1 mg/m^3.

8.10.6.3 Reproductive and Developmental Effects

In rats and mice, dietary nickel (1 mg/kg) reduced the motility of sperm, possibly by oxidative damage. EFSA (2015) reviewed published and unpublished studies in animals demonstrating histological changes in reproductive tissues of male mice exposed to nickel sulfate at a nickel dose of 2.2 mg/kg b.w. Mating of such mice with unexposed female mice gave rise to a decreased number of implantations, an increase in resorptions and decreased fetal weight.

High doses >92 mg/kg per day of nickel chloride gave rise to malformations and skeletal anomalies in the fetuses of pregnant female mice. A number of studies at lower doses reported increased pup mortality—stillbirth or postimplantation loss/perinatal lethality in rats with a LOAEL of 1.3 mg/kg b.w. per day in a study using nickel chloride. EFSA (2015) used a database of unpublished 1- and 2-generation studies in rats exposed to nickel sulfate hexahydrate by gavage to derive a BMDL for 10% increased risk of litters with three or more postimplantation losses. The resulting BMDL-10 value was 0.28 mg/kg b.w. per day for chronic exposure.

8.10.6.4 Genotoxicity and Carcinogenicity

Mammalian cells take up nickel compounds including insoluble nickel subsulfide, crystalline nickel monosulfide, and nickel oxides, and nickel ions are released intracellularly causing cytotoxicity, chromosomal aberrations, and genomic instability. The production of ROS is part of the explanation for such genotoxicity. Inhibition of DNA repair processes is another likely component explaining nickel carcinogenicity. Changes in the methylation pattern of DNA causing silencing of tumor suppressor genes may also be involved.

IARC (2012) summarized available evidence on the carcinogenicity of nickel and its compounds in humans and animals (for specific references see IARC, 2012). The IARC working group noted that there is **epidemiological evidence** for an elevated risk of lung cancer and nasal sinus cancer among nickel refinery workers and for an elevated risk of lung cancer among nickel smelter workers. Epidemiological evidence is also available supporting an elevated risk of cancer in relation to exposures to specific nickel compounds. There is an increased risk of lung cancer in humans exposed to nickel chloride, nickel sulfate and water-soluble nickel compounds in general, insoluble nickel compounds, nickel oxides, nickel sulfides, and mostly insoluble nickel compounds. Studies concerned with lung cancer risks from nickel and its compounds identified both water-soluble nickel and metallic nickel as contributing to risk while other studies addressing nickel metal exposures were uninformative according to the IARC. The SCOEL (2011) summarized data on the risk of sinus cancer and lung cancer in the Kristiansand cohort. They stated that there was an increased cancer incidence after exposure to 1.6 mg/m^3 × years of exposure to water soluble nickel compounds, corresponding to 0.04 mg/m^3 for 40 years. This estimate formed the basis for a proposed exposure limit (see Section 8.10.7).

In **animal experiments,** nickel chloride in drinking water increased the incidence of UV-induced tumors in mice. Nickel subsulfide by inhalation induced lung and adrenal tumors in rats. Nickel oxide by inhalation induced lung tumors and adrenal tumors in rats and female mice. Inhaled metallic nickel increased the incidence of adrenal pheochromocytomas in male rats and adrenal cortical tumors in female rats. Nickel carbonyl inhalation induced lung carcinomas. Transplacental nickel acetate induced malignant pituitary tumors in the offspring of rats. Nickel metal powder and several nickel compounds induced injection site tumors including sarcomas. Section 8.10.7 (below) summarizes the IARC evaluation of available evidence on carcinogenesis.

8.10.7 Risk Assessments and Recommended Preventive Measures Including Exposure Limits Set by International and National Organizations

The IARC, a widely recognized international organization for evaluation of the carcinogenicity of environmental agents, publishes documentation serving as a basis for international organizations and government bodies in various countries, when they formulate decisions concerning preventive measures, provide effective cancer control programs, and decide about public health measures. The IARC (2012) stated that there is sufficient evidence in humans for the carcinogenicity of mixtures that include nickel compounds and nickel metal. These agents cause cancers of the lung and of the nasal cavity and paranasal sinuses.

There is sufficient evidence in experimental animals for the carcinogenicity of nickel monoxides, nickel hydroxides, nickel sulfides (including nickel subsulfide), nickel acetate, and nickel metal. There is limited evidence in experimental animals for the carcinogenicity of nickelocene, nickel carbonyl, nickel sulfate, nickel chloride, nickel arsenides, nickel antimonide, nickel selenides, and nickel telluride. In view of the overall findings in animals, there is sufficient evidence in experimental animals for the carcinogenicity of nickel compounds and nickel metal.

According to the IARC (2012), nickel compounds are carcinogenic to humans (IARC Group 1).

In the EU, the SCOEL (2011) classified nickel compounds as carcinogens in their Group C, i.e., carcinogens with a practical threshold. The reason for this classification is that nickel ions do not interact readily with DNA. As mentioned in Section 8.10.6.4, the genotoxic and carcinogenic effects of nickel are probably due to indirect effects like the formation of ROS and the interaction of nickel ions with cellular DNA repair systems. The SCOEL therefore made quantitative risk assessments based on protection from inflammatory effects in the lungs and stated that the derived OELs should also protect against carcinogenic effects according to available evidence.

A study with inhaled nickel sulfate in rats (Section 8.10.6.2) showed inflammatory reaction in lungs at a nickel mass concentration 0.06 mg/m^3, whereas no effects were observed at 0.03 mg/m^3, and the latter value was regarded as NOAEL. Considering possible species differences in toxicokinetics and toxicodynamics, the SCOEL proposed, an 8-h OEL of 0.005 mg/m^3 (respirable fraction).

Experiments with metallic nickel, Ni_3S_2, or NiO, found inflammatory changes or fibrosis in lungs at the lowest tested dose and a NOAEL could not be established. The SCOEL proposed an OEL of 0.005 mg/m^3 for nickel metal and poorly soluble nickel compounds (respirable fraction). Nickel compounds also cause cancer of the nasal sinuses, and all inhalable nickel-containing particles need to be limited. The SCOEL proposed an OEL of 0.01 mg/m^3 for inhalable water soluble and poorly soluble nickel compounds based on observations of respiratory cancers at slightly higher exposures in the Kristiansand cohort (see above). The SCOEL stated: "Metallic nickel is excluded since neither animal nor epidemiological data point towards a carcinogenic action of nickel metal." The proposed OELs represent the lower daily doses of nickel compounds than those giving rise to reproductive toxicity (see Section 8.10.6.3 and the considerations by the EFSA below). The SCOEL did not consider contact dermatitis, respiratory sensitization, and asthma in their evaluation.

In Sweden, the limit values for occupational environments are the following (AFS, 2015, 2018): nickel metal dust 0.5 mg/m^3; nickel compounds (except nickel carbonyl and nickel subsulfide 0.1 mg/m^3; nickelsubsulfide (trinickeldisulfide) 0.01 mg/m^3; nickel carbonyl 0.007 mg/m^3.

The EFSA CONTAM Panel (EFSA, 2015) cited the evaluation by IARC (2012) and stated "no tumours have been found in the oral carcinogenicity studies in experimental animals. Therefore, the CONTAM Panel considered it unlikely that dietary exposure to Ni results in cancer in humans." The evaluation of oral exposures to nickel compounds by EFSA (2015), therefore, focused on other effects than carcinogenicity. The EFSA Panel selected reproductive and developmental toxicity in experimental animals as the critical effect for chronic effects of Ni and used the BMDL-10 of 0.28 mg/kg b.w. per day (Section 8.10.6.3) as a RP. They derived a tolerable daily intake of nickel in food of 2.8 µg/kg b.w. per day by applying the default UF of 100 to account for extrapolation from experimental animals to humans and for interindividual variability.

The EFSA Panel selected SCD elicited in Ni-sensitive humans after oral exposure to Ni as the critical effect of acute effects of Ni. The Panel used the BMDL-10 of 1.1 µg Ni/kg b.w. as the RP, derived based on the incidence of SCD following oral exposure to Ni of human volunteers (Section 8.10.6.1). The Panel applied a margin of exposure (MOE) approach and considered an MOE of 10 to be indicative of a low health concern. The MOEs calculated considering the estimated mean and the 95th percentile acute exposure levels in EU countries were considerably below 10 for all age groups. Overall, the CONTAM Panel concluded that, at the current levels of acute dietary exposure to Ni, there is a concern that Ni-sensitized individuals may develop eczematous flare-up skin reactions.

In Europe, the Nickel Directive (94/27/EC) was passed in 1994 and was fully implemented in 2001. This *EU-directive* prohibits the sale of products intended to come into direct prolonged contact with the skin that release nickel at rates >0.5 µg cm^2 per week. The maximum nickel release rate for piercing post assemblies is currently 0.2 µg cm^2 per week. All forms of jewelry, watches, buttons, and zippers were initially included, and presently it includes mobile phones as well. The legislation from 1994 is now part of the REACH regulation supervised by the ECHA (https://echa.europa.eu). Nickel is placed on the REACH "restriction list" (see Chapter 7). Several studies in a number of EU countries have documented the efficient prevention of nickel sensitization that has resulted from this legislation (see Garg et al., 2013).

8.11 PALLADIUM (PD)

8.11.1 Properties and Uses

Palladium (Pd), CAS No. 7440-05-3, atomic No. 46, atomic mass 106.42, density 12.0 g/cm^3, melting point 1554.8°C, is a silver white metal belonging to the Platinum Group of Elements. Its most common oxidation states are +2 and +4. Pd can be determined in environmental and biological matrices by ICP-MS methods. The world production in 2015 was 208 tons; it had increased by 100 tons since 2005. In addition to primary production, recycling contributes 70 tons (USGS, 2017). **Uses**: Catalytic converters in automobiles make up a major part of the Pd demand. Because of its catalytic properties, the metal is also used as a catalyst in industrial processes. Pd metal and silver—palladium paste are widely used in the electronics manufacturing industries. Other important Pd uses are in jewelry and coinage. Pd alloys are used in dentistry (crowns bridges).

8.11.2 Dispersion in the Environment and Human Exposure

The **dispersion** of Pd in the **environment** has increased in the last decades because of its use in catalysts for automobiles. Concentrations in road dust up to 390 µg/kg were reported in Germany (Leopold, 2008). The following values were reported in ambient air: 57 ng/m^3 in ambient air in the city Chernivitsi, Ukraine, and 3.3 pg/m^3 in Israel (review Umemura et al., 2015). The reason for the very high value in Ukraine is not known. Tilch et al. (2000) reported 0.2—15 pg/m^3 in Berlin, Germany. Gomez (2002) reported 4.6 pg/m^3 in Göteborg, Sweden, and 55 pg/m^3 in Rome, Italy. Bozlaker et al. (2014) reported 214 pg/m^3 in ambient air in a road tunnel in Boston, Texas, USA. In food, the highest concentrations of Pd occur in bread and nuts (2—3 µg/kg). Intake through food is approximately 1 µg/day (Ysart et al., 1999), and drinking water contributes even less.

Air concentrations of Pd up to 5 µir^3 occurred in **the work environment** of dental laboratories in the 1990s. Workers in those environments had elevated urinary Pd values. Later studies of dental technicians or workers manufacturing catalysts for automobiles, found no increases in urinary Pd. Occupational exposure limits for Pd and its compounds are not available.

The use of Pd in dentistry and in jewelry, including piercing items gives rise to human exposure. There are increased concentrations of Pd in saliva in persons with Pd-containing dental materials. An intake with saliva of 1—15 µg/day is possible (IPCS, 2002). Direct contact between the skin or gingival mucosa and items containing Pd gives rise to uptake in epithelial cells. Such uptake is, as far as we know, not well characterized, but in humans developing sensitization, it can give rise to allergic symptoms (see below Section 8.11.5).

8.11.3 Toxicokinetics and Biomonitoring

The **toxicokinetics** of Pd and its compounds is only partially characterized. The systemic uptake in rats after 3 days was estimated at 0.5% of an orally given dose of a solution of Pd salt. In suckling rats, approximately 5% was absorbed after 4 days. Endotracheal administration gave rise to higher absorption. Of the absorbed amount, the highest concentration was found in the kidneys with lower values in the liver and spleen. Very low concentrations were found in brain tissue. After intravenous injection in rats, only a small proportion of the injected dose was found in the fetuses of dams. Excretion occurred both in urine and in feces after intravenous administration in rats, slightly more in urine (summarized by Umemura et al., 2015). Violante et al. (2005) found a clear relationship between concentrations of Pd in ambient air and concentrations in urine. The authors suggested the use of urinary Pd in **biomonitoring** of exposure.

8.11.4 Toxicity

Acute **toxicity** varies depending on route of exposure and Pd compound (summary by Umemura et al., 2015). In rats, intravenous injection of Pd (II) chloride is toxic in milligram doses, while palladium (II) oxide given orally can be given in grams per kilogram body weight without serious toxicity. Intratracheal application of Pd dust gave rise to inflammatory changes. The lowest intravenous dose of divalent Pd in rats giving rise to an adverse effect (cardiac arrhythmia) was 0.4 mg/kg b.w. A 28-day repeated dose oral study of tetraammine palladium hydrogen carbonate in rats found histological changes in the liver, kidneys, spleen, and stomach at 15 and 150 mg/kg b.w. A NOAEL of 1.5 mg/kg b.w. was established.

Schroeder and Mitchener (1971) studied the chronic toxicity and carcinogenicity of palladium(II) chloride (5 mg/L) given in drinking water to male mice during their whole life span. Pd-exposed mice survived longer and had more malignant tumors than control mice. Because of the longer survival time, the increase in tumors is considered to be related to the longer lives of the exposed animals. Palladium or its compounds are not classified as carcinogenic by the International Agency for Research on Cancer.

8.11.5 Sensitization

Some Pd compounds, for example, $(NH_4)_2PdCL_6$ and $(NH_4)_2PdCl_4$, are strong **skin irritants**, while other compounds like $(NH_3)_2$ Pd Cl_2 and PdO did not produce adverse skin effects when tested in animals. Palladium (II)chloride and tetraammine palladium hydrogen carbonate are strong **sensitizers** in the guinea pig maximization test. $Pd(II)Cl_2$, sodium tetrachloropallidate(II), potassium tetrachloropallidate(II), and ammonium hexachloropallidate(IV) displayed a significant primary immune response in the popliteal lymph node test in mice. Cross reactivity to nickel occurs (summary from Umemura et al., 2015).

Dermal contact and piercing are important human routes of exposure to Pd. Individuals with more piercings have more reactions in patch tests to Pd (and other metals like Ni, Au, and Co). Pd derives also from dental materials and jewelry. Women suffer **sensitization to Pd** much more frequently than men do. Sensitization to Pd is the second most frequent (after Ni) among metals. In a study with patch testing of 906 consecutive patients in dermatology clinics in Europe, 24% displayed a positive test to Pd. Compared to patients without Pd sensitization, the positive patients more frequently had dental crowns. Clinical symptoms related to such sensitivity were skin reactions to metals, oral lichenoid lesions, xerostomia, and metal taste (Muris et al., 2015). Dental materials serve as important sources of exposure with increased concentrations of Pd in saliva (see Section 8.11.2 above). Symptoms related to Pt sensitivity are: swelling of lips, stomatitis, oral lichen planus, itching, dizziness, asthma, and chronic urticaria. Many reports describe recovery from Pd sensitivity after removal of dental materials. In Pd refinery workers, dental technicians, and some other occupations handling Pd, exposure to Pd and its compounds occur. There are reports of individual cases with symptoms such as rhinoconjunctivitis and asthma. However, in occupationally exposed groups, the frequency of sensitization to Pd is low according to available studies (summarized from Umemura et al., 2015).

8.11.6 Human Health Risk Assessment

Gomez et al. (2002) presented a **human health risk assessment** of the concentrations of Pd, occurring is ambient air. These authors summarized available evidence and stated that the present concentrations of platinum and its compounds in ambient air is 15 pg/m^3 or less, and they further stated that palladium concentrations are in the same order of magnitude. Merget and Rosner (2001) estimated a guidance value of 100 ng/m^3 for Pt. Gomez et al. (2002) stated that the toxic potential of Pd is generally presumed to be lower than that for Pt and that traffic-related exposures to Pd would therefore be approximately three orders of magnitude lower than levels were adverse health effects might theoretically occur. A formal risk assessment for Pd in food and drinking water is not available, and it is thus not known whether **human health risks** would result from the exposures reported (see Section 8.11.2 above). Skin or mucosal contact with Pd-containing jewelry or dental materials can give rise to sensitization and subsequent adverse clinical symptoms. Persons with pierced ears or other body parts are at an increased risk. However, limits for release of Pd from material in contact with human tissues are not available. There is an obvious need to better develop TKTD and AOP models and to examine if Pd-induced sensitization and related AOs follow a similar AOP as the general one for skin sensitization discussed in Chapter 3. Possible similarities with the AOP for skin sensitization to nickel (see above, Section 8.10) may be considered. It seems important to define limits of Pd release from Pd-containing items in contact with skin, mucous membranes, dental tissue, and pierced body parts in the same way as for nickel (see Section 8.10.7).

8.12 PLATINUM (PT)

8.12.1 Properties, Uses and Human Exposures

Platinum (Pt), CAS No. 7440-06-4, atomic No. 78, atomic mass 195.084, density 21.5 g/cm^3, melting point 1768.2°C, is a silver grey metal, lustrous, malleable, with common oxidation states +2 and +4 (RSC, 2018). It is resistant to corrosion. It can be determined in environmental and biological matrices by ICP-MS, sector field ICP-MS , and adsorptive voltammetry (this chapter section is a summary of the review by Kiilunen et al. 2015, where specific references are found). The world production in 2011 was 184 tons. Recycling further contributed 58 tons to world supply. **Uses**: A major use of Pt is in catalytic converters in automobiles. It is used as a catalyst in the chemical industry. In the electronics industry, Pt is used in fiber optic cables and for other purposes. It is used in dentistry as crowns, bridges, and in fillings. It is used in jewelry. Pt compounds (cisplatin i.e., *cis*-diamminedichloroplatinum(II)) are used in cancer therapy. Platinum nanoparticles are used as catalysts and have been suggested for use in cancer therapy.

The earth's crust contains around 3 ppm of Pt. The environmental dispersion of Pt has increased in the last decades because of its use in catalytic converters in cars. The levels in ambient air are from <1 to 147 pg/m^3, higher in urban than in rural areas. In the **working environment**, the air levels are usually <2 μg/m^3, but up to 2200 μg/m^3 was reported in a platinum refinery (review by Kiilunen et al., 2015). In the United Kingdom, the intake of **Pt in food** was 0.02 μg/day in 1994; in 2006, it was 2.3 μg/day.

8.12.2 Toxicokinetics

Inhalation experiments in animals showed small lung retention of 1-μm aerosols of platinum metal or Pt compounds. Of the retained amount, longer lung retention was seen with Pt metal and PtO than with soluble Pt compounds. Oral uptake of platinum (IV) chloride was <1% in rats. Injected Pt salts are distributed to the kidney and to a lesser extent in other organs such as the adrenal glands, spleen, liver, and bone. Transfer through the placenta is limited. After inhalation of $(NH4)_2PtCl_4$ in two human volunteers, an initial half-life of urinary excretion was 50 h and a second half-life 24 days. Cis-platinum used in cancer therapy has a biological half-life of 7 days. Elimination of absorbed platinum is to a large extent through urine.

8.12.3 Biomonitoring

It is difficult to use biomonitoring in order to estimate environmental or occupational exposures because of the interference of platinum from dental inlays, crowns, and bridges. However, workers in occupations with increased air levels of Pt had higher biomonitoring values in some studies. Nursing and pharmacy personnel had increased urine or serum platinum from handling cis-platinum cytostatic drugs. Improvements are required in handling routines (Kiilunen et al., 2015).

8.12.4 Acute Toxicity

Metallic platinum dust given orally to rats gave rise to slight necrotic changes in the GI epithelium, and changes in liver cells and in kidneys, but to no lethal effects. The toxicity of orally administered Pt compounds decreased in the following order: $PtCl_4$ > $Pt(SO_4)_2$ $4H_2O$ > PtO_2 Platinum coordination complexes with chloride are more toxic (kidneys being targeted) by the oral route than platinum salts. Nephrotoxicity is the major side effect of cisplatin cytostatic treatment for cancer.

$(NH4)_2PtCl_4$ and Na_2PtCl_6 as well as some other Pt complexes are strong irritants or even corrosive when applied to the eye and are irritants or strong irritants to the skin; platinum (IV)chloride is an irritant to the skin but platinum(II)chloride and platinum oxide are nonirritants (IPCS, 1991b). There are no data on the in vivo toxicity of platinum nanoparticles.

8.12.5 Sensitization and Allergy (Platinosis)

A platinum–related, asthma–like disease named platinosis or platinum salt sensitivity first occurred in photographic studios in the first part of last century and later in platinum refineries. Symptoms include watering of the eyes and asthma–like respiratory manifestations as well as skin symptoms, usually urticaria. The risk of developing allergy to reactive halogen–containing Pt compounds increases with increasing exposure levels and duration. Merget et al. (2000) found that 13/114 workers exposed to hexachloroplatinates (14 $\mu g/m^3$) developed the disease during a follow-up time of 33 months. Decreases in exposure or removal from exposure decreased the prevalence of respiratory symptoms (Merget et al., 2001).

Based on observations in Pt workers, the potency of different Pt complexes to induce positive skin prick test are (in the following order from the highest to the lowest):

$(NH_4)_2$ $[PtCl_6] \cong (NH_4)_2$ $[PtCl_4] > CS_2$ $[PtNO_2Cl_3] > CS_2$ $[Pt(NO_2)_2$ $Cl_2] > CS_2[Pt(NO_2)_3Cl] > K_2$ $[Pt(NO_2)_4]$

The last listed compound is inactive.

Clinical platinum sensitivity, i.e., allergy to platinum compounds with reactive halogen components (platinosis) is a type I, IgE–mediated immune response. Specific platinum salts act as haptens and combine with serum proteins to form a complete antigen. There is an increased level of total IgE, on a group basis, in patients with platinosis compared to nonsensitized persons. Increased levels of Pt-specific IgEs were reported in some studies (review by Kiilunen et al., 2015). Among workers exposed to relatively low levels of hexachloroplatinates (2 $\mu g/m^3$), the risk of developing sensitization was higher among smokers than among nonsmokers (review by Kiilunen et al., 2015). HLA-type DR3 was more common among workers sensitized to Pt than among matched nonsensitized referents, indicating that genetic factors are of importance for the likelihood of sensitization.

Park et al. (2010) exposed mice to platinum nanoparticles intratracheally and found increases in proinflammatory cytokines in bronchoalveolar lavage as well as a cellular inflammatory response in lung tissue. It is difficult to interpret these findings in relation to respiratory sensitization and risk assessment.

8.12.6 Carcinogenicity, Mutagenicity, and Reproductive Toxicity

Data are not available concerning cancer in humans or experimental animals from exposure to metallic platinum, halogenated complexes, or platinum nanoparticles. Based on sufficient evidence in experimental animals, inadequate evidence in humans, and supporting evidence from other relevant data, the IARC determined (IARC, 1981, 1987) that cisplatin is probably carcinogenic to humans (IARC, Group2A). Cisplatin is mutagenic in a variety of test systems; other platinum containing cytostatic drugs are also genotoxic. Some other platinum compounds are mutagenic in vitro but not in vivo (review by IPCS, 1991b; Kiilunen et al., 2015). There is a lack of information on reproductive toxicity of platinum compounds other than cisplatin. High doses of cisplatin given to pregnant rats caused fetal toxicity but no teratogenicity. 1-mM hexachloroplatinate caused decreased sperm motility. Platinum nanoparticles given orally to mice did not cause maternal or fetal toxicity, but increased mortality and decreased growth in the offspring (Park et al., 2010).

8.12.7 Human Health Risk Assessment

No adverse effects are known for human dietary exposure or from exposure through ambient air. Because of the use of catalytic converters in cars, Pt levels are increasing in the general environment. Sensitization is the main health effect of Pt compounds. Hexa- and tetrachloroplatinates are the most potent sensitizers. Reports of a high incidence of platinum sensitivity (platinosis) among platinum workers shows higher risks at higher exposures. These reports also demonstrate higher risks among smokers than among nonsmokers. The SCOEL (2011) reviewed available data and noted that there were suggestions in the scientific literature of a nonsensitizing air level of 10 ng/m^3 for chloroplatinates. However, the SCOEL considered the data too uncertain and determined that available data did not allow an OEL to be set. Also for platinum metal and insoluble platinum compounds, the SCOEL considered that it was not possible to set a health-based OEL based on the available data. In Sweden, there is an OEL of 1 mg/m^3 for platinum metal and poorly soluble compounds. For soluble platinum compounds, they are classified as sensitizing; the limit value is 2 μg/m^3 (AFS, 2015, 2018). A risk assessment for inhalation exposure to platinum nanoparticles is not available.

REFERENCES

AFS, 2015. Hygieniska gränsvarden. AFS 2015:7, p. 74 (Occupational Limit Values, Sweden).

AFS, 2018. Hygieniska gränsvärden. AFS 2018:1, p. 75 (Occupational Limit Values, Sweden).

Ahlmark, A., Bruce, T., Nyström, Å., 1960. Silicosis and Other Pneumoconiosis in Sweden. Scandinavian University Books, Norstedts, Stockholm, Sweden.

Akerstrom, et al., 2013. Environ. Health Perspect. 121, 187.

Akerstrom, et al., 2014. J. Expo. Sci. Environ. Epidemiol. 24, 171.

Akesson, A., et al., 2005. Environ. Health Perspect. 113, 1627.

Akesson, A., et al., 2006. Environ. Health Perspect. 114, 830.

Altman, P., et al., 2007. Kidney Int. 71, 252.

Amzal, B., et al., 2009. Environ. Health Perspect. 117, 1293.

Aoki, Y., et al., 1990. Toxicol. Appl. Pharmacol. 106, 462.

Apostoli, P., et al., 2013. Exp. Toxicol. Pathol. 65, 719.

ATSDR (Agency for Toxic Substances and Disease Registry), 2012. Toxicological Profile for Cadmium. ATSDR, U.S. Department of Health and Human Services, Atlanta, Georgia, pp. 1—430.

Barr, D.B., et al., 2005. Environ. Health Perspect. 113, 192.

Barregard, L., et al., 2016. Environ. Health Perspect. 124, 594.

Berlin, M., Fowler, B.A., Zalups, R., 2015. Mercury. In: Nordberg, G.F., Fowler, B.A., Nordberg, M. (Eds.), Handbook on the Toxicology of Metals, fourth ed. Academic Press, Elsevier, Amsterdam, Boston.

Bernard, A., 2016. Environ. Health Perspect. 124, 1.

Bjerregaard, P., Andersen, C.B.I., Andersen, O., 2015. Ecotoxicology of metals — sources, transport, and effects on the ecosystem. In: Nordberg, G.F., Fowler, B.A., Nordberg, M. (Eds.), Handbook on the Toxicology of Metals, fourth ed., vol. 1. Academic Press, Elsevier, Amsterdam, Boston, pp. 425—459.

Bozlaker, A., et al., 2014. Environ. Sci. Technol. 48, 54.

Brown, R.P., Fowler, B.A., et al., 2015. Toxicity of metals released from implanted medical devices. In: Nordberg, G.F., et al. (Eds.), Handbook on the Toxicology of Metals, fourth ed. Amsterdam, Boston.

Bruce, D.W., et al., 1963. Toxicol. Appl. Pharmacol. 5, 750.

Buchet, J.P., et al., 1990. Lancet 336, 699.

Buchet, J.P., et al., 2003. Int. Arch. Occup. Environm. Health 76 (2), 111.

Budtz-Jorgensen, et al., 2001. Biometrics 57, 698—706.

Burns, L.A., Munson, A.E., 1993. Pharmacol. Exp. Therap. 265, 178.

Bustamente, J., et al., 1997. Toxicology 118, 129—136.

Cassee, F.R., et al., 2011. Crit. Rev. Toxicol. 41, 213.

CDC, NHANES, 2012. 4th National Report on Human Exposure to Environmental Chemicals. US Department of Health and Human Services, Centers for Disease Control and Prevention.

Chaumont, A., et al., 2011. Occup. Environ. Med. 68, 257.

Chaumont, A., et al., 2012. Toxicol. Lett. 210, 345.

Chen, L.C., Lippman, M., 2009. Inhal. Toxicol. 21, 1.

Chen, C.-J., Wang, C.-J., 1990. Cancer Res. 50, 5470.

Chen, X., et al., 2009. Environ. Res. 109, 874.

Choudhury, H., et al., 2001. J. Toxicol. Environ. Health A 63 (5), 321—325.

Conner, E.A., et al., 1993. J. Expo. Anal. Environ. Epidemiol. 3, 43.

Conner, E.A., et al., 1995. Chem. Biol. Interact. 96, 273—285.

Cortona, G., et al., 1992. IARC Sci. Publ. 118, 205.

Dale, J.G., et al., 2017. Environ. Sci. Technol. 51 (4), 1973—1980.

Davidson, T., et al., 2015. Selected molecular mechanisms of metal toxicity and carcinogenicity. In: Nordberg, G.F., Fowler, B.A., Nordberg, M. (Eds.), Handbook on the Toxicology of Metals, fourth ed. Elsevier Publishers, Amsterdam (Chapter 9).

De Boeck, M., et al., 2001. Carcinogenesis 19, 2021.

DECOS (Health Council of the Netherlands), 2012. Arsenic and Inorganic Arsenic Compounds. Health-Based Calculated Occupational Cancer Risk Values. Health Council of the Netherlands, The Hague. Publication No. 2012/32.

Diamond, G.L., et al., 2003. J. Toxicol. Environ. Health A 66, 2141.

Dufresne, A., et al., 1994. Sci. Total Environ. 151, 249.

EC, 1998. European Council Directive 98/83/EC, 1998 on the Quality of Water Intended for Human Consumption.

ECHA/RAC, 2017. RAC Opinion 29 May 2017 ECHA/RAC/A77-O-0000001412-86-148/F Opinion of the Committee for Risk Assessment on the Evaluation of the Occupational Exposure Limits (OELs) for Arsenic Acid and Its Inorganic Salts.

EFSA (European Food Safety Authority), 2009. Scientific Opinion of the Panel on contaminants in the food chain. EFSA J. 980, 1—139.

EFSA, 2015. Scientific opinion on the risks to public health related to the presence of nickel in food and drinking water. EFSA J. 13 (2).

Elinder, C.G., 1986. In: Friberg, L., et al. (Eds.), Cadmium and Health. A Toxicological and Epidemiological Appraisal, vol. 2. CRC Press, Boca Raton, FL, pp. 1—20.

Elinder, C.G., Nordberg, G.F., November 2017. Crit. Rev. Toxicol. 47 (10), 900—901.

EMA, 2017. EMA's Final Opinion Confirms Restrictions on Use of Linear Gadolinium Agents in Body Scans EMA/457616/2017.

Emtestam, L., Olerup, O., 1996. Acta Derm. Venereol. 76, 344.

Engstrom, K., et al., 2011. J. Bone Miner. Res. 26, 486.

Eom, S.Y., et al., 2017. Arch. Environ. Contam. Toxicol. 73 (3), 401—409.

EPA, 2009. In: EPA IRIS (Ed.), Toxicological Review of Cerium and Cerium Compounds.

Ezaki, T., et al., 2003. Int. Arch. Occup. Environ. Health 76, 186.

Fewtrell, L.J., et al., 2004. Environ. Res. 94, 120.

Flanagan, P.R., et al., 1978. Gastroenterology 74, 841.

Fowler, B.A., 2010. Lead. In: Zalups, R., Koropatnik, J. (Eds.), Cellular and Molecular Toxicology of Metals. Taylor and Francis, pp. 113—126.

Fowler, B.A., 2012. Biomarkers in toxicology and risk assessment. In: Luch, A. (Ed.), Volume 3. Environmental Toxicology, vol. 101. Birkhauser-Springer Experientia, pp. 459—470.

Fowler, B.A., 2017. Electronic Waste: Toxicology and Public Health Issues. Elsevier Publishers, Amsterdam, p. 84.

Fowler, B.A., Maples-Reynolds, 2015. Indium. In: Nordberg, G.F., Fowler, B.A., Nordberg, M. (Eds.), Handbook on the Toxicology of Metals, fourth ed. Elsevier Publishers, Amsterdam, pp. 845—853.

Fowler, B.A., Sexton, M.J., 2015. Gallium and semiconductor compounds. In: Nordberg, G.F., Fowler, B.A., Nordberg, M. (Eds.), Handbook on the Toxicology of Metals, fourth ed. Elsevier Publishers, Amsterdam, pp. 787—797.

Fowler, B.A., et al., 1980. Toxicol. Appl. Pharmacol. 56, 59—77.

Fowler, et al., 1983. Lab. Invest. 48, 471—478.

Fowler, B.A., et al., 1993. J. Expo. Anal. Environ. Epidemiol. 3, 441—448.

Fowler, B.A., et al., 2005. Toxicol. Appl. Pharmacol. 206, 121.

Fowler, B.A., et al., 2015. Arsenic. In: Nordberg, G.F., Fowler, B.A., Nordberg, M. (Eds.), Handbook on the Toxicology of Metals, fourth ed. Elsevier Publishers, Amsterdam.

Fransson, M.N., et al., 2014. Toxicol. Sci. 141, 365.

Frenzel, T., et al., 2008. Invest. Radiol. 43 (12), 817.

Frenzel, T., et al., 2017. Invest. Radiol. 52, 396.

Garg, S., et al., 2013. Br. J. Dermatol. 169, 854.

Gessner, B.D., et al., 2015. A systematic review of systemic cobaltism after wear or corrosion of chrome-cobalt hip implants. J. Patient Saf. PDF.

Goering, P.L., Maronpot, R.R., Fowler, B.A., 1988. Toxicol. Appl. Pharmacol. 92, 179.

Gomez, 2002. Sci. Total Environ. 299, 1–19.

Gomez-Aracena, J., et al., 2006. Chemosphere 64, 112.

Haddam, N., et al., 2011. Environ. Health 10, 37.

Hansen, A.F., et al., 2017. J. Trace Elem. Med. Biol. 40, 46.

Harada, Y., 1968. Congenital (or fetal) Minamata disease. In: Katsuna, M. (Ed.), Minamata Disease. Kumamoto University, p. 93.

Hart, A.J., et al., 2014. J. Bone Jt. Surg. Am. 96, 1091.

Health Canada, 2012. Aluminum. www.hc-sc.gc.ca.

Hruba, F., et al., 2012. Environ. Int. 41, 29.

Hultman, P., Pollard, M.K., 2015. Immunotoxicology of metals. In: Nordberg, G.F., Fowler, B.A., Nordberg, M. (Eds.), Handbook on the Toxicology of Metals, fourth ed. Academic Press, Elsevier, Amsterdam, Boston.

IARC, 1987. Overall evaluations of carcinogeniscity:An updating of IARC monographs. IARC Monographs 1-42. (Suppl. 7).

IARC, 2006. Cobalt in Hard Metals and Cobalt Sulfate, Gallium Arsenide, Indium Phosphide and Vanadium Pentoxide. IARC Monograph Number 86. Lyon, France.

IARC, 1981. Cisplatin. IARC Monographs Vol 26.

IARC, 2012. Arsenic, metals, fibres and dusts. In: IARC (Ed.), IARC Monographs, vol. 100C. Lyons, France.

IPCS, 1991a. Nickel. Environmental Health Criteria No 108. UNEP/ILO/WHO, Geneva.

IPCS, 1991b. Platinum. Environmental Health Criteria No 125. UNEP/ILO/WHO, Geneva.

IPCS, 1992. Cadmium. Environmental Health Criteria No 134. UNEP/ILO/WHO, Geneva.

IPCS, 2002. Palladium. Environmental Health Criteria. UNEP/ILO/WHO, Geneva.

Jarup, L., et al., 1998. Scand J. Work Environ. Health 24 (Suppl. 1), 1.

JECFA, 2007. WHO TRS 940. In: WHO (Ed.), Contaminants. Methylmercury and Other. WHO/FAO.

JECFA, 2011a. Aluminum Containing Food Additives. TRS 966 JECFA 74.

JECFA, 2011b. Cadmium Safety Evaluation of Certain Food Additives and Contaminants. WHO Food Additives Series 64, pp. 305–380. http://www.inchem.org/documents/jecfa/jecmono/v64je01.pdf.

Jensen, C.S., et al., 2002. Br. J. Dermatol. 146, 636–642.

Jensen, C.S., et al., 2003. Contact Dermat. 49, 124.

Jensen, C.S., et al., 2006. Contact Dermat. 54, 79.

Jin, T., et al., 2004. Environ. Res. 96, 353.

Kazantzis, G., 1979. Environ. Health Perspect. 28, 155–159.

Kiilunen, M., Aitio, A., Santonen, T., 2015. Platinum. In: Nordberg, G.F., et al. (Eds.), Handbook on the Toxicology of Metals, fourth ed. Academic Press, Elsevier, Amsterdam.

Kjellstrom, T., 1979. Environ. Health Perspect. 28, 169–197.

Klein, C., Costa, M., 2015. Nickel. In: Nordberg, G.F., Fowler, B.A., Nordberg, M. (Eds.), Handbook on the Toxicology of Metals, fourth ed. Academic Press, Elsevier, Boston, Amsterdam, pp. 1091–1111.

Kraus, T., et al., 2006. J. Occup. Med. Toxicol. 1, 4.

Kusaka, Y., et al., 1986. Br. J. Ind. Med. 43, 486.

Lagerkvist, B.J., et al., 1986. Environ. Res. 39, 465.

Lanphear, B.P., 2005. Environ. Health Perspect. 113, 894.

Leopold, 2008. Environ. Pollut. 156, 341—347.

Liang, Y., et al., 2012. Environ. Health Perspect. 120, 223.

Liao, Y.H., et al., 2004. J. Occup. Environ. Med. 46, 931.

Lippi, G., et al., 2005. Br. J. Sports Med. 39, 872—873.

Lison, D., 2015. Cobalt. In: Nordberg, G.F., et al. (Eds.), Handbook on the Toxicology of Metals, fourth ed. Academic Press, Elsevier, Amsterdam.

Liu, Y., et al., 2014. Nano Lett. 14, 1413.

Mechanisms of chemical-induced porphyrinopathies. In: Silbergeld, E.K., Fowler, B.A. (Eds.), Ann. N.Y. Acad. Sci. 514, 352.

Menné, T., 1994. Sci. Total Environ. 148, 275.

Merget, R., Rosner, G., 2001. Sci. Total Environ. 270, 165.

Merget, R., et al., 2000. J. Allergy Clin. Immunol. 105, 364.

Merget, R., et al., 2001. J. Allergy Clin. Immunol. 107, 707.

Meyer-Baron, M., et al., 2002. Arch. Toxicol. 76, 127.

Miyaki, K., et al., 2003. J. Occup. Health 45, 228.

Morgan, D.L., et al., 1995. Environ. Res. 71, 16.

Mortz, C.G., et al., 2002. Acta Derm. Venereol. 82, 352.

Muris, J., et al., 2015. Contact Dermat. 72, 286.

Nakano, M., et al., 2009. J. Occup. Health 51, 513.

NAS/NRC, 1993. Report of the Committee on Measuring Lead Exposure in Infants, Children and Other Sensitive Populations. Fowler BA, Chairman. NAS/NRC Press, Washington, DC, p. 337.

Nawrot, T., et al., 2010. J. Bone Miner. Res. 25, 1441.

Nielsen-Kudsk, 1965. Acta Pharmacol. Toxicol. 23, 263.

Nishijo, M., et al., 2006. Occup. Environ. Med. 63, 545.

Nordberg, G.F., Mahaffey, K.R., Fowler, B.A., 1991. Environ. Health Perspect. 91, 3.

Nordberg, G., et al., 2002. Ambio 31, 478.

Nordberg, G.F., et al., 2015. Cadmium. In: Nordberg, G.F., Fowler, B.A., Nordberg, M. (Eds.), Handbook on the Toxicology of Metals, fourth ed. Academic Press, Elsevier, Amsterdam, Boston, pp. 667—742 (Chapter 32).

Nordberg, G.F., et al., 2018. Pure Appl. Chem. 90, 755.

NTP, 1996a. Toxicology and Carcinogenesis Studies of Nickel Oxide in F344/N Rats and B6C3F1 Mice. NTP Technical Report 451. NTP, US Department of Health and Human Services, Washington, DC, USA.

NTP, 1996b. Toxicology and Carcinogenesis Studies of Nickel Subsulfide in F344/N Rats and B6C3F1 Mice. NTP Technical Report Series 453. NTP, US Department of Health and Human Services, Washington, DC, USA.

NTP, 1996c. Toxicology and Carcinogenesis Studies of Nickel Sulfate Hexahydrate in F344/N Rats and B6C3F1 Mice. NTP Technical Report Series. US Department of Health and Human Services, Washington, DC, USA.

NTP (National Toxicology Program), 2000. Toxicology and Carcinogenesis Studies of Gallium Arsenide (CAS No. 1303-00-0) in F344/N and B6C3F1 Mice (Inhalation Studies). NTP Technical Report 492. Research Triangle Park, NC.

NTP, June 2012. Monograph on Health Effects of Low-Level Lead. https://ntp.niehs.nih.gov.

NTP (National Toxicology Program), 2001. NTP Technical Report on the Toxicology and Carcinogenesis Studies of Indium Phosphide (CAS22398-80-7) in F344N Rats and B6C3F1 Mice Inhalation Studies NTPTR499. NIH Publication No. 01-4433. DHHS, PHS, NIH.

Oberdorster, G., 1992. IARC Sci. Publ. 118. In: Nordberg, G.F., et al. (Eds.), Cadmium in the Human Environment: Toxicity and Carcinogenicity, p. 189.

Oller, A.R., Oberdorster, G., 2010. Regul. Toxicol. Pharmacol. 57, 181.

Oller, A.R., et al., 2008. Toxicol. Appl. Pharmacol. 233, 262.

Park, E.J., et al., 2010. Arch. Pharm. Res. 33, 727.

Patterson, C., et al., 1991. Sci. Total Environ. 107, 205.

Pennington, J.A., Jones, J.W., 1984. J. Am. Diet. Assoc. 87, 1644.

Potolicchio, I., et al., 1997. Eur. J. Immunol. 27, 2741.

Quintanilla-Vega, B., et al., 1995. Chem. Biol. Interact. 98, 193–209.

Ramalho, J., et al., 2016. Magn. Reson. Imaging 34, 1394.

Rand, M.D., et al., 2016. Toxicol. Sci. 149 (2), 385–395.

Rentschler, G., et al., 2014. Metallomics 6, 885.

Res, P., et al., 1987. J. Invest. Dermatol. 88, 550.

Rihimäki, V., Aitio, A., 2012. Crit. Rev. Toxicol. 42, 827.

Roels, H., et al., 1987. Ann. Occup. Hyg. 31, 135.

Rogosnitzky, M., Branch, S., 2016. Biometals 29, 365.

RSC, 2018. Periodic Table. www.rsc.org/periodic-table/element/.

Ruiz, P., et al., 2010. Toxicol. Lett. 198, 44.

Sauni, R., et al., 2010. Occup. Med. (Lond.) 60, 301.

Schmidt, M., et al., 2010. Nat. Immunol. 11, 814.

Schroeder, H.A., Mitchener, M., 1971. J. Nutr. 101, 1431.

Science Lab, 2013. MSDS Gallium AA Standard. ScienceLab. Com. Inc., Houston Texas.

ScienceLab.Com. MSDS, 2013. Indium Webpage. ScienceLab.Com. Inc., Houston, Texas.

Scinicariello, F., et al., 2007. Environ. Health Perspect. 115, 35.

Scinicariello, F., et al., 2010. Environ. Health Perspect. 118, 259.

SCOEL, 2007. Recommendations from SCOEL for Elemental Mercury and Inorganic Mercury Compounds. In: SCOEL (Ed.), 84: SCOEL.

SCOEL, 2010. Recommendations from the Scientific Committee on Occupational Exposure Limits for Cadmium and Its Inorganic Compounds. SCOEL/SUM/136.

SCOEL, 2011. SCOEL/SUM/85. In: European Commission — SCOEL (Ed.), Recommendation from the Scientific Committee on Occupational Exposure Limits for Nickel and Inorganic Nickel Compounds.

Shaver, C.G., Rydell, A.R., 1947. J. Ind. Hyg. Toxicol. 29, 145–157.

Signes-Pastor, A.J., et al., 2017. Environ. Res. 159, 69.

Simic, A., et al., 2017. J. Trace Elem. Med. Biol. 41, 91.

Sjogren, B., et al., 2015. Aluminum. In: Nordberg, G.F., Fowler, B.A., Nordberg, M. (Eds.), Handbook on the Toxicology of Metals. Academic Press, Elsevier, Amsterdam, Boston, pp. 549–564.

Skerfving, S., Bergdahl, I., 2015. Lead. In: Nordberg, G.F., Fowler, B.A., Nordberg, M. (Eds.), Handbook on the Toxicology of Metals, fourth ed. Elsevier Publishers, Amsterdam, pp. 911–967.

Smith, D.R., Khang, M.W., Quintanilla-Vega, B., Fowler, B.A., 1998. Chem. Biol. Interact. 115, 39.

Song, H., et al., 2017. Chemosphere 172, 155.

Sorahan, T., Esmen, N.A., 2004. Environ. Med. 61, 108.

Spasovski, G.B., et al., 2006. Nephrol. Dial. Transplant. 21, 2217.

Spencer, A.J., et al., 1997. Toxicol. Pathol. 25, 245.

Stayner, R., et al., 1992. IARC Sci. Publ. 118, 447.

Suwazono, Y., et al., 2000. Environ. Res. 84, 44.

Suwazono, Y., et al., 2010. Toxicol. Lett. 197, 123.

Takenaka, S., et al., 1993. J. Natl. Cancer Inst. 70, 367.

Tallkvist, J., et al., 2001. Toxicol. Lett. 122, 171–177.

Thomas, L.D., et al., 2011. J. Bone Miner. Res. 26, 1601.

Thun, M.J., et al., 1985. J. Natl. Cancer Inst. 74, 325.

Tilch, J., et al., 2000. Fresenius J. Anal. Chem. 367, 450.

Tower, S.S., 2010. J. Bone Jt. Surg. Am. 92, 2847.

Trzcinka-Ochocka, et al., 2009. Environ. Res. 110, 286.

Umemura, T., et al., 2015. Palladium. In: Nordberg, et al. (Eds.), Handbook on the Toxicology of Metals, fourth ed., vol. II. Academic Press, Elsevier, Amsterdam, Boston, pp. 1113–1123.

UNEP, 2013. Global Mercury Assessment 2013. UNEP, Geneva, Switzerland.

Unice, K.M., et al., 2012. Food Chem. Toxicol. 50 (7), 2456.

U.S. National Research Council, 2000. Toxicological Effects of Methylmercury. National Academies Press, Washington, DC, 344 pp.

USEPA, 2012. Arsenic, Inorganic. IRIS, Washington, DC. www.epa.gov.

USGS (US Geological Survey), 2015. Minerals Yearbook. Indium. Advance Release, pp. 35.1–35.5.

USGS, 2017. Mineral Commodity Summaries, p. 135.

USGS (U.S. Geological Survey), January 2018. https://minerals.usgs.gov (mercury), Commodity Summaries, p. 63 Gallium, p. 95 Lead.

Violante, N., et al., 2005. J. Environ. Monit. 7, 463.

Wallander, M., Lofgren, P., Rydén, M., 2015. Lakartidningen 1124–1226.

Wallin, E., et al., 2005. Osteoporos. Int. 16, 2085.

Wang, H., et al., 2003. J. Bone Miner. Res. 18, 553.

Wang, Y.H., et al., 2009. Toxocol. Appl. Pharmacol. 241, 111–118.

Wappelhorst, O., et al., 2002. Nutrition 18, 316.

Wedeen, R.P., Berlinger, B., Aaseth, J., 2015. Lanthanum. In: Nordberg, G.F., Fowler, B.A., Nordberg, M. (Eds.), Handbook on the Toxicology of Metals, fourth ed. Elsevier Publishers, Amsterdam, pp. 903–909.

Weisser, K., et al., 2017. Regul. Toxicol. Pharmacol. 88, 310.

WHO, 2009. Global Health Risks: Mortality and Burden of Diseases Attributable to Selected Major Risks. www.who.int/healthinfo/global_burden_disease/.

WHO, 2011. WHO Drinking Water Guidelines 2011. WHO, Geneva.

Ysart, G., et al., 1999. Food Addit. Contam. 16, 391.

Appendix

GLOSSARY OF TERMS AND ACRONYMS

8-OHdG 8-hydroxydeoxyguanosine

A1M α-1-microglobulin

AAS Atomic absorption spectrometry

ACGIH American Conference of Governmental Industrial Hygienists

Absorbed dose See below under dose

ACSL Advanced Continuous Simulation Language

ADI Acceptable daily intake (of substances in food)

ADME Absorption, distribution, metabolism, and excretion

AFS Arbetsmiljöverkets författningssamling (regulation by the Occupational Environment Authority, Sweden)

AI Adequate intake

ALA δ aminolevulinic acid

ALAD δ aminolevulinic acid dehydratase

AO Adverse effect or outcome

AOP Adverse outcome pathway

AROI Acceptable range of oral intake

ART Advanced REACH Tool (ECHA)

As3MT Arsenic-3-methyl transferase

AsB Arsenobetaine

ATSDR Agency for Toxic Substances and Disease Registry, US

B2M β_2-microglobulin

BCd Cadmium in whole blood

BE Biomonitoring equivalents (Chapter 3, Section 3.4.4; Chapter 7, Section 7.3.3)

BEI Biological exposure index (ACGIH)

Biomonitoring By biomonitoring or biological monitoring, we mean a continuous or repeated measurement of any naturally occurring or synthetic chemical, including potentially toxic substances or their metabolites or biochemical effects in tissues, secreta, excreta, expired air, or any combination of these, in order to evaluate occupational or environmental exposure and health risk. Evaluation is performed by comparison with appropriate reference values based on knowledge of the probable relationship between ambient exposure and resultant adverse health effects (after IUPAC, 2007, see Duffus et al., 2007).

BMCL Benchmark concentration, lower confidence limit

BMD Benchmark dose

BMDL Benchmark dose, lower confidence limit

BMD$_{or}$ Benchmark dose according to the original definition by Crump (1984).

BMR Benchmark response

BPR Biocidal Product Regulation (Regulation EU 528/2012 concerning the use of biocidal products)

Bw Body weight

CAS No Chemical Abstract Service Number

CDC Centers for Disease Control and Prevention (US)

CdMT Metallothionein complexed with cadmium

CERC Crisis and Emergency Risk Communication

CFR Code of Federal Regulations (US)

CLP regulation Classification, Labelling and Packaging regulation: EC 1272/2008 (EU).

CMR Carcinogenic, mutagenic, reprotoxic (ECHA)

CNS Central nervous system

CPS Carcinogenicity potency slope

Critical effect For deterministic effects, the effect that occurs when the threshold (critical) concentration is reached in the critical organ. It is the adverse effect that occurs at the lowest exposure, and this effect is therefore used in risk assessment as the basis for preventive measures.

Critical organ The organ that attains the critical concentration of a substance and exhibits the critical effect under specified circumstances of exposure and for a given population. It is the organ where the critical effect is expressed.

CSA Chemical Safety Assessment (ECHA, EU)

CSAF Chemical Specific Assessment Factor (used instead of default factor in risk assessment)

CSF Cerebrospinal fluid

DALY Disability-adjusted life years

DECOS Health Council of the Netherlands

Deterministic effect Term applied to health effects, the severity of which varies with the dose and for which a threshold exists. Synonym: threshold effect

Dose According to IUPAC (see Duffus et al., 2007), the *dose* is the total amount of a substance administered to, taken up by or absorbed by an organism, organ, or tissue. The proportion of the given dose that is absorbed systemically is the *absorbed dose*, also named *internal dose* (see Duffus et al., 2007, 2009, 2017)

Dose descriptor A description of toxic effects in relation to dose, e.g., NOAEL (ECHA)

DMA Dimethyl arsenic acid; cacodylic acid

DMT1 Divalent metal transporter 1

DNEL Derived no-effect level (ECHA)

DRI Daily reference intake (EU, see Chapter 6)

DRI Dietary reference intake (US). A general term including RDA, AI, and UL

DRV Dietary reference values

D$_t$ Threshold dose

EBC Exhaled breath condensate

EC European Community (previously used term, now EU)

EC European Commission

ECG Electrocardiogram

ECHA European Chemicals Agency (EU)

ECHA/RAC ECHA Risk Assessment Committee

ECVAM European Center for Validation of Alternative Methods (see EURL)

ED-10 Effect dose 10%, i.e., the dose giving rise to a specific effect in 10% of individuals in a group or population

EFSA European Food Safety Authority (EU)

EM Essential metal

EMA European Medicines Agency (EU)

EPA Environmental Protection Agency (US)

ESOD Erythrocyte superoxide dismutase

ETM Essential trace metal

EU European union

EU-INCO DC European Union, International Collaboration with Developing Countries

EURL ECVAM The EU Reference Laboratory for Alternatives to Animal Testing

EUSES The EU computerized system for the evaluation of substances

Exposome According to Wild (2012), the exposome complements the genome by providing a comprehensive description of lifelong exposure history.

FAO Food and Agriculture Organization (UN)

FDA Food and Drug Administration (US)

FeNO Fraction of exhaled nitric oxide

FEV-1 Forced expiratory volume in 1 s

FFQ Food Frequency Questionnaire

GBCA Gadolinium-based contrast agents (used in MRI)

GdCA Gadolinium containing Chelating Agent

GGT Gamma-glutamyltransferase (glutathione transpeptidase)

GHS Globally Harmonized System of Classification and Labelling of Chemicals (UNECE)

GSHPx Glutathione peroxidase

GST Glutathione-S-transferase

GTMM Generalized toxicokinetic modeling system for mixtures

Hazard A set of inherent properties of a substance, mixture of substances, or a process involving substances that, under production, usage, or disposal conditions, make it capable of causing adverse effects to organisms or the environment, depending on the degree of exposure; in other words, it is a source of danger (IUPAC glossary, Duffus et al., 2007, 2017).

HBGV Health-based guidance value

HG-AAS Heated graphite atomic absorption spectrometry

HGV Hygieniskt gränsvärde (hygienic limit value, Occupational Exposure Limit, Sweden)

HI Hazard index. An index used for calculation of the joint action of mixed exposures (Chapter 6)

HLA Human lymphocyte antigen system

HLA-DPB1 Glu69 Genetic variant of human lymphocyte antigen

HMLD Hard metal lung disease

i.v. Intravenous (into a venous blood vessel)

IACUC Institutional Animal Care and Use Committee (US)

IARC International Agency for Research on Cancer

iAs Inorganic arsenic

IC-ICP-MS Ion chromatography inductively coupled plasma mass spectrometry

ICOH International Commission on Occupational Health

ICP-AES Inductively coupled atomic emission spectroscopy

ICP-MS Inductively coupled plasma mass spectrometry

ICRP International Commission for Radiological Protection

ILO International Labour Organization

Intake The amount of a substance that is taken into the body, regardless of whether or not it is absorbed: the total daily intake is the sum of the daily intake by an individual from food, drinking water, and inhaled air (according to IUPAC: Duffus et al., 2007, 2017).

Internal dose See above under dose

IOM Institute of Medicine (associated with the National Academy of Sciences), US

IPCS International Programme on Chemical Safety. A joint venture of UNEP, ILO, and WHO

IQ Intelligence quotient

IRB Institutional Review Board (US rules for research)

ISO International Standardization Organization

IUPAC International Union of Pure and Applied Chemistry

JECFA Joint FAO/WHO Expert Committee on Food Additives

KI Karolinska Institutet (Stockholm, Sweden)

LBMD Lower confidence limit of benchmark dose

LC$_{50}$ Median lethal concentration dose

LCA Life cycle analysis

LD$_{50}$ Median lethal dose

LLNA Local lymph node assay

LMM Low molecular mass

LOAEL Lowest observed adverse effect level

MeHg Methylmercury

MIE Molecular initiating event

MMA Monomethylarsonic acid; methylarsonic acid

MMAD Mass median aerodynamic diameter

MMT Methylcyclopentadienyl manganese tricarbonyl

MOA Mode of action

MOE Margin of exposure

MoM Metal-on-metal orthopedic prosthesis

MOS Margin of safety

MRI Magnetic resonance imaging

MRL Minimal risk level (ATSDR, US)

MSDS Materials safety data sheet

MT Metallothionein, a small, sulfur-rich protein

NAEL No adverse effect level (ECHA)

NAG N-acetyl-β-ᴅ-glucosaminidase

NAS National Academy of Sciences (US)

NAS/NRC NAS/National Research Council (US)

NCATS National Center for Advancing Translational Science

NDA Scientific Panel on Dietetic Products, Nutrition and Allergies (EU-EFSA)

NexGen Next Generation Risk Assessment: Incorporation of Recent Advances in Molecular, Computational, and Systems Biology (USEPA, 2018)

NHANES National Health and Nutrition Examination Survey (US)

NIEHS National Institute of Environmental Health Sciences

NIH National Institutes of Health (US)

NIOSH National Institute of Occupational Safety and Health (US)

NOAEL No observed adverse effect level

NOEL No observed effect level

NSF Nephrogenic systemic fibrosis (Chapter 8, Lanthanides)

NTP National Toxicology Program (US)

OECD Organization for Economic Cooperation and Development

OEL Occupational Exposure Limit

OSHA Occupational Safety and Health Administration (US)

PbB Lead (Pb) level in blood

PBG Porphobilinogen

PBPK Physiologically based pharmacokinetic models

PBT Persistent, bioaccumulative, toxic (REACH, CLP)

PCC Population critical concentration

PCC-50 The concentration in the critical organ at which 50% of a population has the critical effect

PEL Permissible exposure limit (OSHA).

PGE Platinum group elements

PIC Prior Informed Consent Regulation (EU 649/2012)

$PM_{0.1}$ Particulate matter less than 0.1 μm in diameter

PM_{10} Particulate matter less than 10 μm in diameter

PMTDI Provisional maximum tolerable daily intake

POD Point of departure

ppm Parts per million

PRI Population reference intake

PTDI Provisional tolerable daily intake

PTMI Provisional tolerable monthly intake

PTWI Provisional tolerable weekly intake

PUFA Polyunsaturated fatty acids

QAQC Quality assurance and quality control

QSARs Quantitative structure activity relationships

RBP Retinol-binding protein

RDA Recommended dietary allowance (nutrients in food) (US)

REACH Registration, Evaluation, Authorization and Restriction of Chemicals. EC 1907/2006 (EU)

REE Rare earth elements (Chapter 8).

REO Rare earth oxides, oxides of REEs

REL Recommended exposure limit (NIOSH, US)

RfC Reference concentration

RfD Reference dose (US EPA)

Risk According to IUPAC (see Duffus et al., 2007):
1. Probability of adverse effect caused under specified circumstances by an agent in an organism, a population, or an ecological system.
2. Probability of a hazard causing an adverse effect (based on Duffus et al., 2007, 2017).

Risk characterization Outcome of hazard identification and risk estimation applied to a specific use of a substance or occurrence of an environmental health hazard (Duffus et al., 2007, 2017)

ROS Reactive oxygen species (intracellular toxic chemical species)

RP Reference point (EFSA)

RSC Royal Society of Chemistry (UK)

SAR Structure—activity relationships

SCD Systemic contact dermatitis

SCF EU Scientific Committee on Food

SCOEL Scientific Committee on Occupational Exposure Levels (EU)

SCTM Scientific Committee on the Toxicology of Metals (ICOH)

SF-ICP-MS Sector field inductively coupled plasma mass spectrometry

S-PUFA Serum polyunsaturated fatty acids

SRPMI Safe range of population mean intake (WHO, see Chapter 6)

SVHC Substances of very high concern (ECHA)

Target dose Dose or concentration of a toxic agent at the site of action

Target organ An organ in the body affected by the toxic agent.

TD Toxicodynamic

TD-10 Toxic dose 10%; the dose that causes a toxic effect in 10% of individuals in a group

TDI Tolerable daily intake

TGMA Task Group on Metal Accumulation (TGMA, 1973)

TGMI Task Group on Metal Interactions (TGMI, 1978)

TGMT Task Group of Metal Toxicity (TGMT, 1976)

Threshold effect Dose or concentration below which a defined effect will not occur ()

TK Toxicokinetic

TKTD Toxicokinetic-toxicodynamic

TLR4 Toll-like receptor 4

TLV Threshold Limit Value (ACGIH, US)

Total absorption Absorption by various uptake routes added together

Tox21 Toxicology in the 21st Century, see USEPA (2018). Tox21 is a federal collaborative effort between the USEPA, NIH, NTP at the NIEHS, NCATS, and the US FDA to utilize the tools of modern toxicology, share toxicology information across agencies to improve chemical risk assessments for public health.

ToxCast Toxicity Forecaster, see USEPA (2018). A publically available high-throughput toxicity database on thousands of chemicals. ToxCast is a component of the US Federal multi-agency Tox 21 collaboration.

Toxicovigliance (According to the IUPAC, Duffus et al., 2007, 2017) Active process of identification, investigation, and evaluation of various toxic effects in the community with a view to taking measures to reduce or control exposure(s) involving the substance(s) which produce these effects.

TRACY International project for producing reference values for concentration of trace elements in human blood and urine, see, Vesterberg et al. (1993).

TSCA Toxic Substances Control Act (US)

TTC Threshold of Toxicological Concern (Chapter 7)

TWA Time weighted average

UF uncertainty factor

UL Tolerable upper intake level

UN United Nations

UN GHS United Nations Globally Harmonized System of Classification and Labelling of Chemicals (UNECE)

UN HQ UN Headquarter (Geneva, Switzerland)

UNECE United Nations Economic Commission for Europe

UNEP United Nations Environment Programme

US United States of America

USDA U S Department of Agriculture
USEPA US Environmental Protection Agency
USGS US Geological Survey
vPvB very Persistent, very Bioaccumulative
WHO World Health Organization (UN)
ZPP Zinc protoporphyrin

REFERENCES

Crump K. 1984. Fundam. Appl. Toxicol. 4, 854.

Duffus, J.H., et al., 2007. Pure Appl. Chem. 79, 1153—1344.

Duffus, J.H., Templeton, D.M., Nordberg, M., 2009. In: Concepts in Toxicology in IUPAC. RSC Publishing, Cambridge, p. 179.

Duffus, J.H., Templeton, D.M., Michael, S., 2017. Comprehensive Glossary of Terms Used in Toxicology. RSC Publishing.

USEPA, 2018. In: EPA (Ed.), Next Generation Risk Assessment: Incorporation of Recent Advances in Molecular, Computational, and Systems Biology. https://www.epa.gov/.

Vesterberg, O., et al., 1993. Scand. J. Work. Environ. Health 19 (Suppl 1), 19—26.

Wild, C.P., 2012. Int. J. Epidemiol. 41, 24.

TGMA, Task Group on Metal Accumulation, 1973. Accumulation of toxic metals with special reference to their absorption, excretion and biological Half-times. Environm. Physiol. Biochem. 3, 65—107.

TGMI, Task Group on Metal Interaction, 1978. Factors Influencing metabolism and toxicity of metals: a Consensus Report. Env. Health Perspect. 25, 3—41.

TGMT, Task Group on Metal Toxicity, 1976. A Consensus Report from an International Meeting Organized bu the Subcommittee on the toxicology of metals of the Permanent Commission and International association on occupational health. In: Nordberg, G.F. (Ed.), Effects and Dose-response Relationships of Toxic Metals. Elsevier, Amsterdam, pp. 1—111.

INDEX

'*Note:* Page numbers followed by "f" indicate figures, "t" indicate tables.'